DENTAL PATHOLOGY AND SURGERY

LONDON: PRINTED BY
SPOTTISWOODE AND CO., NEW-STREET SQUARE
AND PARLIAMENT STREET

DENTAL

PATHOLOGY AND SURGERY

BY

S. JAMES A. SALTER, M.B., F.R.S.

MEMBER OF THE ROYAL COLLEGE OF SURGEONS, AND EXAMINER IN DENTAL SURGERY AT THE COLLEGE; DENTAL SURGEON TO GUY'S HOSPITAL

NEW YORK

WM. WOOD & CO., PUBLISHERS

56 AND 58 LAFAYETTE PLACE

PREFACE.

It is just twenty-three years since I determined to devote myself to the practice of Dental Surgery as the profession of my life. Having previously practised surgery in its general and broader aspect, both in private and with hospital appointments, I was at once impressed by the too narrow and circumscribed view, which was comprehended by the literature of the speciality I had adopted.

It had appeared to me that even eminent hospital surgeons were scarcely aware how serious are some of the maladies directly dependent on tooth-disease, and how largely the pathology of the teeth is associated with serious morbid changes in contiguous structures. The fairness of these remarks may be briefly illustrated by saying that 'Warty teeth' had been mistaken for Exostoses of the jaw; that Dentigerous Cysts had scarcely been recognised, and that the external orifice of an outward-pointing alveolar abscess, dependent on a carious tooth, was still constantly attributed to necrosed bone.

These are a few examples of a general imperfection of knowledge among surgeons. On the other hand, the pathology of the teeth themselves was very imperfectly investigated by dentists. The many morbid changes, both chronic and acute, which occur in the tooth-pulp, were either undescribed, or but imperfectly known. The same may be said of the series of tumours of the hard tissues of the teeth, now grouped together under the title 'Odontomes.' And many more instances of the like kind might be enumerated. It appeared to me that there was a considerable field of surgery and pathology—a sort of debatable ground between that occupied by the surgeon and by the dentist—which was open to further research, and which would amply repay the labour of investigation.

My appointment to Guy's Hospital, as Dental Surgeon, gave me abundant opportunities for prosecuting such researches. The population tributary to Guy's Hospital is immense, and the poor patients, whom I have there attended, have given me a rich reward in cases and pathological specimens—an ample return for any services I may have rendered them.

The records of these, and those furnished by private practice, supplemented by communications and specimens sent me by kind friends, have constituted many single and serial papers, which have been published in the Transactions of learned Societies and in medical periodicals.

The Medical and Chirurgical Society have published

some of my papers. Several have appeared in the 'Transactions of the Pathological Society,' and more numerous communications have found publicity in the pages of the 'Guy's Hospital Reports.' Others have been given to the profession in the 'Archives of Dentistry' and the 'Dental Journal.'

When it was determined, some fifteen years since, to publish a large concrete work on Surgery, consisting of essays written by different authors, and which ultimately assumed the shape of the *System of Surgery*, so ably edited by Mr. Holmes, I was solicited to contribute the article on 'Surgical Diseases connected with the Teeth.' This again appeared in 1870, much enlarged, in the second edition of that work.

The present volume is a digested collection of all my previous essays and papers, arranged in the form of chapters; and several more chapters have been added to previously published matter.

I have ventured to think that, after the many years devoted, not without some diligence, to the study of the pathology and surgery of the teeth, I should be justified, without presumption, in publishing my views in a distinct and authentic form; and I have thought it the more desirable to do so, as I have been incorrectly quoted by high authority, and in some instances my scattered writings have been used without acknowledgment.

In the following pages it will be found that some subjects are not considered which may perhaps be fairly held to belong to dental surgery. It would have been easy to have supplied chapters on such subjects by compilation; but it has been my desire as far as possible only to express views and to record observations where I could do so with authority; or, at least, as the result of independent thought and investigation. And I have wished, too, that my book should be on Dental Surgery rather than on Dentistry proper.

How far this work may be of benefit to others, I leave for them to decide. For myself, the researches upon which it is based have been a constant source of pleasure and of mental profit.

My obligations are due to Mr. Christopher Heath for some of the illustrations in this book; and to Mr. Charles James Fox for much kind assistance in the revision of the proofs.

S. J. A. S.

CONTENTS.

CHAPTER I.

CHAPTER II.

CHAPTER III.

CHAPTER IV.

CHAPTER V.

CHAPTER VI.

CHAPTER VII.

CHAPTER VIII.

CHAPTER IX.

CHAPTER X.

CHAPTER XI.

CHAPTER XII.

CHAPTER XIII.

CHAPTER XIV.

CHAPTER XV.

CHAPTER XVI.

CHAPTER XVII.

CHAPTER XVIII.

CHAPTER XIX.

CHAPTER XX.

CHAPTER XXI.

CHAPTER XXII.

CHAPTER XXIII.

CHAPTER XXIV.

CHAPTER XXV.

CHAPTER XXVI.

CHAPTER XXVII.

CHAPTER XXVIII.

LIST OF ILLUSTRATIONS.

DENTAL PATHOLOGY

AND

SURGERY.

CHAPTER I.

GENERAL ANATOMY OF THE TEETH AND CONTIGUOUS STRUCTURES.

THE dentition of man is diphiodont; that is to say, there are two sets of teeth, the *temporary* and *permanent*, numbering respectively twenty and thirty-two teeth.

In the temporary set there are four incisors, two canines, and four molars in each jaw; in the succeeding set these are replaced by others—incisors succeeding incisors, canines succeeding canines; the temporary molars are replaced by premolars or bicuspids, and behind these are developed in succession, as the maxillæ elongate, three permanent molars on each side of each jaw.

The formulæ of human dentition may be thus expressed.

The temporary set:—

$$I\frac{2\ 2}{2\ 2};\ C\ \frac{1\ 1}{1\ 1};\ M\frac{2\ 2}{2\ 2}=20$$

The permanent set:—

$$I\frac{2\ 2}{2\ 2};\ C\ \frac{1\ 1}{1\ 1};\ P\ \frac{2\ 2}{2\ 2};\ M\frac{3\ 3}{3\ 3}=32.$$

In histological development, in structure, in physiology, and in their diseases, the teeth have certain resemblances to bones, and, at the same time, characteristic differences from them.

A considerable portion of each tooth is naked, whilst bones are wholly clothed by periosteum; the hard tissues of human teeth are destitute of blood-vessels—bone is highly vascular; teeth are perishable, and may be shed—bones last the life-time of the individual; lost substance of two of the tissues of teeth, enamel and dentine, is never restored, though in the latter there is a curious process of internal repair, in this resembling some bones and differing from others.

Teeth certainly are not extraneous organs, as suggested by Hunter, but have a distinct vitality: they undergo nutritional changes by virtue of a plasmic circulation in their tubular structure, and two of their hard tissues manifest sensibility, which, in disease, may be exalted to extreme painfulness.

The teeth are not parts of the true skeleton, but may be considered as elements of a dermal skeleton. They are developed from the tegument of the mouth; and though closely embraced by the alveolar processes of the maxillary bones, are never, in man, united to them.

It is not my intention to enter upon a description of the development, the structure, and the physiology of the teeth, further than as illustrating their diseases.

Human teeth are composed of three hard elementary substances, enclosing a soft fleshy mass in the centre.

The three sclerous substances are enamel, dentine or ivory, and crusta-petrosa or tooth-bone.

Enamel is the hardest tissue in the body; it contains above 95 per cent. of earthy matter. In structure it consists of a series of dense fibres, running with a somewhat wavy course, but generally at right angles to the dentine surface of the crown of the tooth upon which they rest, radiating outwards, and ending free upon the masticating surface of the crown of the tooth. Close to the dentinal surface the fibres are frequently separated from each other by the protrusion between them, for a short distance, of the dentinal tubes, and the latter are sometimes large and bulbous in that situation.*

There is every reason to believe that enamel is totally destitute of vitality; that it undergoes no nutritional changes after

* This may account for the fact, stated by Retzius, that the enamel close to the dentine contains more animal matter than elsewhere.

it is once formed, and that it is only influenced by the physical and chemical agencies to which it is exposed.

Dentine or *ivory*, which constitutes the bulk of a tooth, is a tissue of bony hardness; it consists of earthy matter to the extent of not less than three-fourths of its weight. Histologically it is composed of a series of minute tubes about $\frac{1}{9000}$ of an inch in diameter, radiating from the central hollow chamber or pulp-cavity, in which is lodged the soft vascular organ, the pulp, which is mainly concerned in the nutrition of the tooth. Between the dentinal tubes is a hyaline structure called the intertubular tissue. The tubes pursue a wavy course, and branch more or less, especially in the crowns of the teeth near the surface, and occasionally they exhibit dilatations somewhat like bone-lacunæ.

The dentinal tubes have extremely thin walls, which can scarcely be said to be visible in the hard tissue when seen in profile, but which, in transverse section, as viewed by high powers of the microscope, display a broad brilliant ring of considerable thickness around each. This appearance is an optical illusion, and has given rise to much error in interpreting the histological elements of dentine. Whether the broad ring is the result of the curious phenomenon, *irradiation*, or the *diffraction of light* by the thin cut edge of the tube, I am not prepared to say; but the appearance is not without parallels, which are thus explained. This fact was first pointed out by Henle,* in 1841, and is easy of confirmation. It can be demonstrated both by analysis and by synthesis. In some fractures of sections of dentine these fine tubes are seen standing out rigid and calcified from the broken edge. The animal basis of the dentinal tubes and that of the intertubular substance are different; the former is considerably denser, and, after decalcification, strong hydrochloric acid will remove the intertubular substance, or render it absolutely transparent—thus the tubes can be isolated, and their minute diameter, corresponding with the dark dentinal tube as seen in the profile view of hard sections, is at once recognised.

If tubes, thus distinctly free from all surrounding *walls*, be

* *Allgemeine Anatomie*, von J. Henle; constituting the sixth volume of Sömmerring's *Baue des menschlichen Körpers*. Leipsig, 1841.

traced along their course, occasionally some are seen turning their broken ends towards the observer; the rings in question are apparent, and the illusion is manifest. The accompanying diagram will explain this perhaps better than a description.

Fig. 1.

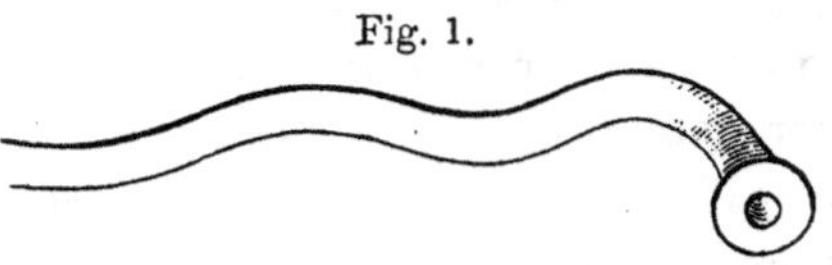

Synthetically this question of histology is demonstrated with equal clearness. In studying the development of dentine, it is found that upon the formative pulp there is arranged a series of columnar cells constituting the *membrana eboris*, from the distal extremities of which minute tubular threads project; and, as the dentine forms from without inwards, these are prolonged centripetally, a homogeneous blastema separating them and being calcified with them. These prolongations are the dentinal tubes,* and the calcified blastema is the intertubular tissue. No other elements hitherto discerned enter into the formation of dentine, and the minute tubes, freed by the decalcification and the solution of the intertubular tissue in dentine, through the action of hydrochloric acid, are identical with the thread-like prolongations seen on the ends of the columnar cells of the dentinal pulp. These minute tubules of dentine, when free and soft, have a certain resemblance to nerve fibres, and this circumstance, combined with the belief that the luminous rings around the tubes represent the walls of comparatively large hollow canals, has led a distinguished microscopist to conclude that they are nerves, or the equivalents of nerves, occupying the cavities of such canals. And, unaware that the histological facts had been recorded both in description and illustration by Henle long previously, he presented to the Royal Society a memoir "On the Presence of Fibrils of Soft Tissue in the Dentinal Tubes," † and in that memoir he speaks of them as "organs of sensation." But the truth is they are the dentinal tubes themselves, and

* This was discovered by Lent, "Ueber die Entwickelung des Zahnbeins und des Schmelzes," in Siebold and Kölliker's *Zeitschrift*, 1854, p. 121.

† By John Tomes, F.R.S. In the *Philosophical Transactions of the Royal Society*, vol. cxlvi., 1856.

there is nothing whatever separating these bodies from the intertubular substance. In the observations made by this author, great stress was laid upon the examinations being made on perfectly fresh specimens, so that the soft structures may not have suffered injury or decay. The minute tubules may, however, be demonstrated just as well in the oldest specimens of dentine. The accompanying illustration (fig. 2) is from a specimen, prepared by myself, of a portion of decalcified dentine from the tooth of an Ancient Briton, that had been entombed probably for not less than two thousand years; all soft uncalcified tissues must have perished for ages.

Fig. 2.

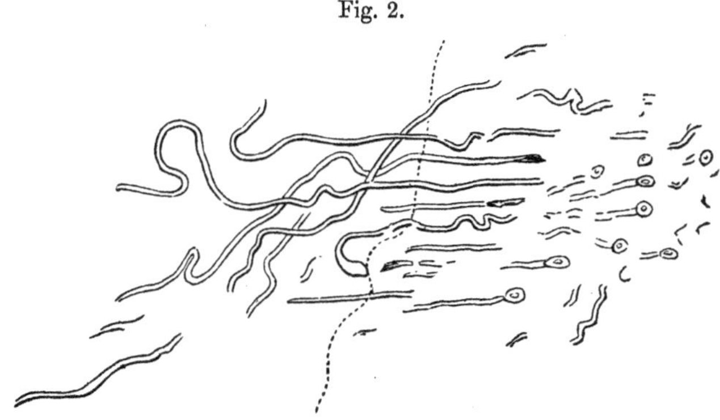

In this figure the dentinal tubules are free to the left of the dotted line, but to the right they are still held in position by the intertubular substance, which, though perfectly hyaline and transparent, has not yet dissolved away.*

The dentinal tubules are hollow and appear to contain a dense plasma.

Mr. Tomes has contributed a valuable record in support of this view: "When accidentally stretched between two masses of dentine the diameter of the fibril (decalcified tube) becomes much diminished, and, when broken across, a minute globule of transparent but dense fluid may sometimes be seen at the broken end, gathered more or less into a spherical form." The axis of the tube, therefore, whatever may be its disputed nature, being occupied by fluid.

* For a more lengthened discussion of this subject, the reader is referred to a paper by the author "On some Points in the Anatomy and Physiology of the Dentinal Tubes," in Truman's *Archives of Dentistry*, 1865.

Human dentine is non-vascular, that is, it is destitute of blood-vessels; though occasionally, as an abnormal condition, erratic vascular canals are seen in its substance. This will hereafter be referred to, as well as that peculiar form of secondary dentine, osteo-dentine, which is produced by the intrinsic calcification of the tooth-pulp, and which is abundantly vascular.

Dentine exhibits vital phenomena, which show it to be part of the living body.

I. It is sentient.

II. It is susceptible of nutritional changes.

III. It takes cognisance, so to speak, of injuries done to its outer surface, leading to a renewal of ivory-growth on the surface of the pulp.

Hunter* denied that dentine is sensitive, and that view was long entertained. I believe it was M. Duval† who first prominently pointed out that the ivory of human teeth is endowed with sensation; and he particularly mentioned that the external layer, just beneath the enamel, and which he named "Dictyodont," manifests the most acute sensibility. This circumstance may arise from the fact that the outer layer is often imperfectly calcified, and that some of the tissue here remains soft and more impressible; for it is found that the same exalted sensibility is displayed when the surface of any exposed dentine is acted upon by acids, and again it is seen in pale soft decay.

I believe that both the periosteum around the fangs of the tooth and the pulp itself have a nervous connection with the substance of ivory. The destruction of the pulp very much reduces the sensitiveness of dentine, and generally seems to destroy it; but in not a few instances I have found masses of dentine still intensely sensitive when their direct connection with the pulp has been severed by lesion of intervening tissue; and it has occurred to me as probable that the sentient perception has, in such cases, been through the periosteum. It does not necessarily follow, however, that the nervous connection

* *The Works of John Hunter*, Palmer's edition, vol. ii. p. 50. London, 1835.

† *Observations Pratiques sur la Sensibilité des Substances Dures des Dents*, par J. R. Duval. Paris, 1833. This paper was originally read before the Royal Academy of Medicine of Paris, 1831.

between the pulp and the dentine should be by a direct radiation in the same course as the tooth-tube structure: it may be diffuse and circuitous, and thus an outlying mass of dentine may still maintain a sentient connection with the pulp. I am inclined, however, to believe that the periosteum shares in this function, as it does in the nutrition and general vitality of the teeth; and this opinion is supported by the fact that Czermak has found a large supply of nerves in the periodontal membrane, and has traced them to the hard substance of the fangs.* The mode in which the hard tissues of the teeth are supplied with nerves is still an enigma; but that there is some supply is certain, on physiological grounds.

Tomes mistook the decalcified tubes for nerves, or their equivalents. Other anatomists, especially Neumann, have described cylindrical processes as projecting from the ends of the tubes (sheaths); and Boll has figured the same with clear definition.† It is assumed that these are nerves. It should be remembered, however, that minute branches of the tubes might easily be mistaken for emanations from within the tubes, as I have myself seen; and, further, that the viscid contents of tubes, drawn out especially after induration by chromic acid (as employed by Boll), might readily be mistaken for fibrils, and, indeed, might so appear.

The nerves of the tooth-pulp form loops towards its periphery, which may be readily demonstrated by the action of caustic alkali, and from these, according to Boll, large numbers of very minute fibrils proceed outwards, passing between the ivory cells and their tubular prolongations. It is highly probable that these are the nervous elements distributed to the dentine; but whether they pass into the intertubular substance, or, fastening upon the tube walls, are so piloted into the ivory structure, is quite uncertain. It is, however, highly improbable that they pierce the wall of the ivory cell, and occupy the axis of the tube.

The sensibility of dentine has some peculiarities: it is exalted

* "Beiträge zur mikroskopischen Anatomie der menschlichen Zähne," von Dr. Johann Czermak, in Kölliker and Siebold's *Zeitschrift*, p. 317. Leipsig, 1850.

† "Untersuchungen über die Zahnpulpa," von Franz Boll, in Schultze's *Archiv für Mikroskopische Anatomie*, p. 73, Tafel v. fig. 45. Bonn, 1868.

to pain (especially when softened in early decay) by certain sapid bodies, which have no particular effect upon nerves of ordinary sensation, such as salt and sugar, especially the latter, which is remarkably irritating in its low uncrystallised forms. Again, the sensibility is numbed in a singular degree by some of the pungent hydrocarbons, such as creasote and phenole, which, *à priori*, would not have been expected to produce such a result.

Fig. 3.

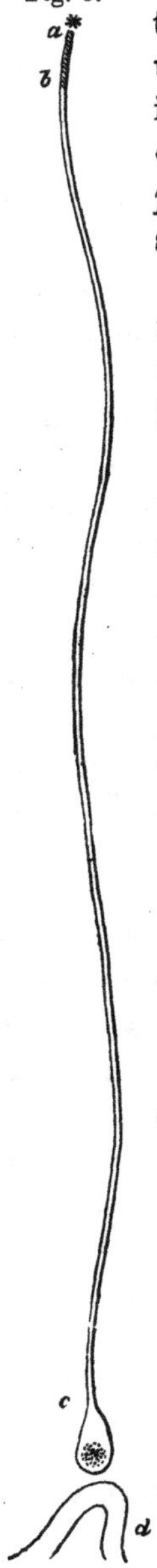

Dentine, that is matured, afterwards undergoes nutritional changes under certain circumstances as far as the tubes are concerned, but apparently not in regard to the intertubular tissue.

It is very common for dentinal tubes, leading from the pulp to a slight superficial decay, or an abrasion, in the crown of a tooth to be sealed up by a deposit of calcified material for a short space at the distal end of the tube, while the whole of the rest of the tube has remained patent. A section of a dry tooth, in which this has occurred, shows the tissue around the decay, or abrasion, clear and transparent, the tubes being filled with material apparently of the same, or nearly the same, density as the surrounding structure, while leading to the pulp the tubes are opaque and air-filled. Now, where this occurs in the crown of a tooth, the only source of nutrient material is the vascular supply of the pulp; and the calcific matter must traverse the whole length of the tube before deposition at its terminal extremity. This will be more intelligible by reference to the accompanying diagram. The asterisk represents the spot of decay, or abrasion; *a b*, that portion of the tube closed by calcific deposit; *b c*, that portion of the tube filled with air in a dry specimen, and with plasm in the living state; *d*, a capillary loop. This may seem too diagrammatic and mechanical a method of expressing what occurs; but it is not so. A figure illustrative of this is seen under the head "Dentine of Repair," where the clear tissue, close to the carious surface, has been thus produced.

The tube in the diagram is drawn as terminated towards the blood-vessel by the persistent developmental cell, which appears to remain through life, and ever ready to resume a continued growth by centripetal elongation, when the outer surface of the dentine is injured, producing "dentine of repair." The entrance of nutrient material into the tube must therefore be by endosmosis through this cell-wall.

A similar filling-up of the tubes by calcified material takes place in the fangs of teeth, especially after inflammatory action. This produces a semi-transparency; the dentine looks like horn.

In jaundice the plasm in the tubes is stained yellow by the bile; and where the pulp becomes disorganised, the colouring matter of the blood often imparts a red or purple hue to the contents of the tubes.

The development of dentine of repair is another indication of vitality. When the surface of the dentine is injured either by decay, by friction, or by fracture, an impression is conveyed to the formative pulp, by which a fresh growth of dentine is started, having a definite relation to the external injury. This will be further illustrated in the chapter on Secondary Dentine. When dentine is removed by absorption from the external surface or the end of the fang of a tooth, it is never restored; but the erosion may be filled up by a deposit of crusta petrosa.

Crusta petrosa, or *tooth-bone*, is a structure closely resembling the bone of the skeleton; and it clothes the dentine of the tooth's fang just as the enamel covers the crown.

The tissue contains about 70 per cent. of earthy matter.

Crusta petrosa consists of bony laminæ, which in transverse section constitute a series of rings around the dentine of the tooth's fang, and in vertical section display elongated wedge-shaped processes, broad towards the apex of the fang. Among these are interspersed true bone lacunæ, large and oval, with their long axes parallel to that of the fang: they usually have a profusion of canaliculi mostly passing from within outwards, and from without inwards. Among the lacunæ are frequently seen tubes, sometimes numerous and parallel to each other, radiating from centre to surface, and much resembling dentinal tubes. These when cut across present the same broad ring as is seen in a similar section of dentinal tubes.

The lacunæ are wanting towards the neck of the tooth, where

the crusta petrosa is a thin, nearly transparent layer, and they appear and increase somewhat rapidly about the middle of the fang and towards its extremity. The tooth-bone is not always an even layer on the dentine, but is often thick at places, obliterating the folds of the latter, and not infrequently uniting fangs together.

Crusta petrosa is normally non-vascular, but towards the apex of the fang it is occasionally pierced by a few blood-vessels in the teeth of old people, where the tissue is often much thickened. These constitute Haversian canals, which generally terminate in blind extremities. The tubes of the dentine and those of the tooth-bone, as well as the canaliculi of the latter, frequently anastomose. Tooth-bone is very liable to absorption and re-deposition.

This tissue is sensitive, and, when exposed by the recession of the gum and alveoli, is irritated to pain by the same sapid bodies as affect dentine, especially by salt. The manner in which nerve-tissue enters the substance of tooth-bone, and is distributed among it, is unknown. Its chief source of supply is probably from the periosteum; but it may have some connection with the nerves of the pulp, just as dentine seems to have with the nerves of the periosteum.

Fig. 4.

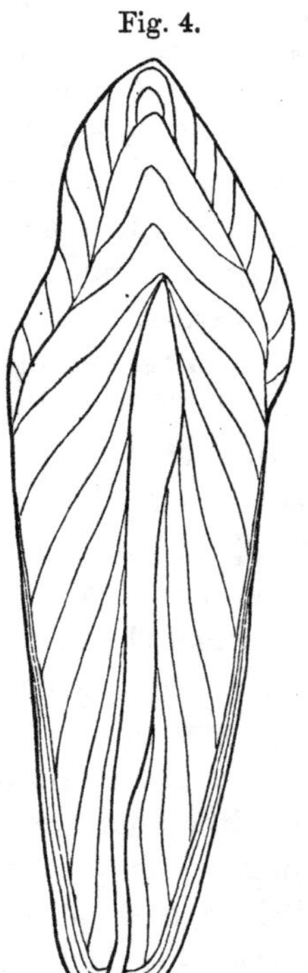

The hard tissues of the teeth have a general radiating character in their structure, and are at the same time laminated. The radiation indicates the ultimate histology and the structure as associated with the nutrition of the tissues: the lamination indicates the increments of their development—the successive portions by which the tooth is built up. These indications may be fairly called *incremental lines*, and are indicated in the accompanying diagram.* Theoretically, the process of a tooth's growth is continuous,

* Professor Owen has called these markings in dentine "contour lines." The term is scarcely admissible, as they only approximate remotely the contour of the tooth.

the three hard tissues being evenly produced upon the surface of the formative pulps; but really that is not so, the enamel, dentine, and crusta petrosa indicating, by a sort of lamination, a distinctly repeated periodicity, as though the tissue were formed perfectly and imperfectly, or of different density, at intervals of time more or less evenly repeated. This is especially the case with dentine. This repetition of different nutritional conditions, a sort of alternate plus and minus, so to speak, is a phenomenon of very general existence in the growth and nourishment of tissues; but it has been scarcely dwelt upon by physiologists with the importance that it deserves. As regards the tissues of the teeth, it is of extreme interest from the clearness of its demonstration in them, and from the fact that they retain through life a permanent register of alternate growth-complete and incomplete.

This alternation of developmental force is most marked in the dentine, and manifests itself in the matter of calcification. That is to say, a layer of dentine will form over the entire area of the pulp, and its calcification will be complete; and then another layer will form, in which the calcification is incomplete, the earthy impregnation being partial and defective, either from the growth of the animal basis being too rapid, or the supply of calcareous matter being deficient. And so on alternately. Now this imperfect calcification of the alternate layers is demonstrable from the fact that the animal matter of dentine is not evenly impregnated by the earthy in a general and progressive manner; but as the histological elements are formed on the surface of the pulp, the earthy matter impregnates the soft mass at a series of isolated points, which gradually enlarge into spheres of perfectly calcified dentine, while the intermediate portions remain unchanged. It is by the progressive enlargement and fusion together of these spheres—"calcification globules"—that normal dentine is completed. If, however, the animal matter is imperfectly supplied by the calcareous, while the tissue progresses in growth, the calcification is permanently imperfect; the matured structure remains as a series of hard globules with soft interspaces. And when such specimens of dentine are dried, these interspaces become air-filled, from the shrinking of the very soft tissue occupying them, and are white and opaque as seen with reflected light, and dark with transmitted light. These interspaces have been often mistaken for lacunæ. Now this layer of imperfectly formed dentine occupies the area of the pulp at a given time throughout, though most marked near the margin of the forming tooth-cap where the tissue is forming fastest, and it illustrates the successive increments of which the tooth is built up. See fig. 43, where this is shown in the vertical section of a canine tooth. The histological characters, as seen with the microscope, are displayed in fig. 44, where they are treated among the vices of original tooth development.

A somewhat similar effect is produced in enamel by these alternations of nutritional force: the enamel is calcified first as a cap on the summit of each tooth-cusp, and then in a series of rings down the crown of the tooth; and the markings, more in colour and transparency than in difference of structure, which are thus produced, display at the summit an arch and then a series of rhomboidal forms, as shown in figure 4. Where there is any grave fault in the structure of the enamel, it is usually found to abut upon the extremity of a severely marked incremental line in the dentine.

The lamination of crusta petrosa is likewise, in all probability, a manifestation of periodicity and alternation.

The *Soft Structures* connected with the teeth have a very important bearing on Dental Disease. They are the Pulp, the Gum, and the Periosteum.

The *Pulp* is a soft mass, which exactly fills the chamber in the fang and crown of the tooth; it is of a pinkish colour, and rather translucent. It contains a large amount of fluid, and dries to a mere film. Nerves and blood-vessels are very abundant throughout the structure.

The blood-vessels form long plexuses, the larger vessels in the centre of the pulp giving off irregular loops towards the surface. They are extremely numerous, and a pulp treated with acetic acid shows the nuclei of vascular muscle in all directions. Indeed, the structure of minute blood-vessels is well exhibited for study in the pulp.

The nerves form a large element of the mature pulp; they enter the apex of the fang in small bundles of various size and number, and these divide and subdivide in plexuses forming long meshes, which ultimately, near the surface, break up into primitive fibres. Here they form very distinct loops immediately beneath the *membrana eboris.* From these loops, according to Boll, very minute fibrils pass outwards between the cellular elements of the extreme surface of the pulp.

There appear to be no lymphatics in the tooth-pulp.

A very pale ill-defined areolar tissue, pervaded by numerous round and oval cells, or nuclei (the granules of Purkinje) occupies the spaces between the vessels and nerves. These cellular bodies towards the surface are enlarged and more oval, increasingly so as they become more superficial, where they assume the form of columnar epithelium. From the extremities of these project minute tubular prolongations which constitute the animal basis of the dentinal tube wall, and are in direct continuity with the calcified dentinal tubes of the indurated dentine.

The *Gum* is the mucous membrane which surrounds the necks of the teeth, and is continuous with that of the rest of the mouth; it has no exact limit, but may perhaps be said to be from a quarter to a third of an inch broad from its free edge.

In structure it consists of an elastic layer of fibrous tissue intimately connected and continuous with the periosteum of the jaw; upon this is placed a regular and strongly marked papillary structure, covered in by a dense epithelium. The papillæ are long and cylindrical near the edge of the gum, like the fingers of a glove, and they become shorter and expanded in passing towards the jaw and palate. Each papilla contains a single capillary loop.

The epithelium is soft and small and round immediately upon and between the papillæ, becoming larger and flatter towards the surface, where it is squamous and cuticular, and completely covers in the papillæ, forming an even surface. The change in form and size of the deep and superficial epithelium is very gradual, and there is no distinct line of demarcation—nothing like a *rete mucosum*, as in the skin.

Where the gum is in contact with the necks of the teeth, the structure is very much modified; the papillæ cease and the hard squamous epithelium is wanting. The surface is here soft and clothed with a smaller and rounder epithelium: there are no true glands, such as Serres described, but the surface is cupped and folded between the ramifications of a beautiful capillary network. This surface emits a profusion of those globular cells which are constantly found in the fluids of the mouth, and which are called by authors *mucous corpuscles.* Whether they all come from this source I cannot say; but they are certainly largely produced here and constitute the bulk of that yellow oozy material which collects around the necks of the teeth in uncleanly people.

The accompanying illustration shows the vascular arrangement of the gum on the dental surface; and the sudden change from the papillary loops to the gland-like plexus is very manifest. The alteration in the disposition of the vessels exactly coincides with the modification of the surface and of the epithelium. This is probably a truly glandular structure, but of the simplest kind.

Fig. 5.

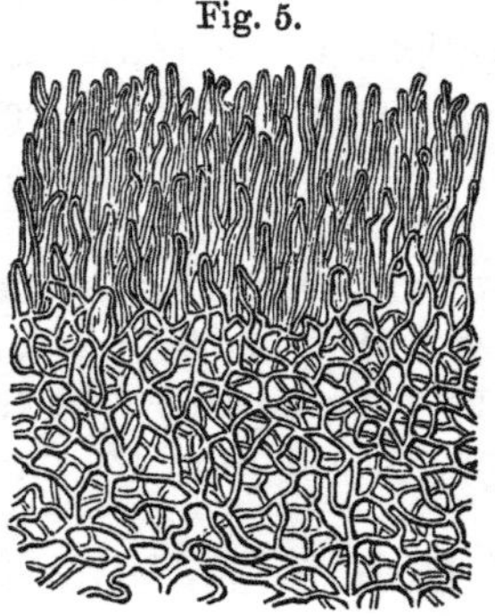

The supply of nerves to the gum is small, and it is insensitive unless the surface is ulcerated, when, like some other tissues slightly furnished with nerves, it is intensely painful.

The *Periosteum* lines the socket of the tooth and ministers to its nutrition, and to that of the surrounding alveolar process. It has been customary to take too artificial a limit, and to make too exact a definition of the fibro-vascular tissues surrounding the fangs of the teeth, and to divide them into periodontal membrane, periosteum, endosteum, and gum. With exception of the mucous membrane of the gum, they are really one and continuous; they share, to a great degree, the same vascular supply and the same general influences of health and disease. The membrane which intervenes between the alveolus and the tooth-fangs has, however, some characteristics which distinguish it from ordinary periosteum. It is entirely devoid of fat cells, it consists of connective tissue in which the elastic element is wholly wanting, and it has a very large supply of nerves.

CHAPTER .II.

FUNCTIONS OF THE TEETH.

Mastication is the most important of the functions of the teeth, and is so obvious that it need not be dwelt upon. The teeth have, moreover, a tactile faculty which is exercised in detecting the texture of food and the presence of foreign bodies.

Another function of the teeth, hitherto too little dwelt upon, is that they play a very important part in the formation of articulate sounds: they constitute an essential element in the organs of speech. Without them the precise and clear pronunciation of a great many letters, particularly consonants, would be impossible, and the resources of the oral cavity, as an organ of speech, greatly circumscribed. Accordingly we find that, when the teeth are lost, certain imperfections in articulation are immediately entailed; and thus the knowledge of the particular way in which the teeth help to form articulate sounds is of much practical importance to the dentist, as it is only by this knowledge that the imperfections of articulation will enable him to tell what is amiss, how to correct it, and, indeed, whether the teeth are in fault or not.

With the formation of many articulate sounds, both vowels and consonants, the teeth have nothing to do, and, therefore, into the discussion of the mechanism by which these are produced it will not be necessary to enter. Nevertheless I think it well, before describing how the sounds are effected in which the teeth are immediately concerned, to say a few words on the mechanism of articulation generally, as it will render the more special part of the subject clearer and more intelligible.

Articulate sounds are essentially produced by the passage of air through the oral canal. . Now, there are chiefly three parts of the oral canal that may severally impress certain characters on air passed through them, and these are the three points where closure, *perfect*, *imperfect*, and *modified*, may be produced at will—namely, the soft palate, the front teeth and gums just behind them, and the lips. Certain characters are also given to the sounds by the relation of the size of the oral cavity to the size and shape of these orifices.

Articulate sounds have been divided into *vocal* and *consonantal* sounds, or vowels and consonants, and to a certain extent the distinction is a good one and based on physiological truth; but as it is usually understood, and as we find it explained in grammars, it is quite incorrect. It is usually stated that vowel sounds are the true voice sounds, and that consonants are merely the method of commencing and terminating vowels; that vowels are open sounds, and consonants closed sounds; that vowels are capable of prolonged utterance, and that consonants are incapable of pronunciation without the aid of vowels. We see this implied in the very names themselves—vowels (*vocales*), voice sounds; consonants (*con sono*), something necessarily sounded with something else.

Now, this error has arisen, as shown by Müller, from the supposition that voice sounds were necessary to articulate utterance; that articulation was, in fact, nothing more than the modification of laryngeal vibrations; whereas in truth almost all articulate sounds, both vowels and consonants, may be pronounced in a whisper without any vocalisation, as anyone may satisfy himself in a moment; thus, V or S may be pronounced as well in a whisper as with the superaddition of the voice, and the sound prolonged with as much facility as the vowel sounds E or O. Indeed, in following my remarks on this subject and verifying for himself my description of the way in which the sounds of the different letters are produced, I should advise the reader to pronounce them in a whisper, and not to speak them "out," as by eliminating the laryngeal vibrations he will get the oral element of the sounds more unmixed and simple, and their analysis will be easier and more precise.

In what, then, does the essential difference between vowels and consonants consist? I think mainly in this—that while vowel sounds depend on the relation of the size of the oral cavity to the size of its orifices, consonantal sounds depend on some superadded condition of orifice quite independent of size. To take an example—in *far* and *fear* the difference is in the vowel sound, and the difference of condition is in the *size* of the oral cavity and aperture, both being more capacious in *far*; but in *oth* and *oss*, where the difference of sound is consonantal and the vowel sound the same, we find the size of the cavity and its relation to the orifice to be unchanged, but that the dental orifice is modified by the altered relations of the tongue to the teeth.

I am aware that this definition can only be stated approximatively; for as there is no real physiological distinction between some vowels and some consonants, so no definition can be laid down that would separate the whole of the one class from the whole of the other. This is illustrated in the accom-

Fig. 6.

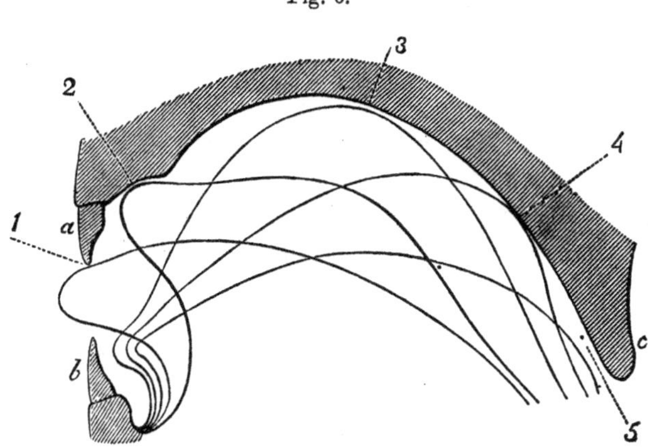

This diagram is intended to illustrate, by section, the relation of the tongue to the teeth and palate in the production of several sounds.

a. Superior incisor tooth.
b. Inferior incisor tooth.
c. Uvula.
1. Application of tongue to incisor tooth in producing the sound "*th.*"
2. Tongue to palate, sound "*d*"—closure complete; sound "*s*"—closure incomplete.
3. Sound "*ch*" (*German*), as in "Liebchen."
4. Sound German and Scotch guttural, as "Och!"
5. Sound "*g*" hard and "*k.*"

panying diagram. It represents a vertical section, in the middle line, of the upper jaw, the soft palate, and the tongue in various positions, and shows that the apposition of different parts of the upper surface of the tongue along the under surface of the soft or hard palate, or to the gum behind the teeth and upper incisors, produces the sounds of various letters, five of which are consonants and one a vowel. Thus, if the back of the tongue is applied to the soft palate, the sound of K is produced; if the sound of the Scotch *Och* is pronounced, it will be seen that the apposition takes place a little further forwards; for the pronunciation of the German *ch*, as in *Liebchen*, the apposition is still further in front; if, now, the upper surface of the front of the tongue is brought close against the front of the palate, whilst the tip is pressed against the back of the lower incisor teeth, so that a narrow horizontal chink is formed, on breathing through it the sound of E is produced; if the tip of the tongue is placed close against the gum behind the upper incisors, we get S; lastly, if we carry it a little further forwards and place it against the edge of the incisors themselves, projecting the tongue a little beyond the teeth, we get *th*. Thus, the apposition of the tongue to the upper wall of the mouth at six successive points, from behind forwards, gives six definite articulate sounds, one of which is a vowel.

Thus, while the teeth have far more to do with the formation of consonants than vowels, the associated distinction between oral cavity and orifice, as connected the one with the formation of vowel sounds, the other with that of consonants, is lost.

The principal way in which the teeth assist in the production of articulate sounds is by acting as an arch, or horseshoe-shaped ridge, within which and against which the tongue may act as a valve, and by pressing against which it may produce modified and variously-placed partial or complete closure.

The outline of the tongue, when flaccid and in a state of rest, coincides with that of the alveolar arches both in size and shape; and as its border is on the same level as the line of meeting of the upper and lower teeth, the teeth and the edge of the tongue are always, when this natural condition of rest is not disturbed, in close juxtaposition. This is not strictly and absolutely true with regard to the anterior extremity of the tongue, which is slightly depressed, so that the tip of it rests, not against the line of meeting of the incisors of the two jaws, but against the back of those of the lower one. It is this approximate coincidence of shape and close propinquity that make the instantaneous application of any part of the edge of the tongue to the corresponding part of the dental arch of either jaw so easy, and this it is also that makes any considerable dental irregularity or deficiency destroy, by preventing this application, the power of producing certain articulate sounds. Hence (to state this proposition conversely) we may lay down the practical rule that all measures taken with a view to restore imperfect articulation due to the teeth must have for their object to restore this coincidence between the entire dental arch and the entire border of the tongue.

Although the tongue is so placed that its edges may be pressed with equal facility against the teeth of *either* jaw, it is against various parts of the dental arch of the *upper* jaw that it is, in actual fact, pressed in the formation of most of the dental consonants.

Whenever the border of the tongue is closely applied to the inside of any of the teeth, then closure is produced, and air cannot pass; whenever this closure is not produced, then air can pass, and then it is that the particular sound produced by this modification of aperture is generated. Thus, the seat of the sound is always, not where the tongue is in contact with the teeth, but where it is *not* in perfect contact with them. This is a point that it is of importance to bear in mind in drawing an inference, as to the whereabouts of a deficiency in the teeth, from the particular defect of speech that the patient may exhibit.

Upon the principles that I have laid down I have endeavoured to construct what may be called a physiological alphabet. The arrangement is based upon the situation of the closure by which the sound is produced, upon the completeness or incompleteness of the closure, and upon whether the breathing is soft or aspirate, and the table shows how completely symmetrical the whole subject is, and what a parallelism runs through it. It shows, too, to the formation of how large a number of letters the teeth contribute.

TABLE.

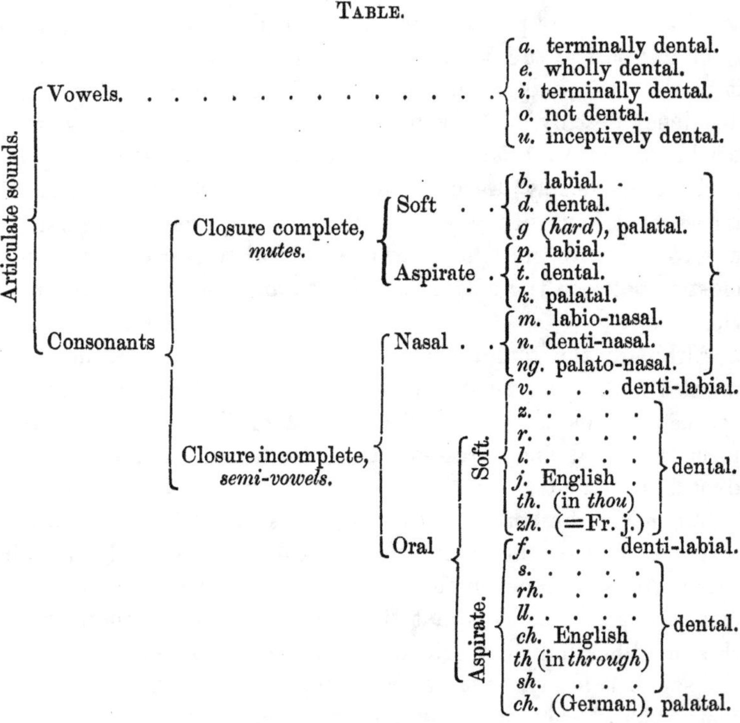

Of the consonants it will be seen that nine—B, D, G, P, T, K, M, N, NG—are subdivisible into threes in a very orderly and regular way. Three are labials, B, P, and M; three are dentals, D, T, and N; three are palatals, G hard, K, and NG (as in *thing*). Of the labials, one, B, has a soft breathing; the other, P, an aspirate breathing; and in the third, M, the sound is continued through the nose after the labial closure, and I therefore call this a "labio-nasal." In the same way the dental has a soft, an aspirate, and a denti-nasal; and the palatal a soft, an aspirate, and a palato-nasal; so that there are three with a soft breathing, three corresponding ones with an aspirate breathing, and three nasal, in which the sound is continued through the nose after the oral closure. In all these nine the oral closure, whether at lips, teeth, or palate, is complete, and those of them (the first six) in which the sound is not continued through the nose are therefore called *mutes*, because they produce complete arrest of sound.

In all the other consonants the oral closure is incomplete, and the characteristic sound of the letter is produced, not by the method of closure, as in the others, but by the particular shape and seat of the orifice or constriction produced by the partial closure. The sound in these is therefore continuous, and may be protracted any length of time, and the letters are thence called "semi-vowels," or continuous consonants. Putting aside the German *ch* (in English we do not possess it), they are fourteen in number, and may be coupled two and two, seven having the soft and seven the aspirate breathing, and each aspirate letter corresponding to one with a soft breathing. Thus V corresponds to F, Z to S, &c.; so that there are really only seven distinct consonantal sounds of this class and seven modifications of the parts engaged in their production, each of these sounds being doubled by the substitution of one breathing for the other. Two of the letters, V and F, are produced by certain relations of the teeth and lips, and I therefore call them "denti-labial;" the other twelve depend upon the relation of the teeth and tongue, and I therefore call them "dentals;" perhaps with more correctness they might be called "denti-linguals."

Let me now analyze more particularly and in order the way in which all these letters are formed. As my object is only to show the part which the teeth play in their formation, I shall not say anything about the labials and palatals.

In pronouncing D the tip of the tongue is placed firmly against the gum behind the upper incisors, and its edges against the upper alveolar arches and teeth, so as to produce complete closure, and these parts are then suddenly opened. In T exactly the same is done, only the breathing accompanying the opening is more forced. In N the method of oral closure is exactly the same, only after the closure is established the sound is continued through the nose. Thus T may be said to be D-aspirate, and N may be said to be D with nasal prolongation. This is how it is that when the nose is obstructed by cold or otherwise, N becomes D; thus, "nonsense" pronounced "dodsedse" gives an idea of cold in the head.

Conversely, in cases of cleft palate, in which the posterior nares cannot be closed, and the sound is therefore not prevented from prolongation through the nose, D cannot be sounded, but is pronounced like N, so that a person with cleft palate, instead of saying "How do you do?" says, "How noo you noo?"

In the pronunciation of V and F the upper front teeth are brought against the lower lip, and the air is driven through them—in V gently and in F forcibly. For this sound therefore the uppers incisors are necessary. In old people who have completely lost all their upper incisors the gum answers nearly or quite as well; but the loss of a single incisor or of the two central incisors materially interferes with the pronunciation of these letters. It is perhaps in consequence of being unable to bring the thick and prominent lower lip against the upper teeth that Africans (negroes) are unable to say these letters.

In the pronunciation of consonants in which the sound depends upon air driven through a chink between the tongue and the teeth, the closure may be lateral and the aperture mesial, or *vice versâ*: thus, in TH and S the aperture is mesial; in L the closure is mesial and the aperture is lateral.

In the pronunciation of TH the tip of the tongue is brought against the upper teeth, and the air is driven through the chink thus formed; in TH, as in "thou," with the soft breathing; in TH, as in "thick," with the aspirate.

If now the tip of the tongue is a little retracted and brought close against the gum behind the upper teeth, and a slight chink still permitted while the sides of the tongue are firmly applied to the side teeth of the upper jaw (especially, as it seems to me, the bicuspids), and the air driven through this chink, the sound of S will be produced; if we substitute the soft breathing for the aspirate, we shall have Z.

Let the tip of the tongue be still further retracted, so as to be brought against the edge of the gum where it makes an angle to pass up and form the roof of the palate, we shall get the sound of R; but in this case, from the way the tip of the tongue is twisted up, I think the lateral closure is not perfect, or at any rate that the chink is more laterally extended than in the pronunciation of S.

In sounding L, the closure is mesial and the aperture lateral. We make it by applying the tip of the tongue firmly against the gums behind the upper incisors, but exercising no lateral opposition—in fact, leaving a space open on each side: through these two lateral apertures the air is driven, and so the sound is generated. Thus the difference between D and L is, that in the former there is lateral closure, in the latter lateral aperture, but the mesial closure is the same in both; and in pronouncing D and L in succession, as in "candle," we merely have to liberate the sides of the tongue from their contact with the upper alveolar arch and teeth.

SH is perhaps the most purely dental sound of any; for in its formation the air is simply driven through the closed or nearly closed teeth. In S the chink through which the air is driven is exceedingly slender and also laterally circumscribed. In SH we have a larger or coarser sibilation, the tongue not narrowing the chink, nor being concerned in the production of the sound at all. I think it is only through the teeth in front of the bicuspids that the air is driven in this sound (SH), and that it is prevented from lateral escape through the bicuspids and molars by the pressure of the cheeks, by means of the buccinator muscle, against the outsides of the teeth. Anyone pronouncing the sound will feel that his cheeks are pressed against the outsides of his teeth, and that his buccinators are in a state of action; and this, no doubt, is how it is that the lips are protruded in uttering it; for, to fix the commissures of the mouth, that the buccinators may act from them with advantage, the orbicularis oris contracts, and when this is the case either the mouth must be closed, or, to prevent this, the lips must be protruded. In the lateral apertures between the teeth being closed, and the air prevented escaping through them by the pressure of the cheeks against their outsides, instead of the edges of the tongue against their inside, the formation of this sound differs from that of all others. That the lateral escape of air between the molars interferes with the firmness and integrity of the sound may be shown by introducing the finger between the cheeks and the teeth, and so holding the former out; the lateral escape of air at once alters the sound. The French J, which would be spelt in England ZH, is the soft breathing of which SH is the corresponding aspirate. The English J is really a compound sound, and begins with the sound of D; it is, in fact, DJ. Anyone analysing in his own person how the J in "judge" is sounded, may satisfy himself of this, and that the movements of the parts concerned are those that would produce D and the French J in succession. CH, as in "church," is the correlative aspirate of the English J, and might be spelt TSH.

Of the five English vowels, A, E, I, O, U, together with the additional vowel sounds in AH, AU, OO, only one can strictly be said to be dental. In the pronunciation of E it will be observed that the tip of the tongue is pressed against the back of the lower incisor teeth, so as to be flattened and expanded, and the air driven through a horizontal chink formed between the upper surface or the front of the tongue thus flattened out and the gum behind the upper incisors; and it would be extremely difficult to pronounce this vowel without thus pressing the apex of the tongue against the lower front teeth. But, if the pronunciation of the vowels A, I, and U be analysed, it will be observed that the sound of E enters into them all—A and I terminating with the E sound, and U commencing with it. Thus E is a pure dental vowel; A and I terminally dental; and U inceptively dental. To these must be added Y, which so commonly has the sound of E, as in "yes," and "joy."

Now, the loss or injury of any of the passive organs of speech produces a corresponding defect in the articulation of the sufferer; and, if the teeth are the organs affected, then dental sounds are interrupted or interfered with. This is always very manifest, and by far most manifest immediately after the loss of a tooth or teeth has taken place; for by degrees the loss is, to a certain extent, compensated by the adaptation of the soft parts, and the cultivated skill of the speaker. The injury inflicted on the speech is always more marked when the loss consists of a few teeth, and especially those towards the front of the mouth—there being thus produced a marked gap between teeth still standing. The loss, for instance, of the superior central incisors while the laterals remain, puts an end to the F's and V's of the speaker, and a blowing sound through the opening takes their places, or is superadded. When, however, several teeth are removed, and a considerable surface of gum is left free, the tongue or the lips, as the case may be, can be applied to it somewhat as they had been previously to the teeth; thus, if all the upper incisors and canines are gone, the upper gum rests on the lower lip, so as to imitate the sounds of F and V; but the want of the teeth with the little intervals between them deprive those sounds of the slight sibilant accompaniment which properly attends them, and which is produced by the passage of air between the teeth; the sound is dull and short; thus, V has somewhat the sound of B, and F of P: still the sound is approximately correct.

When lateral teeth (molars and bicuspids) are lost, the flattening out of the tongue, and the in-sinking of the cheek remarkably fill up the gap and compensate for the loss; and thus, to a considerable extent, the consequent defect in articulation is remedied.

These compensating changes in the soft parts are not sudden, but progress by time. After a gap or a lateral vacancy has existed some months, the tongue, if the loss of teeth be on one side, loses its symmetry and bulges so into the hiatus as to fill it —at least so as to meet the cheek.

Everyone who has supplied artificial teeth in such a case must have observed what is the consequence—how frequently the tongue and cheek are at first bitten by the substitutes for those natural teeth, the removal of which has allowed the soft parts to enlarge and expand.

These changes in the soft parts are merely instanced as some of the compensatory conditions by which the effects on speech of the loss of teeth are remedied.

Without carrying this subject further, it may be stated in general terms that, though the loss of the teeth will injure or destroy those elements of sound which it is their office passively to assist in forming, the plasticity of the soft parts will greatly relieve or remedy such injury. Further, that an individual adapted by habit and long use to speech without teeth, is at first incommoded by their artificial restoration. But that those persons will ultimately have the best articulation who, having lost teeth, are supplied artificially by that which is the nearest approach to a perfect dentition.

CHAPTER III.

SUPERNUMERARY TEETH—THIRD SETS OF TEETH—DEFICIENCIES OF TEETH.

The number of the human teeth being definite and fixed, a departure from that number is an abnormality. This more often occurs as an excess than a deficiency.

Supernumerary teeth occur as additions to the temporary set; as additions to the permanent set; but more commonly than either as superadditions to the permanents—superadded, that is, as regards both time and character. The only instances with which I am personally acquainted, where this condition has affected the temporary teeth, have consisted in a repetition of one of the lower milk incisors, ranging with the others, and not to be distinguished from them. Many years since, I saw this in a young cousin of my own; and it was impossible to say which of the two left lower lateral temporary incisors was the supernumerary, and which the normal tooth. They were nearly or quite coincident in time of advent, and ranged in unbroken arch.*

In one instance the supernumerary tooth was organically united to its normal neighbour.

I am not aware that supernumerary teeth of the character of temporaries, ever follow upon the milk set as others do upon the permanents.

Where supernumerary teeth occur in connection with the first set, I believe it may be stated that they are coincident with those that are contiguous to them and similar in form and general characters; ranging, moreover, in the same arch.† They are usually found in the lower jaw. When the supernumerary

* The permanent lower incisors were afterwards normal in number.

† An interesting exception to this has occurred in the practice of Mr. Ibbotson. The temporary supernumeraries were followed by supernumerary teeth.

teeth appear later in life, they are generally, though not always, behind the range of the normal teeth. And as to time of advent, they may appear *just before*, *with*, or *soon after* the true teeth which are near them, and with which their genesis has been associated. Most often they follow the normal teeth in date of eruption: least often they antecede them.

In their relation to the proper teeth of the permanent set, they are by far the most commonly connected, both by proximity and apparent resemblance, with the incisors; less commonly with the molars; and still more rarely with bicuspids and canines. They are far more common in the upper than in the lower jaw.

These permanent supernumeraries, if they may be so called, are divisible into—

Conical teeth—canine-like;

Cubic-crowned, resembling lower bicuspids; and

Teeth mimicking those of the true set in their immediate neighbourhood.

The *conical* supernumerary teeth are usually found towards the extreme front of the upper jaw, and frequently single between the two superior central incisors, as seen in the accompanying illustration (fig. 7). When behind the arch of

Fig. 7.

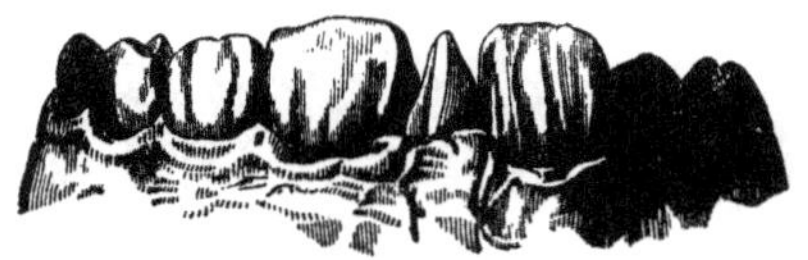

the true teeth they are still generally well forward; but instead of being single, are sometimes in pairs. Or rather, it should

Fig. 8. Fig. 9. Fig. 10.

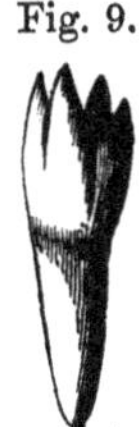

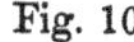

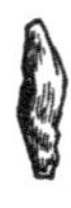

be said, they are in twos, which often differ considerably in form. Thus, one will be a single conical cusp, while the fellow tooth will be broken up into several small cusps: as is illustrated by the left and central figure in this series (figs. 8 and 9).

These canine-like supernumeraries usually consist of a short conical crown and a long conical root, and there is seldom any distinct indication which is the front and which the back of the tooth.

It is uncommon to find supernumerary teeth in the lower jaw associated with the permanent set. The minute figure to the right (fig. 10) represents a central supernumerary tooth which I extracted from deep down in the front of the lower jaw: it was projecting forwards, and had pierced a hole in the lower lip. This example occurred in a boy, ten years old, at Guy's Hospital. The point of the supernumerary tooth had appeared a few months after the permanent incisors were cut. The incisors were not separated, as the little supplemental tooth pierced the gum nearly half an inch below their necks.

The *cubic-crowned* teeth, resembling lower bicuspids, are, I believe, always found in the upper jaw immediately behind the central incisors or slightly to their outer edges, and usually in pairs. The accompanying illustration (fig. 11) shows their general situation. The form of these teeth is very characteristic, and pretty constant. In front the crown presents a smooth oblong surface; behind it is lumpy and corrugated; while at the summit the enamel surface is bulged-in in the form of a pit. The roots are usually long, cylindrical, and straight.

Fig. 11.

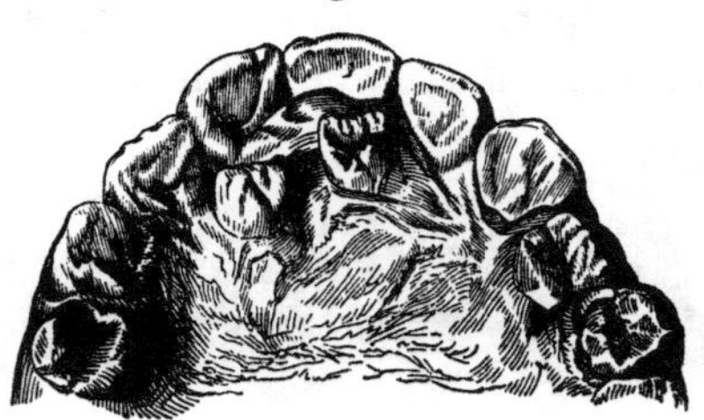

Fig. 12. Fig. 13.

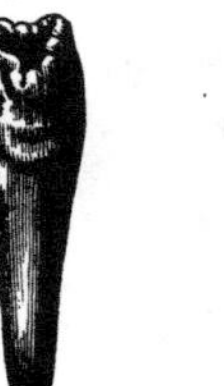

The accompanying figures (12, 13) represent the left tooth taken from the mouth, which is illustrated by the foregoing woodcut. The left figure represents the back of the tooth when *in situ*, the right its front. The tooth was extracted before the end of the fang was completely formed.

The supernumerary teeth which mimic those in their own immediate neighbourhood are the most interesting, involving the practical question as to which of two teeth, close together and just alike, should be considered the normal tooth, and so retained; and as bearing upon the curious theoretical question, how far their formation may be considered as an effort to produce a third set of teeth; or at least how far their presence may explain those reputed instances in which a third set has been said to have occurred.

The only supernumerary teeth which resemble the normal form of the true teeth, are those which sometimes occur towards the front of the mouth.

The superior incisors sometimes; more often the laterals than the centrals: the upper canines very rarely, and still more rarely the bicuspids. Further back in the mouth, and associated with the molars, the supernumeraries are usually but small conical cusps, and sometimes appear to be actual cusps belonging to the neighbouring teeth, as if thrown off by fission.

I have seen three instances in which the superior permanent central incisor has been mimicked. They were all three exactly alike. Upon the shedding of the temporary incisors one of the apparent permanent successors was cut in advance of its fellow: this was followed by the tooth on the other side; and then appeared a third incisor over the first that had come. The event proved that the second and third were the normal central incisors; the first that was cut being a supernumerary tooth, but like the true tooth on the same side, excepting that the back of the crown was more corrugated, and the serrations at the edge rather deeper than usual. As I have said, I have seen this three times, with scarcely any variation of the circumstances. I have in my collection one plaster cast, and two teeth illustrative of this condition.

The supernumerary *lateral* incisor, however, completely imitates the true tooth. I have seen five instances of this, and in two cases both laterals were thus repeated. I have four such supernumerary laterals in my possession. One of the cases in which both laterals were repeated was very interesting. A young lady about twelve years of age was brought to me respecting the irregularity of the teeth in the front of her mouth, and this consisted in the presence of four superior lateral incisors—two very prominent, and two backward. When the mouth was shut, the lower incisors divided the two in front from those behind. I extracted the latter, and those in front soon fell back into their places. The teeth I had extracted were perfect lateral incisors, and could not be distinguished in any way from those that remained. In the other instance, where two supernumerary laterals were present, they were in the true dental arch, and they were rather smaller than those which I took to be the normal teeth. In the other three instances the imitation was on one side only—there was one supernumerary lateral incisor.

A very remarkable example of supernumerary incisor development came under my notice some time since, which can be best understood by reference to the accompanying figure taken from

Fig. 14.

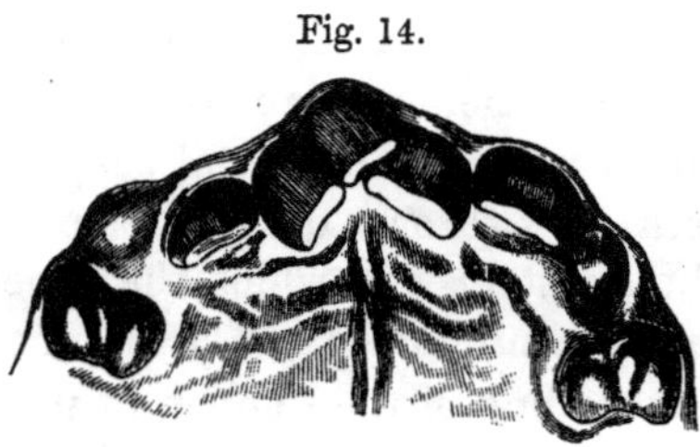

a plaster cast of the boy's mouth. The patient was about twelve years old. Describing the front of this patient's mouth, and beginning from the left (the right of the figure), there was first the anterior bicuspid, then the left canine just through the gum, then a large broad incisor tooth, then a similar one just a trifle smaller; after that two small incisors of the form of central incisors united together organically, then another incisor wider than either of the two latter, and smaller than either of the first two, but still resembling a central rather than a lateral. Still further to the right (the left of the figure) is seen the projecting gum over the right canine just about to pierce, and then the right anterior bicuspid.

It is difficult to interpret the incisor elements of this dentition; all the teeth resembled centrals. Their edges were faceted by direct application to the summits of the lower teeth. The patient was to have come to me again; but he did not return.

Supernumerary canines are far less common than incisors. It does not follow that a supernumerary tooth, because it is opposite a canine, is therefore a supernumerary cuspidatus. Again, many of the supernumerary teeth are pointed, and resemble to some extent canine teeth; still they have none of the moulding of a true eye-tooth.

However, genuine repetitions of the cuspidatus do occur. I have seen two in the same individual. In the autumn of 1866, a German gentleman applied to me on account of the annoyance which his tongue (in a state of syphilitic ulceration) experienced by contact with two teeth projecting from the palate on either side, just within the eye-teeth. Upon examining the mouth, I found two supernumerary pointed teeth in the situation indicated. I extracted them, and found that they were exactly like the true cuspidatus that remained in the normal position. The patient claimed one of these teeth, and I have retained the other. The supernumerary teeth were cut a few years after those in proper place.

The only example of a supernumerary bicuspid tooth which has come within my knowledge is the specimen here figured. There is a minute tooth with two cusps attached to a second upper bicuspid. The crown is free, but the root fused to the larger tooth. This little supernumerary is truly bicuspid, inasmuch as its crown presents two eminences with an intervening depression; but it cannot be said that the form of the crown is exactly like that of a full-sized normal premolar.

Fig. 15.

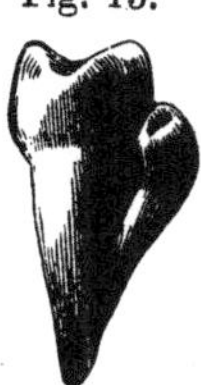

Such, then, are the supernumerary teeth which mimic those of the true set; and they add, as far as their number and similitude go, a certain weight in favour of the authenticity of those instances of third sets of teeth which are reputed to have occurred. Of this more will be said presently.

I have never seen or heard of an instance in which a supernumerary tooth had more than one fang. The structure of the tooth is generally very compact, and the enamel thick. Where the surface is irregular, it is usually produced by tubercular masses of enamel. In one instance only have I seen the enamel rocky and pitted: in this instance, there were two supernumeraries in the same mouth, and both similarly affected. In one instance, in which I made a section of a supernumerary tooth for the microscope, I found the dentinal tubes passing into the enamel to a remarkable extent; and those sacculated, club-shaped cavities sometimes seen extending from the dentine into the enamel, were extremely numerous.

As regards the treatment of supernumerary teeth, I know but of one plan—*extraction*. Excepting where a supernumerary tooth is organically connected with a normal tooth, it is, I believe, always in the way, and better removed. In the front of the mouth they usually dislocate the incisors, protruding them, and even altering the expression of the face, and, when central, separating them in the middle line. They should therefore be extracted as soon as possible, when it will be found that the normal teeth soon assume their proper position.

Third Sets of Teeth.—The doubtful question as to the occurrence of third sets of teeth may well be considered here. It is of small practical importance, but is very interesting physiologically; and the uncertainty which attaches to the disputed circumstance is not a little remarkable as a matter of scientific observation and evidence.

There is no recorded instance of the occurrence of a third set of teeth in the writings of any modern observer of scientific repute; but the authorities of earlier date, who have asserted the fact, are so respectable, that it is difficult altogether to discard from one's mind the idea that the circumstance has occurred in some shape. At the same time, it must appear to any scientific reasoner as most remarkable, that in the immensely increased population of more recent times, subjected far more than formerly to acute professional scrutiny, no such occurrence has been seen.

The fallacies by which a mistaken judgment may happen in this matter (at least, as regards partial third sets of teeth) are such as would be not unlikely to lead to errors. *Supernumerary teeth*, and still more *impacted teeth*, which, though belonging to the normal set of permanents, have not been previously missed, and have, late in life, pierced the gums from the prolonged absorption of alveolar process, would be, and probably have been, considered as representatives of a third set of teeth. These fallacies would not, however, explain those instances where complete third sets have been recorded.

Hunter has had the credit of stating that he himself saw one instance in which a complete third set of teeth was developed.

He has, however, recorded no such observation; but, having expressed himself rather ambiguously, Dr. Mason Good misunderstood his remarks, and incorrectly attributes to him this statement. Subsequent writers,* copying Dr. Good's *résumé* of the subject, have repeated the error, until Hunter has been regularly accredited with the assertion.

All that Hunter did assert on his own observation was, that he once saw an instance in which "two fore teeth shot up in the lower jaw." These he supposed to be portions of a third set.

The following instance of a complete third dentition is thus recorded, in the third volume of the "Edinburgh Medical Commentaries," † on the authority of the editor:—"A country labourer, who was an inhabitant of the town of Hawick, in the south of Scotland, lost all his teeth by the time he arrived at the sixtieth year of his age. But, about half a year afterwards, a new set made their appearance. All of them appeared within the space of twenty days; but during this time he suffered the most excruciating pain. His new set of teeth continued fresh and firm for a period of thirty-four years. He is still alive, has entered the ninety-sixth year of his age, and has all his teeth except three, which he has lost within these two years, one of them very lately."

In another instance, recorded by Dr. Bisset, a physician at Knayton, in Yorkshire, in a letter ‡ to Dr. Duncan, an old woman of ninety-eight is stated to have cut twelve molar teeth, and two upper incisors. Six months afterwards, four molars had been shed, and the remainder were somewhat loose.

Dr. Mason Good § saw a lady, seventy-four years of age, who cut "several straggling teeth." And he records another instance that occurred to him:—"A lady of seventy-six, mother of the late Henry Hughes, Esq., printer of the Journals of the House of Commons, cut two molars, and at the same time completely

* Dr. Harris in his *Dental Surgery* has repeated this assertion in edition after edition. (*Dental Surgery*, by C. A. Harris, Philadelphia. Several editions.)

† *Edinburgh Medical Commentaries*, vol. iii. pt. i. p. 105. Lond. 1784.

‡ Published in *Edinburgh Medical Commentaries*, vol. viii. p. 371. Lond. 1787.

§ *The Study of Medicine*, by John Mason Good (4th edit.), vol. i. p. 40. Lond. 1834.

recovered her hearing, after having been for some years totally deaf."

This latter case was probably an instance of impacted teeth being laid bare through the prolonged absorption of jaw-bone in old age. No such explanation, however, can apply to the marvellous history, which Dr. Stare has recorded in an early volume of the "Philosophical Transactions of the Royal Society," and of which the following is an abstract.*

The subject of this curious abnormality was "a Bedfordshire gentleman of an old English family," and he was grandfather of Dr. Stare, who records the case. When eighty years of age all his teeth were sound and firm: at eighty-two he lost first one, and then a second front tooth. After this, in the succeeding three years, the whole of the front teeth were shed. They were subsequently replaced by an entire new set of teeth, which, it seems, he retained till his death in his hundredth year. This singular history is narrated in a letter to Sir Hans Sloane, with earnest assurances of its truthfulness, by Dr. Stare, who refers to the circumstance, not only from his own observation and inspection, but as notorious at the time.

Deficiencies of Teeth.—It is by no means rare to find certain of the teeth wanting from the set; and this may arise from the tooth being embedded in the jaw, and not projected; or from its not being formed: to the latter I now refer. This is more common with the permanent than the temporary teeth. The latter may be complete, and the succeeding set deficient.

The superior lateral incisor is more often absent than any other tooth. I have no right permanent upper lateral; but the temporary was present. Deficiency, like all other congenital peculiarities of the teeth, is very apt to run in families. I have three near relatives in whom the superior laterals are wanting; and in some others they are small and imperfectly formed.

I am acquainted with three sisters, two of whom have no upper wisdom teeth; in the third they are very minute.

I had a patient whose mouth contained no inferior incisor teeth, and no upper laterals. The wisdom teeth were absent

* Letter from Dr. Frederick Stare to Sir Hans Sloane, "Concerning a person who had a new set of teeth after eighty years of age." In *Phil. Trans.* vol. xxviii. p. 273.

from both jaws; but as the patient was only twenty years of age, the latter might still appear.

Two other examples show the hereditary character of these defects. A young lady, thirteen years of age, was brought to me by her father. She had no central incisors of the lower jaw, but the laterals were separated to the full extent. The temporary centrals had come out, but from the condition of the alveolar border it was clear that their successors were totally wanting. The father, fifty-six years old, also had no lower central incisors; neither had he the second molars or wise teeth on either side of the lower jaw; the second bicuspids were wanting, and their place held by the second temporary molars, still sound and firm. In the upper jaw the wisdom teeth were absent. This gentleman had never had a permanent tooth extracted.

Two interesting cases, in which great deficiency of teeth was associated with almost complete alopœcia, are recorded in the thirty-first volume of the "Transactions of the Medico-Chirurgical Society" (p. 71). The subjects of these peculiarities were cousins, and each had four molars in the upper jaw, and no other tooth.

Otto * mentions, on the authority of others, two cases in which teeth were wholly wanting. The first occurred in a woman who at sixty years of age had never had any teeth.† The other two were brothers, adults, members of a Jewish family. Neither of them had teeth or hair.‡

* *Lehrbuch der Path. Anatomie, &c.*, von Dr. A. W. Otto. Berlin, 1830.

† Borelli, *Hist. et Obs. Med. Phys.*, Cent. II. Obs. XI. i., p. 144. 1676.

‡ Daaz, in Stark's *Archiv. f. d. Geburtshülfe*, vol. iv. p. 684. Jena, 1792.

CHAPTER IV.

IRREGULARITIES IN THE POSITION OF THE TEETH.

Irregularities of the teeth, as regards their relation to each other and to the jaws containing them, constitute some of the most important considerations in the practical treatment of the teeth, and they are not without interest theoretically.

Irregularities of the temporary teeth are uncommon, and are not of much importance. The incisors sometimes have a distorted position, but the commonest form of irregularity in the teeth of the first set is that which is relative in the two jaws. It is not very rare in families, where there is a strong tendency to what is known as an "underhung bite," for the temporary incisors, or even the canines of the lower jaw, to project beyond those of the upper. And though this may not be attended by any irregularity of the relative position of the teeth in either jaw, it still constitutes a serious irregularity of the teeth as taken collectively.

These irregularities of the temporary teeth may not require immediate interference, but they indicate the propriety of most careful superintendence during the advent and progress of succession.

Irregularity of the teeth appears to be one of those conditions induced by artificial life, and progressing in degree during the lapse of time in successive generations. It is almost unknown among the lower animals in a wild state; but it has been induced in some through domestication.

This subject may be treated with almost endless extension, and with profuse illustration, as the conditions of irregularity are almost without limit in their variety, and may be complicated in cause.

I propose to consider them here briefly and practically, and principally by illustrative cases that have occurred in my own practice.

The *causes* of irregularities may be (1) congenital and hereditary, (2) the prolonged retention of temporary teeth, (3) accidental mechanical influences, (4) disproportion of the size of the teeth and jaws, (5) faulty development of the jaw-bones.

There are few conditions in which hereditary influences are more manifest than in the irregularities which occur in the teeth; and these show themselves often in minute particulars, and are displayed with distinctness by collateral relations. The prolonged retention of temporary teeth is frequently associated with irregularity in their successors or their permanent neighbours, and is probably often the cause of such irregularity; though perhaps the imperfect or tardy growth of the permanents may be at least partially the reason why the temporary teeth are so retained. Accidental mechanical influences, such as thumb-sucking or hypertrophy of the tongue, will cause certain irregularities. But by far the most common cause of irregularities in the teeth is their being disproportionately large in comparison with the jaws. This is a condition which has been progressing in development for a long period of time and very many generations, and appears in some way dependent on civilised life. The disparity is such as to lead to the crowding of teeth so constantly seen, and which is sometimes so excessive as to altogether exclude some member of the dental series from eruption, and hold it permanently impacted in the substance of the jaw.

This condition is not infrequently induced by the premature extraction of the temporary teeth, which permits contiguous permanent neighbours to approximate each other to the displacement or partial exclusion of the successor of the extracted tooth.

Malformation of the jaws is much less common, and is only certainly displayed in some peculiar irregularities, as in the V-shaped jaw.

In considering irregularities of the teeth in regard to their treatment, they may be divided with much practical advantage into (1) *Simple* and (2) *Compound* or *Contingent.*

Simple irregularities are those in which the misplacement is absolute as regards the jaw affected, and independent of the position of the teeth in the opposite jaw. They may affect both jaws in the same individual, but they are uninfluenced by each other.

Compound irregularities are contingent on the position of the teeth of the opposite jaw, as to cause or maintenance, and are dependent on the "*bite.*"

The importance of these distinctions will be manifest in considering the treatment of these cases. In curing irregularities it will be necessary to remove all obstructions which prevent the teeth from assuming a regular arrangement; and it may be necessary to apply mechanical elastic force to complete that result. Both these elements of treatment may be requisite in a single case. Again, there is a peculiar method of applying mechanism where no force is involved, namely, in those cases in which the irregularity is contingent on the bite, and where the closure of the mouth causes its maintenance. In such cases the jaws must be kept apart during treatment, and this is accomplished by the passive mechanism of gagging.

Very much depends on the age of the patient when the irregularity comes under treatment. For instance, where it is brought about by crowding, the mere removal of some tooth or teeth in a *young* patient may allow the remainder to assume the natural arch, and this they will generally do without assistance; whereas the same condition in an older patient will require mechanical pressure to place the teeth in proper range, and it may be necessary to maintain them in this position by similar means for a considerable period, as when once firmly established they have a tendency to return to their original relations.

It has appeared to me that this subject may be conveniently treated by the consideration of typical examples of irregularity; and the accompanying figure (16) illustrates one of the commonest forms—where the upper canine tooth, from insufficient room, makes its appearance high up, and in front of the range of contiguous teeth. I refer to this form of irregularity, first, not only from its frequency, but because its consideration involves many general

Fig. 16.

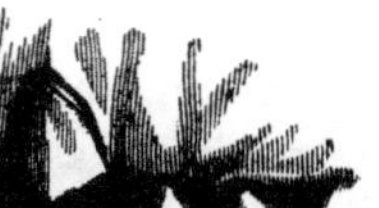

questions of importance bearing on the whole subject. It may arise from the premature removal of the temporary canine tooth, thus allowing the bicuspid and lateral incisor to approach close to each other.

This condition usually manifests itself between ten and thirteen years of age, and, if uncomplicated, it is readily cured by the extraction of a tooth behind the coming canine; and in the simplest cases the removal of the first bicuspid effects the remedy at once. Circumstances, however, may suggest the desirability of sacrificing another tooth, the second bicuspid, or even the first molar; and this point requires careful consideration. And it should further be remembered that much may be done by nature, through the expansion of the jaw itself; and this is especially the case where the permanent teeth make their appearance very early, and at a time when the jaw, from the age of the patient, may be supposed to be too soon invaded by its large and many occupants. I have sometimes known bicuspid teeth removed to make room in young patients with much crowding, when afterwards it has been apparent that such a proceeding was unnecessary,—the jaw growing to such an extent that considerable spaces were developed between the remaining teeth—spaces which in the aggregate would have accommodated the teeth that had been extracted. It is a question, therefore, with young patients to consider how much may be done by nature in time, before a sacrifice is entailed which cannot afterwards be remedied.

In estimating which of the three teeth (first or second bicuspid, or first molar) should be extracted in any given case, many points arise which should be carefully balanced in the mind of the operator before he makes his selection. The respective value of the teeth must be considered as *features*, as *organs of mastication*, and in relation to their *prospective durability* and their *soundness* at the time. These are all important points for consideration, irrespective of the cardinal question as to which tooth would, by its removal, best effect the required object, furnish the needed room, and allow the misplaced anterior tooth, or teeth, to range in proper order with the others. Unquestionably the bicuspid teeth are superior as features to the molar; indeed, the farther forward in the mouth a tooth is situated, the more does it modify the form of the lips, the more is it seen in expression, and consequently the more would its absence be remarked. It must be recollected, however, that there are two bicuspids, so much alike that when one is lost the other takes its place as far as appearance goes. As an organ of mastication a molar is of greater value than a bicuspid. The present *soundness* or otherwise of the bicuspids and molar is a question of the greatest importance, and must often decide finally and peremptorily the question under consideration. Provided the loss of either a bicuspid or a first molar would give the necessary space with equal ease and certainty, or nearly so—one being carious and the other sound—there can be no hesitation as to which should be extracted. The decayed tooth should be taken out, and a double good will thus be effected, the regulation will be achieved, and a source of future or perhaps present pain will be removed. It must be recollected, however, that it will take a far longer time for the crowding of the canines and incisors to obtain relief by the removal of a molar tooth than by the loss of a bicuspid; and in patients who have reached some fourteen or fifteen years of age, or in whom the irregularity has existed for some time, it may even be doubtful if the loss of a molar will extend forward the required relief. And this leads to the consideration of another very important point. The ' 'te" of the bicuspids in the two jaws may be interlocking; the cusps of the lower bicuspids may so abut, when the mouth is closed, upon the posterior aspect of the cusps of the upper bicuspids as to prevent the latter from moving backwards after the removal of the first molar; and thus, though the room may be furnished, the crowded upper front teeth are mechanically prevented from obtaining the benefit of it. The operator, therefore, should well look to this point before deciding on the removal of a molar. I urge this, not on theoretical grounds, but because I have more than once seen a molar removed under these circumstances; and, the bite keeping the upper bicuspids immovably forwards, no improvement in the irregularity took place. Finally, the question of relative *prospective durability*, as between the bicuspids and first molar, supposing each to be sound, is a point the importance of which cannot be over-estimated. This matter is not so easily decided by the statistical records regarding the decay of the two teeth as has been imagined. No doubt first molars are more prone to decay than bicuspids, and it may be prognosticated as probable that at the time any particular first molar is cut its term of soundness will be shorter than that of any particular bicuspid, when *it* first comes into the mouth. But that does not state the case fairly. The question is, which tooth, supposing both to be sound at the time when the regulation is required (say at about twelve years of age), has the best prospect of prolonged soundness and usefulness? It should be remembered that a first molar tooth at that time has been in the mouth some *six* years, and if then sound, it has for that long period resisted the influences of decay. The bicuspid, though also sound, has only been exposed to like influences for a year or a few months. The existing evidence therefore, though negative in its nature, is, as a matter of probability, altogether in favour of the molar on the score of prospective soundness; and my own experience is that if a first molar is free from decay at twelve years of age, it is nearly as likely to remain sound as any other molar; whereas no such estimate can be formed of the prospective durability of a bicuspid that has been in the mouth only a few months. This is the real question as between a sound bicuspid and first molar at the usual time for removing one of them to make room, and it is in favour of the retention of the molar.

I would, therefore, say, as a summary of these arguments: Provided the removal of either tooth would be equally efficacious, or nearly so, remove a decayed tooth rather than a sound one; this will lead to the very frequent extraction of the first molar. If both the bicuspids and first molar are sound, extract one of the former; and the regulation, though not more effectually perhaps, will be more speedily accomplished than by removing the molar.

The foregoing observations have been written with special reference to the upper teeth, but they may be applied to those of the lower jaw. The greater durability of the inferior bicuspids, however, and the more easy cutting and more forward position of the lower wisdom-tooth which result from the removal of a first molar, would tend to balance more evenly the claims of the two teeth respectively; still, where both are sound at twelve years, I would remove a bicuspid and retain the molar. As regards the first and second bicuspids respectively, the removal of the former I consider preferable.

This crowding of the canine tooth in the upper jaw upon the lateral incisor, entailing the loss of a tooth to remove unsightly irregularity, not infrequently involves another question of much nicety and requiring a judicious balance of opposing arguments. The question I refer to does not relate to the loss of a bicuspid or a molar, to make room for more forward teeth, but it is this: In a *confirmed* irregularity in a patient of more advanced years, when posterior room cannot be expected to allow the canine and lateral incisor to range in proper arch, the disfigurement being great, which of the teeth in question ought to be sacrificed? Such cases constantly occur. Take the following as an example: A young lady eighteen years of age has been entirely neglected as to her teeth. The first bicuspid tooth of the right side, upper jaw, is almost in contact with the lateral incisor; the canine is in front, high up, and rather to the outside of the lateral, while the latter tooth is so far forced back as to shut behind the lower teeth when the mouth is closed, having an intersecting bite. Such cases, with or without the latter complication, are but too common.

Now, the lateral incisor is of the first importance as a *feature* tooth; its loss makes a marked deficiency; its replacement by the large pointed canine is a disfigurement. On the other hand, the lateral incisor is a perishable tooth in comparison with the canine. The cuspidatus is also a marked feature tooth; but the large pointed cusp of the bicuspid makes a fair substitute for it in that respect. There are many points, therefore, to be balanced in the mind before deciding which tooth to sacrifice, lateral incisor or canine. Another circumstance occasionally arises in these cases of much importance. The fang of the lateral incisor becomes absorbed from the pressure of the canine; it is very common to a slight degree, occurring then upon the outer and front surface of the fang, about the sixth or eighth of an inch from the neck of the tooth. I have at least a dozen such specimens, and they were all removed in cases similar to those I am now discussing. But sometimes the whole root is absorbed, the crown of the lateral incisor merely adhering loosely to the gum. I have known an instance in which the operator was manipulating the canine and lateral incisor, in doubt which to remove, when the crown of the latter tooth came off in his hand, the whole fang having been absorbed. Before, therefore, removing a canine tooth to make room for the lateral incisor in such irregularities as these, it should be clearly ascertained that the incisor holds its place in the jaw by a firm root. My own practice, in these confirmed cases, is to remove the canine, when the lateral is sound and bites in front of the lower teeth; to remove the lateral when it is either carious or loose, or bites within the lower teeth. If the canine be retained, the point of its cusp should be rounded off by the file, so as to resemble as much as possible the lateral incisor of the other side. On the ground of symmetry, where interference is necessary on both sides, it will be well (unless there are positive indications to the contrary, such as much difference of position or soundness of the respective teeth) to sacrifice the same tooth on the right as on the left.

An *overlapping* and *crowding* of the upper incisor teeth is

Fig. 17.

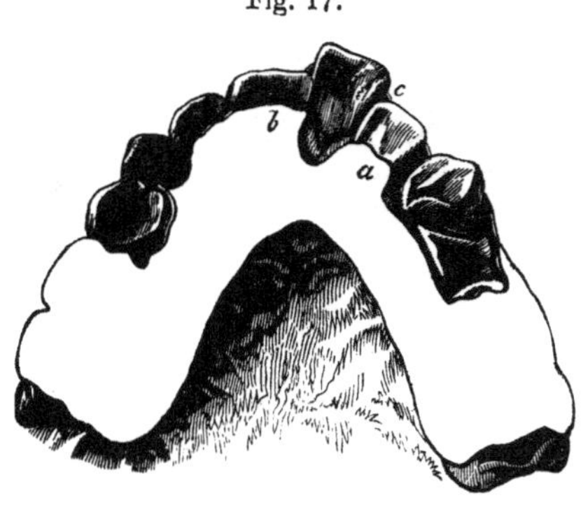

Fig. 18.

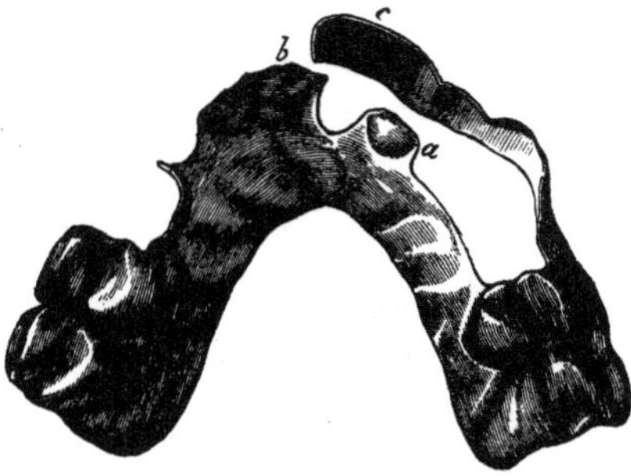

not uncommon, and may exist in very various degrees and forms. The accompanying illustrations are of a sufficiently characteristic example (figs. 17, 18), and show the treatment which rectified the irregularity in this instance. The left central incisor projected beyond the normal arch, while the right central and both laterals were within it. To obtain room the first left bicuspid was extracted, and then a plate (fig. 18) was adapted, in which processes *a* and *b* pressed out the in-standing teeth, while a band of hard elastic gold, *c*, drew in the projecting incisor.

An incisor tooth being twisted and placed more or less across the line of the maxillary arch, is another not uncommon irregularity.

The accompanying figure (fig. 19) illustrates this condition, where the right lateral incisor was thus placed. The tooth was

Fig. 19.

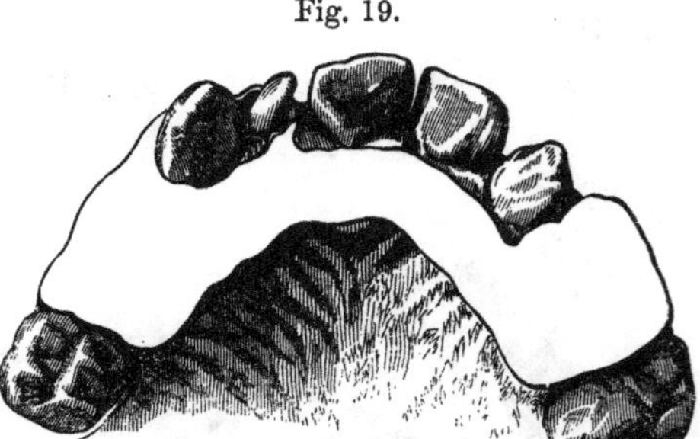

readily restored to its normal position by the plate (fig. 20), the small process, *a*, pressing out the receding angle of the tooth,

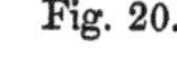

Fig. 20.

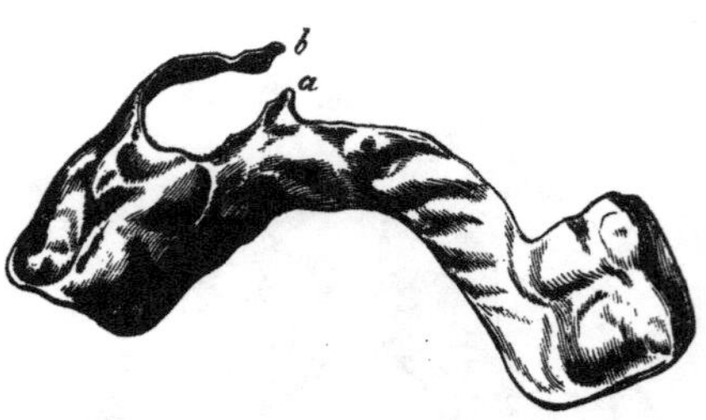

and the elastic band, *b*, forcing in the projecting angle, the points of pressure being increased from time to time, following up the movement of the tooth.

The sudden, forcible twisting of the tooth into its right position, by means of forceps, has been adopted in many of these cases with better results than could have been anticipated; but necrosis and loss of the tooth sometimes follow; and I think the proceeding scarcely justified, when the same result can be accomplished safely by gradual pressure.

Simple separation of the central incisor teeth is not uncommon, and they may be readily drawn together by an india-rubber ring; but they are very prone to return to their former position, even after prolonged and repeated use of the appliance. This plan of treatment, moreover, is not free from serious risk: the india-rubber ring is apt to pass up far on to the neck of the tooth, peeling the gum from the tooth, which, if continued, leads to its loosening and may even entail its loss. I have known an instance in which a young lady lost both the central incisor teeth from this cause. Where the separation of the incisors is

Fig. 21.

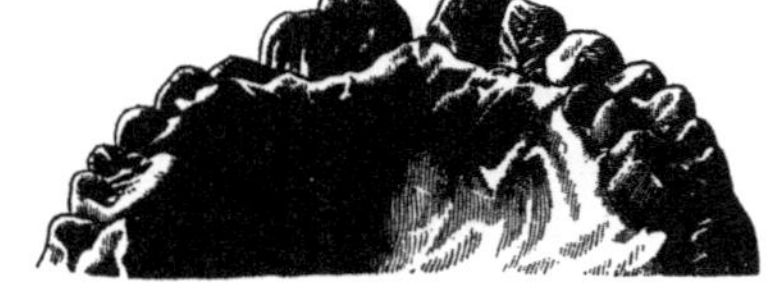

attended with obliquity of axis, as in the accompanying illustration (fig. 21), it is desirable to apply a plate with processes pressing the projecting angles and edges towards the centre, adding increased length to the processes as the teeth yield. The case here figured was thus treated with the best results.

In *contingent* irregularities, where the bite is intersecting, or altogether "underhung," where some or all of the upper six front teeth shut behind the lower in closing the mouth, it will be necessary to adopt the passive mechanism of gagging, either alone or in combination with elastic pressure; for, if the jaws are not separated somewhat, the misplaced teeth are persistently held in their wrong position every time the mouth is closed. The accompanying illustration (fig. 22) shows how this occurred with the superior lateral incisors on each side. If such a case as this is taken early, say from seven to ten years of age, and there is sufficient room for the backward laterals to come forward, or if room be made by extracting the temporary canines, it is generally quite sufficient to separate the jaws by a

Fig. 22.

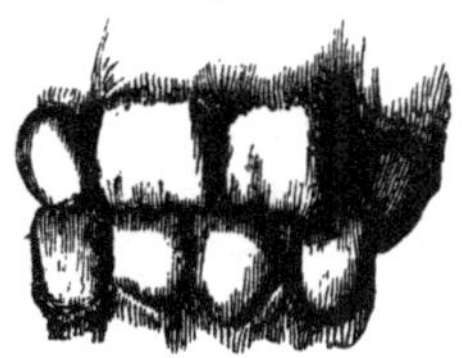

gag, and the teeth then spontaneously come forward in proper range. This passive mode of treating these cases originated with Mr. Bell, and it is wonderfully successful as well as simple. The gag consists of a little 'cap' (fig. 23) made to a model of one of the molar teeth, and upon it are soldered thicknesses of

Fig. 23. Fig. 24.

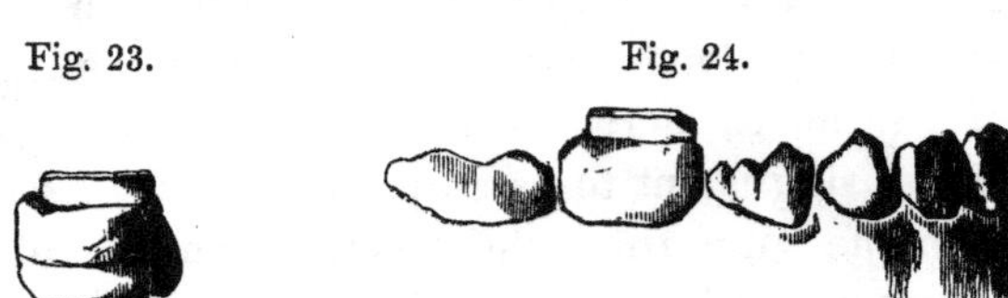

metal enough to separate the front teeth ; it is made to clip firmly the neck of the tooth, and it remains on permanently. In fig. 24 the cap is seen embracing the second temporary molar tooth, which is the one I usually fasten it to. When the displaced upper teeth have advanced sufficiently to allow the lowers to shut behind them, the gag should be removed, and then closure of the mouth completes the cure, by forcing forward the teeth which had been too backward.

If the upper tooth obstinately remains in its wrong position, it will be necessary to force it forward by pressure, and this may be accomplished by a plate such as is represented in fig. 18.

Another and very powerful method of bringing forward upper teeth in an underhung, or an intersecting bite, is by placing upon the lower incisor teeth a plate from the upper edge of which a process passes obliquely upwards and backwards, so that when the patient closes his mouth the upper teeth rest on the sloping surface and are pushed forwards. This may be done for one particular tooth, as shown in the accompanying illustration (fig. 25), or it may be applied to all the front teeth, as in a complete underhung jaw. In the latter cases I have found it very efficacious. It should be applied early—before the lower permanent canines have appeared. It will be necessary generally to remove the lower temporary canines, so as to get fastenings around the permanent lateral incisors. The force thus exerted on the upper teeth is very great, and I have by

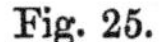

Fig. 25.

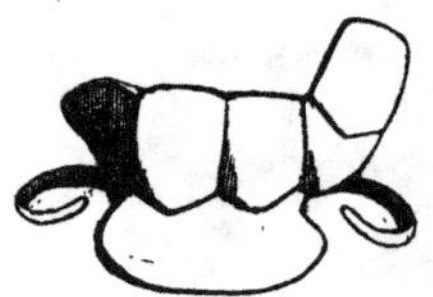

this method completely rectified the underhung condition, even where it was a marked inherited condition.

Crowding and overlapping of the inferior incisor teeth is a common form of irregularity. It very frequently occurs as a transient condition in changing the teeth; but, when it threatens to become permanent, treatment should be adopted, either by giving lateral relief, removing a bicuspid tooth, or by extracting one of the irregular incisors, and of these it is usually desirable to remove the most prominent. The gap readily fills up, and the loss of the tooth is scarcely to be observed.

The *canine* teeth are very prone to assume a *wrong position* and *direction*, and this is frequently associated with retention of their temporary predecessors. This displacement may vary from the slightest departure from a correct position to a complete impaction in the substance of the jaw. The accompanying illustration (fig. 26) shows the permanent canines occupying a

Fig. 26.

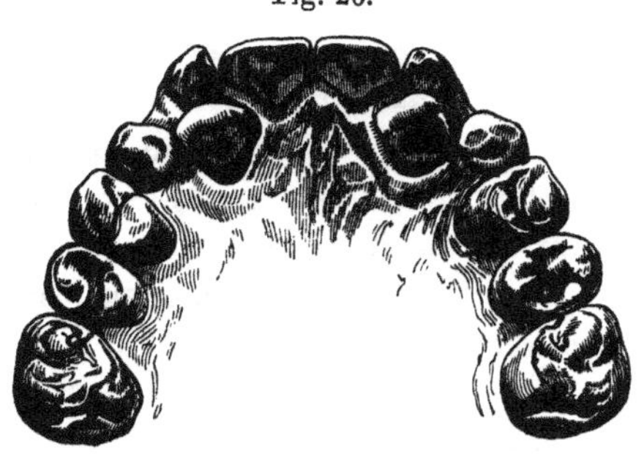

place in the palate, with the temporaries remaining in the arch. In this case I removed the temporary teeth; and, though the patient was seventeen years of age, I succeeded with a plate in forcing the permanent teeth into their proper place, and they were retained there by the bite.

Irregularities of the *bicuspids* are not uncommon, and they usually consist of a too inward position or direction. Persistence of a temporary molar or its fangs may be a cause, or a general crowding of the teeth. Not infrequently an upper bicuspid, usually the second, is found in the palate, resting against the lingual surfaces of the contiguous teeth, and sometimes twisted on its axis. In the lower jaw a bicuspid may lean inwards, so as to present its masticating surface to the tongue. In any case, if inconvenience is experienced, it is better to extract the irregular tooth; and it will be most readily accomplished by operating from the opposite side of the mouth, and drawing the tooth towards the operator.

Of the *molar* teeth the first and second very seldom present irregularity of position, but it is common with the wisdom-tooth. These latter misplacements are of much surgical importance, and are treated of in a separate chapter on "Difficult Eruption of the Wisdom-teeth."

The position assumed by the third molar is sometimes very singular. It has been found imbedded in the ascending ramus of the lower jaw; and in another instance it pierced the cheek and the crown was exposed on the surface of the face.

Separation of the teeth of the two jaws in the front of the mouth, while the molars are in contact, is occasionally met with.

It may arise from (1) congenital malformation of the lower jaw. It may be induced (2) by contraction of the cicatrix of a burn in the throat, pulling down the front of the lower jaw; or (3) by the protrusion of an hypertrophied tongue. I have seen cases from all three causes, and have treated both the first and last varieties. The plan consisted in placing a padded leathern cup under the chin; this was connected by tightening bands with a cap on the head. In each case there was slight temporary improvement; but the least suspension of the pressure allowed a return of the deformity, and no ultimate benefit resulted.

In the case produced by hypertrophy of the tongue, a large portion of that organ was removed by the galvanic *écraseur,* and this was followed by a slow, but considerable spontaneous improvement in the form of the lower jaw, the front teeth ultimately approximating the uppers very closely.

The *V-shaped jaw,* or "*rabbit-mouth,*" as it has been called, from the prominence and exposure of the incisor teeth, constitutes an irregularity of a most serious character, and one which is difficult of treatment. It is a condition which is apt to affect many relations of the same generation, especially the brothers and sisters of one family, and in a certain sense is *inherited*; but I have frequently observed (as is the case with harelip) that many children of the same parents will exhibit the V-shaped jaw, while neither the father nor mother have it.

This is an irregularity which has developed with the progress of civilisation. It did not exist in the earlier races of mankind (Mummery), and it is now especially seen among those of refined and delicate organisation (Coleman). It is generally associated with enlarged tonsils, spongy gums, and offensive breath; and Dr. Langdon Down has pointed out that it is very frequently concurrent with congenital idiocy. It must be observed, however, that this form of jaw is often seen in persons of the highest intellectual capacity.

The altered form of the jaw and position of the teeth consists of a lateral flattening of the arch and a projection of its centre; the bicuspids and molars, especially the former, approach each other, and the incisors project. It mostly affects the upper jaw, the roof of which is narrowed and much vaulted.

Not infrequently the lower jaw is shorter than usual, with a peculiarly close bite, the lower incisor teeth resting on the palate behind the upper incisors. Not only do the incisors of the upper jaw project, but they assume an oblique direction, so as to rest on and overlap the lower lip.

The treatment of these cases is tedious and often unsatisfactory. It may be sought to obtain two results—an increase in the width between the bicuspid teeth, and a diminished projection of the incisors and their sockets. The first object may be accomplished more or less by a palatal plate pressing the teeth outwards, the force being established and maintained by the width of the plate being in excess of that of the interval between the teeth, and the pressure kept up by increasing the width as the teeth yield. This may be accomplished either by a metal plate, or by vulcanite or ivory, with the addition of compressed wooden pegs.

The drawing in of the incisor teeth and a rectification of their direction of growth is, as it seems to me, of more importance, and in my experience is more easy of attainment. This may be achieved by keeping up persistent pressure on the teeth in front, and removing all resisting influence behind.

A plate fastened to the first molar and second bicuspid may be the fixed attachment, from which the force is applied, and this may consist of metal bands extending round the front of the teeth, bent in from time to time as the teeth yield; or, what I prefer, an apparatus such as is here figured (fig. 27). In this a frame, *c*, fits over the incisor teeth, and from this a spiral spring, *b*, extends to a swivel and screw, *a*. The elasticity of

Fig. 27.

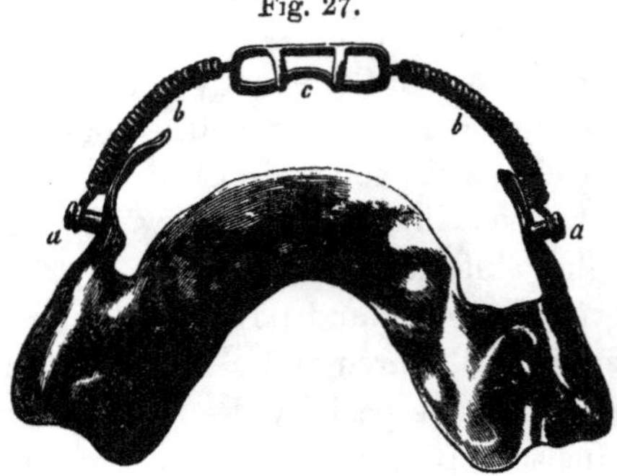

the spring soon brings in the teeth, and it should be tightened by shortening as the case progresses. Care should be taken that the bar across the palate does not obstruct the recession of the teeth and alveoli.

As the incisors come in it will be desirable to prevent any hindrance which further-back teeth might occasion. It may be necessary to extract a bicuspid on either side. In a severe case I have extracted both bicuspids on each side, and have subsequently drawn the front teeth and their sockets so as to closely approximate the canines to the first molars. The teeth have a tendency to go back to their former position, and it is often necessary to wear the apparatus for a long period to prevent this. As long as the incisors project beyond the lower lip this will happen, and an intelligent patient will much assist the

Fig. 28.

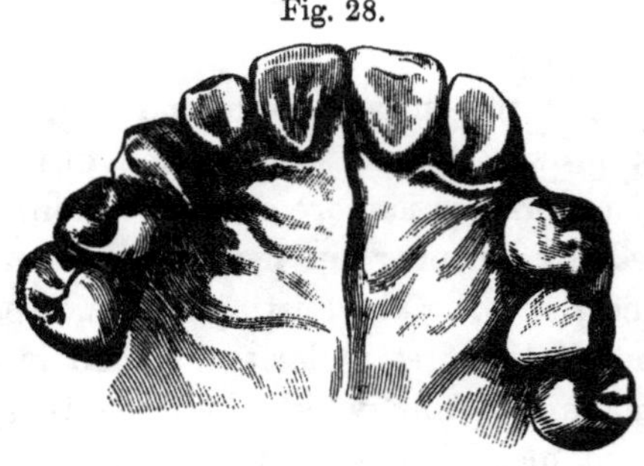

treatment by pressing in the teeth with the lower lip, and taking care that they never rest upon it.

Transposition of teeth is an occasional though rare form of irregularity. It is confined, when complete, to the upper canine tooth, which may occupy a position between the bicuspid teeth, as in the accompanying figure (fig. 28), or it may separate the central from the lateral incisor. The former case is of no importance, but the latter may be somewhat unsightly. Still, no treatment is available.

I have seen an incomplete transposition, in which the lateral incisor was nearer the mesial line of the mouth than the central; but it was behind it, and out of the alveolar arch.

Inversion of the teeth is another and very rare form of irregularity. I have seen both the superior lateral incisors completely inverted and growing upside-down; the crowns of the teeth appeared in the nostrils, from which I removed them.

CHAPTER V.

UNITED TEETH.

CONTIGUOUS teeth are sometimes united together. This fact, though now not called in question, was seriously disputed and denied after its publication by Mr. Fox, who was, I believe, the first to describe it in a systematic work on dental surgery. In 1803 Mr. Fox wrote, "Sometimes in the formation of the teeth two pulps unite, and upon their surfaces appear as two distinct teeth; but upon attempting to remove one it is discovered to be united to the next." * It is this statement that was called in question.

M. Maury † (1828) described united teeth, speaking of them as "soldered together," and he figured six examples of this condition.

The next observation that was made upon this subject was by my relative, Mr. Bell, in 1829: "The intimate and inseparable connection of two teeth by means of a true bony ‡ union of their roots and sides, though not a frequent occurrence, is too well established by facts to admit of a moment's doubt. I have met with six instances of it in my own practice." §

But though this circumstance appears to have escaped the notice of previous writers on dental surgery (even that of Hunter), it was nevertheless recognised by some early anatomists:

* *The Natural History of the Human Teeth*, p. 29. By Joseph Fox. London, 1803.

† *Traité Complet de l'Art du Dentiste.* Paris, 1828.

‡ It is evident that the term "*bony union*," used by Mr. Bell, was not intended to convey the idea that the union was effected by crusta petrosa, or by true bone. At the time Mr. Bell wrote, what we now know as *dentine* was considered *dense bone* of a peculiar kind.

§ *On the Anatomy, &c. of the Teeth*, p. 107. London, 1829.

thus, instances are mentioned by Rhodigius,* Eustachius,† and Haller.‡

Where teeth are united together it is usually confined to two contiguous individuals, but sometimes more are involved. Otto § mentions three, and Eustachius four, in a state of union.

There are two distinct kinds of united teeth: two methods by which the union is effected: the one congenital, in which the pulps are originally fused together, and in which the dentine is continuous in the two teeth; the other in which the union is secondary, occurring in after life, and brought about by an exuberant growth of crusta petrosa, encircling and coupling contiguous fangs which have ceased to be separated by alveolar plates. The minute structure and the development of these two forms of united teeth will be considered more fully presently. I allude to them now before detailing instances so as to point out which are congenital and which secondary.

It is not a little remarkable that, considering how comparatively few cases are on record, almost all classes of teeth appear to have been subject to this condition; a circumstance which shows that there is nothing in the form or development of any particular teeth, or any region of the mouth, more calculated to produce it than any other.

Otto saw three incisive teeth in a child united together: this was probably congenital: indeed, I believe whenever the temporary teeth are united, it is an ivory and congenital, and not a cemental or secondary union.

Of the three cases that occurred to Mr. Fox, one consisted in a union of the central incisors of the lower jaw by their fangs and the sides of their necks and crowns (congenital). In another, the second and third molars of the upper jaw were united by their fangs (probably secondary). In the third, the fangs of the second lower bicuspid and first molar were completely fused together (congenital). These specimens are still to be seen in the Museum at Guy's Hospital.

The six instances described and figured by Maury are—

* *Lectiones Antiquæ.* Basel, 1517.

† *De Dentibus: Opuscula Anatomica.* Venet., 1574.

‡ *Elementa Physiologiæ, &c.* Bernæ, 1764.

§ *Lehrbuch der Pathologischen des Menschen und der Thiere.* Berlin, 1830.

1st. Two superior central permanent incisors, union throughout and congenital. Planche VIII. fig. 4.

2nd. Second and third lower molars united at the roots; probably cemental and secondary. Fig. 7.

3rd. First upper molar and second bicuspid; the latter embraced by the roots of the former, and the union probably cemental. Fig. 12.

4th. Inferior temporary central incisors; union congenital. Fig. 15.

5th. Two inferior bicuspids, the roots fused into one and clearly congenital. Fig. 18.

6th. First upper molar and supernumerary tooth; apparently congenital. Fig. 23.

In the six examples referred to by Mr. Bell, three consisted in the lateral union of the temporary superior central incisors. The other three are undescribed; but I am informed by Mr. Bell that they were in one case the permanent superior central incisors; in another the permanent inferior central incisors (all these congenital); and the second molar and *dens sapientiæ* of the upper jaw: the nature of this union I cannot say.

I have myself seen nine examples of dental union: a permanent lateral and canine of the upper jaw; a permanent *dens sapientiæ* of the lower jaw and supernumerary tooth; superior second bicuspid and supernumerary tooth, the latter being itself a miniature bicuspid (see fig. 15, p. 31); right central and lateral permanent incisors of the lower jaw; two supernumerary teeth, mimicking permanent upper incisors (see fig. 14, p. 30); two examples in which the temporary superior central incisors were anchylosed their entire length, crowns and fangs, with common pulp-cavity; temporary lateral of the lower jaw fused to a similar supernumerary tooth: all these being *ivory* union and congenital. One other case of union of teeth has occurred to me, to be more fully described elsewhere. It consisted in a coupled pair of bicuspid teeth, the uppers of the right side: these were soldered together by an excessive development of crusta petrosa embracing the fangs of the two as one.

Thus, in these few examples, we see that individual teeth of each kind have been the subjects of this peculiarity: temporary and permanent teeth; regular and supernumerary; teeth of the upper and of the lower jaw; molars, premolars, canines, and incisors. Considering how few instances have been reported, this diversity is remarkable.

I now describe more particularly two of my specimens, one congenital, the other secondary.

The first consisted in a united cuspidatus and lateral incisor. The teeth were completely united by a very-broad union. When viewed superficially, the crowns of the teeth appeared distinct: the division on the surface which separated them down to the necks was so marked that a casual observer or careless operator would probably be unaware of their junction. Below the necks the fangs were completely united together; and though the junction of the roots at the upper two-thirds was indicated by a groove, the rest of them was so completely fused as to obliterate all indication of a double origin (see fig. 29). On dividing the teeth at the points indicated by the transverse lines in the figure, it was seen that there were two pulp-cavities in the crowns, and but one in the fused roots, as is shown in the accompanying little diagrams (see figs. 30 and 31).

Fig. 29.

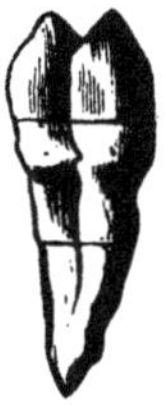

Fig. 30.

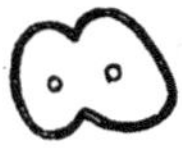

Fig. 31.

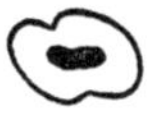

I made sections of these teeth for the microscope, by which I had an opportunity of observing, what I believe had never been seen before, the histological character of the uniting medium (fig. 32).

A section through the crowns of the teeth, made transversely midway between the summit and the neck, exhibited the form of the figure 8, and it displayed to the naked eye a mass of dentine surrounded by enamel, and interrupted only by a small pulp-cavity in each of the teeth. Between these pulp-cavities, where the union existed, there was no break of surface, and nothing in the aspect of the dentine to indicate that the teeth were distinct individuals. The enamel did not appear to pass between them. The question was settled by microscopical scrutiny.

A thin section of these teeth, viewed with low magnifying powers, displays within the enamel a mass of dentine, consisting of tubes radiating from each pulp-cavity, and passing across the union, without interruption. Near the edges of the teeth this continuity of tissue is most obvious: the tubes from one pulp can be followed across the line of junction, and are seen to end upon the inner surface of the enamel of the opposite tooth.

In the centre, however, between the teeth, the section divides the tubes in an oblique direction: they are thus seen more or less cut across, and cannot be traced in lines; but there is clearly no interruption of tissue. This will be better understood by referring to the accompanying illustration (fig. 32).

Fig. 32.

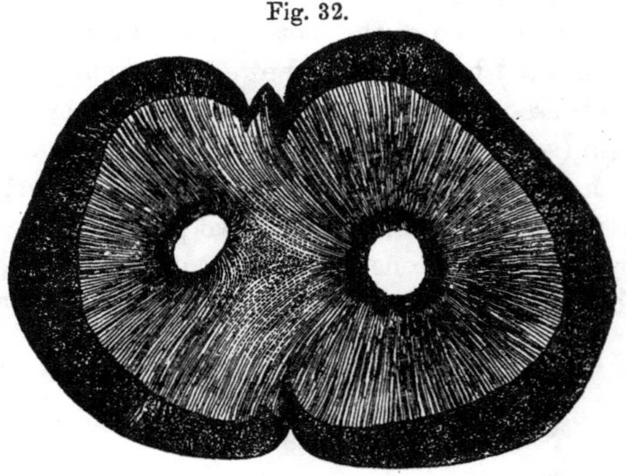

There is one point in this section which is curious and interesting: it is, that at the margin of the teeth, where they come in contact—at the extremities of the line of union—there are two small mammillary projections, one on each side, occupying the interval left by the curving inwards of the outline of the teeth. These appearances suggest the idea that, when in a soft and plastic condition, the pulps were firmly pressed together within their sac, and that where they met they were pressed out, as it were, into these little eminences. I sacrificed another specimen of teeth, united congenitally, to make sections for the microscope: the union was here also by continuous dentine.*

These specimens then establish the fact, not only that the

* The description and illustrations of these specimens were published by me in the *Transactions of the Medico-Chirurgical Society*, vol. xxxv. p. 201. Plates I. and II., 1852.

teeth are occasionally united together, but that the union is effected, in certain instances, by a fusion of the dentinal tissue of the two individuals.

As regards the development and formation of teeth thus united, it can but be concluded that the two pulps were within one and the same sac; and that though they were distinct at their summits, they were as one, except outward moulding, through most of the crown and the whole of the fang. Although the congenital union of two contiguous teeth is an abnormal condition, it can scarcely be considered pathological: it can simply be considered as the result of some modifications in the papillary and follicular mouldings of the surface which occur in the earliest stages of tooth-development. And considering that the near proximity of two pulps, or the imperfect formation of the septa between the sacs, would furnish circumstances favouring, if not determining, its production, it may rather be a matter of surprise that this deviation from the natural condition is not much more frequent. The union of distinct teeth, formed upon separate pulps, and exhibiting the outward anatomical form of certain recognised teeth, is merely an exhibition of the same sort of process on a large scale, as is seen in miniature in the formation of every tooth with more than one cusp. Each cusp commences, as each tooth, by a separate calcific centre, upon a single eminence of pulp—upon, in fact, a miniature tooth-pulp: and when these become confluent, they show through a very short space, near the summit of the crown of the teeth, the same relation in section as I have just described in these united teeth: it only needs a deeper fissure between the cusps to render the analogy more complete.

The *secondary* union of contiguous teeth—that which occurs in after life—is brought about by the encasement of mature tooth-fangs within a common growth of crusta petrosa. Normally, each fang is separated from every other fang by a tube of alveolar bone, a portion of the true skeleton bone. Many morbid conditions of the fangs of teeth occasion absorption of the alveolar plates, and this occurring immediately between two, may place them in a common socket. It is but necessary for this apposition of neighbouring fangs and a union of the periodontal membranes of the two teeth to occur, when a fusion of the cemental blastema from the two sources, in active development, would accomplish the encasement of the two teeth-fangs as one. This secondary union of contiguous teeth is perhaps scarcely as frequent as the congenital form, though, from its affecting the fangs of the teeth, it is less likely to be observed when present. It more often affects the molar teeth than others, and I believe is seen, when present, in those who are affected with a general excess of cemental formation on the teeth.

The accompanying illustrations (figs. 33, 34) represent two fangs—those of the two superior bicuspids, before alluded to. The figure on the left represents them in face; that on the right

Fig. 33.

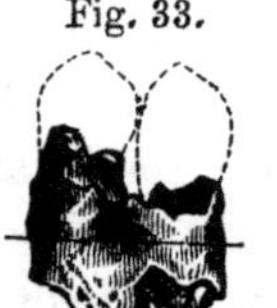

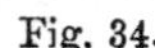

Fig. 34.

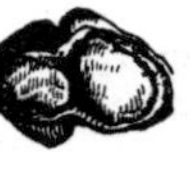

shows the extremities of the fangs seen endwise. These fangs were separate at both extremities, but united in the middle by a band of crusta petrosa, enveloping the two in a common sheath, very clearly shown in the right figure. The dotted lines in the left figure indicate the crowns of the teeth, which had long been decayed and broken away. I extracted several other stumps and decayed teeth from the patient on the same day (preparing for artificial teeth), and they all presented an immense amount of general crusta-petrosal hypertrophy.

I have made a section for the microscope of the two united bicuspid fangs—the plane of section being indicated by the line in the foregoing fissure. The illustration (fig. 35) shows the arrangement of the fang-tissues in this specimen, and implies the method and sequence of their formation. In this instance, as is common, the first bicuspid had two roots, and the second but one. Starting from each narrow pulp-cavity, there is first a ring of dentine; then rings of crusta petrosa belonging to each fang, and then a belt of the same tissue involving the whole. The dentine circles, with a certain amount of cement, were the original fangs: the enlarged cemental rings indicate the progressive hypertrophy of the tooth-fangs, and the contingent atrophy of the alveolar plates, which issued in a common socket, and a structural fusion of the two teeth.

Fig. 35.

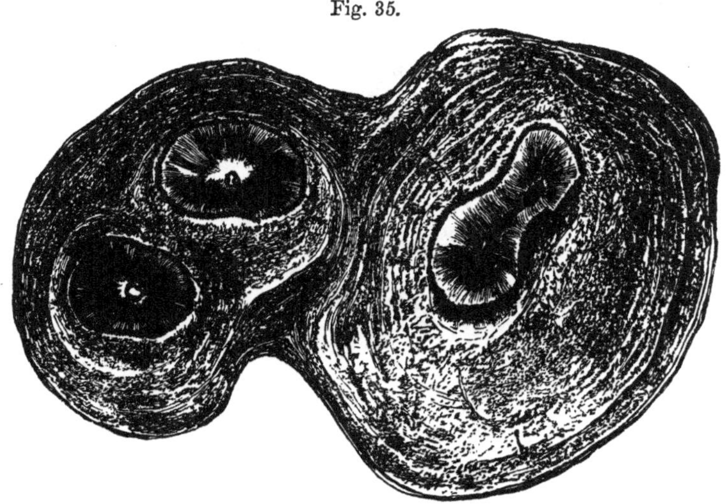

The anatomical condition, which I have now described, is not without important *practical* bearing. Two teeth may be united side by side, though apparently distinct organs: one may be diseased, and require extraction, and the other be sound: or one may be out of place, and (in a young mouth) may suggest the propriety of its removal for regulation. Now, in many of the recorded cases, perhaps the majority, it would have been *impossible* to have ascertained the union of the teeth while in the jaw: in the *great majority* it would surely have been overlooked by an ordinary observer. In *all* the recorded instances it would have been impossible to have separated the attached teeth before extraction. These propositions involve an inevitable accident; and the rarity of that accident, and the fact that it has not yet been recorded, results from the abnormality, which would induce it, being itself so rare. *Two teeth may be extracted where one was intended, because they are joined together.* On the 24th of June 1867, a maiden lady, about forty years of age, came to me to have her jaws cleared of stumps and decayed teeth, preparatory to wearing artificial substitutes. I had extracted several, all coated about the fangs with excessive cement, when I removed the first upper bicuspid root on the right side: with it came away the root of the second bicuspid:

they were united together by a common cemental sheath, and are represented in the previous figures. The gum was so full, and the tongues of gum passing up between the two buried fangs were so complete, as to mask this union entirely.

The possibility of such an event as this must have occurred to every one in contemplating united teeth; but I am not aware of any recorded instance where it has occurred in actual practice.

CHAPTER VI.

SECONDARY DENTINE.

When a tooth is completely formed, but as yet has never been subjected to wear of the ivory, or inflammation or irritation, the pulp remains a soft, vascular, nervous mass. This fleshy body then contains no schlerous elements,* but it does contain elements which are capable of transformation into ivory of essentially the same nature (both chemical and anatomical) as the dentine previously formed. Such fresh growth differs, however, in some of its anatomical characters; it is, moreover, an after-growth, or secondary formation, and it is divisible into varieties.

The terms "Osteo-dentine," and "Secondary Dentine," have been applied respectively by Professor Owen and Mr. Tomes to designate some of those forms of dentine which are thus found within the primary single system of the tooth,—formed from the one original pulp. The former referring, and being applied to structures normal and abnormal, both in man and other animals, and the latter being used by its author in relation to those quasi-morbid, or truly morbid products, which are found in the injured and diseased teeth of the human subject.

The two terms have been applied by anatomists, in respect to human teeth, as synonyms and parallel expressions, but really they are not so; for whereas *osteo-dentine* refers to an inconstant anatomical condition, *secondary dentine* has a general physiological meaning, and refers to period of formation. "Secondary dentine" is, as it were, *generic* of the whole; "Osteo-dentine" is specific, and applies to that one form of secondary

* A few calcification islands are said occasionally to be present in the pulps of developing teeth; but I have not met with them.

dentine, in which the new tissue consists of a series of dentine systems arranged around isolated blood-vessels, or secondary pulpules.

This nomenclature is not only incomplete, but inaccurate.

Considering *Secondary Dentine* as applicable to all the after-formations of dentine by which the pulp-cavity is diminished or obliterated, subsequent to the tooth having attained a mature and adult condition, I would subdivide it, according to the anatomical distinctions which the different forms exhibit, into *Dentine of Repair*, *Dentine Excrescence*, and *Osteo-dentine*. I first suggested this arrangement in the "Guy's Hospital Reports" for 1853.

The accompanying diagram (fig. 36) shows these three forms of Secondary Dentine. The tinted triangle at the top of the pulp-cavity represents a mass of Dentine of Repair compensatory for the wear of the summit of the cusp. The nodule projecting from the side into the pulp-cavity is a Dentine Excrescence; and the dark cylinder in the axis of the pulp shows where the intrinsic calcification of that organ usually commences in the formation of Osteo-dentine. The illustration must be considered as simply diagrammatic.

Fig. 36.

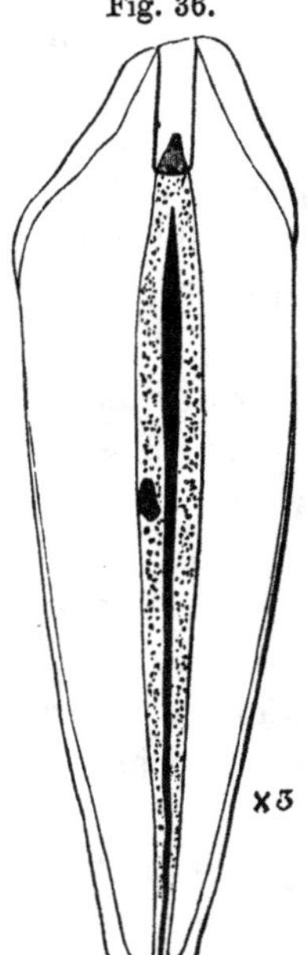

Dentine of Repair has been recognised and described by Hunter and subsequent writers; and its meaning, as a remedial effort of nature, has been understood; but recent observers, even with the assistance of the microscope, have not described many interesting points concerning its anatomy. The amount of knowledge till recently obtained has scarcely been added to since the time of Hunter. He remarks: "A tooth very often wears down so low, that its cavity would be exposed, if no other alteration were produced in it. To prevent this, nature has taken care that the bottom part of the cavity should be filled up with new matter, in proportion as the surface of the teeth is worn down." *

* *Hunter on the Teeth*, 4to, 1771, p. 108.

Mr. Bell, with rather more definition, observes: "It is first deposited in that part of the cavity towards the worn surface, and becomes gradually more and more filled as the tooth becomes abraded." *

The circumstance of repair, as thus generally expressed, had not received a more exact description until 1853, though the microscope discloses the laws which regulate its development; laws which are exact, regular, and intelligible.

Before the publication of Mr. Tomes's Lectures on the Teeth, the filling up of the pulp cavity by new dentine was only recognised as the result of abrasion from wearing. Mr. Tomes, however, has shown that decay of the tooth may produce the same result, and I have had many opportunities of verifying the correctness of this observation. I have also found that fracture of the crown of a tooth, so long as it does not open the pulp-cavity, causes a similar result: there is an internal repair in proportion to the external lesion.

Correctly to understand the laws which are followed in the formation of dentine of repair, it is necessary to examine sections of teeth variously worn and variously broken. Sections should be made carefully, so as to cut the dentine parallel with the radius from the centre of the pulp cavity to the point of injury, and not obliquely or on one side. The injury and the corresponding point in the pulp cavity should be disclosed at once. A very slight magnifying power, from ten to twenty diameters, will suffice to exhibit the general arrangement.

Fig. 37.

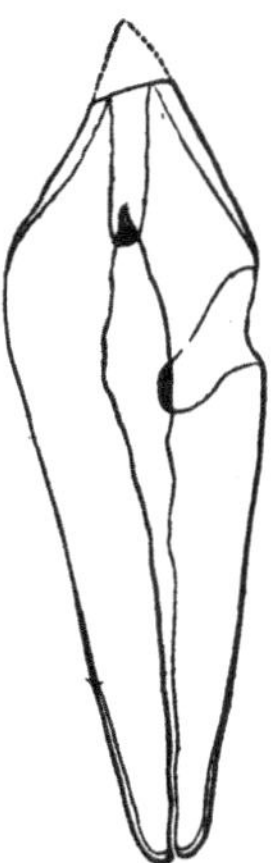

Those teeth which are partially worn at the summit of their cusp, or cusps, and are likewise grooved at the neck, when cut vertically and so mounted, are the most illustrative; and, on that account, I have selected a tooth thus worn for the subject of an outline figure.

The accompanying drawing (fig. 37) represents a section of a superior canine tooth, of which the apex of the crown is worn by attrition in mastication; and by friction of the tooth-brush it has been

* *Bell on the Teeth*, 8vo. 1835, p. 193.

grooved along the anterior surface of the neck. This amount, and this position of wear are extremely common, and are, in all cases where the tooth is a living one and the dentine pulp is alive, accompanied with a development of dentine of repair. In this specimen it is seen that the friction at the apex of the crown has removed all the enamel from the summit, and a small amount only of the dentine. In the section some ten or fifteen tubes correspond to the worn surface; a large mass of tissue intervenes between the wear and the repair, but yet the latter (in the shape of a triangular mass of secondary dentine in the summit of the pulp cavity) has appeared, and in proportion to the former. Wear, which is the mere result of mechanical friction, has no relation to the structure of the dentine—it occurs simply in the place and in the direction of the rubbing—but the consequent repair has a direct relation to its intimate anatomy. Now, of the tubes that abut upon the worn surface, the central would correspond to those most worn down; those which in the entire tooth had reached the extreme point of the cusp, and had consequently, by the removal of the top, been more shortened than any others. The contiguous tubes have been reduced next in amount, whilst those at the extremity of the worn surface have been least shortened. Upon tracing the tubes which have thus been rubbed down, from their outer extremities to the pulp cavity, it will be found that the amount of secondary dentine laid on, so to speak, upon their inner extremities, is in proportion to the amount removed externally. Thus, in this specimen, the central tubes abut upon the apex of the triangular mass of secondary dentine, while those at the sides of the wear, and next to the yet unbroken enamel, terminate internally at the edges of the new repair tissue. And it should be observed that, not only does the repair tissue correspond with the amount of injury done to each tube, but that it is generally limited by the internal abutment of those tubes which are at the edge of the worn surface.

And this correspondence of the repair with the individual tubes injured is illustrated with peculiar clearness by the situation which the secondary dentine obtains where the injury has consisted in a groove in the neck of the tooth. The tortuous direction of the dentinal tubes in this situation, and their elevation out of the horizontal line, as they pass from within outwards, present circumstances which admirably test and illustrate the manner in which the structural direction of the tissue determines the position of the repair. By tracing the curves and the convergence of the tubes as they pass inwards to the pulp cavity, they are found on the interior to correspond to the dentine of repair far below the horizontal line of lesion.

The next figure, 38, represents a central incisor of the upper jaw, in which one of the angles has been broken off. The section is vertical and from side to side. The fracture has injured at the extremity a large number of tubes, but, by their convergence as they approach the pulp cavity, it will be seen how much smaller is the area of resulting repair.

Fig. 38.

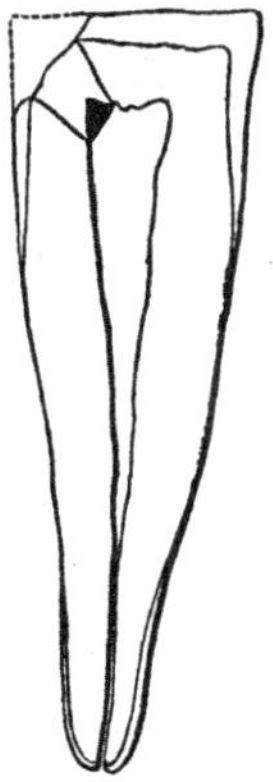

Now, in all these instances, it will be seen that the dentine of repair has a very close relation both in amount and position to the injury that has caused it. When, however, the amount of wear, or fracture, or decay, is great, there ceases to be that exact and proportionate recompense, the new tissue forming over a large surface of the pulp-cavity, and often much in excess: and it may be stated, as a general rule, that even where the injury is slight, if the repair be not in accurate proportion, the difference is on the side of excess, and corresponds to a larger surface than is indicated by the internal abutment of the injured tubes. The next illustration (fig. 39) is an accurate representation of an interesting specimen, a vertical section of an inferior canine tooth, in which dentine of repair is seen in three situations—in two developed as the recompense or repair for lesion, the result of mechanical friction, and in one as a compensation for the inroads of superficial caries. At the summit of the cusp and the front of the neck the dentine has been worn into by friction; at the back of the neck there is a crescentic cavity eaten out by caries.

In making the section, from the bending of the fang, it was not possible to open the pulp cavity from end to end. The upper half is exposed in about its centre; in the lower half the dentine of the fang is exhibited, just on one side of the pulp-cavity. The external injury, and the plano-convex masses of dentine of repair in the pulp cavity are so clearly defined, that the specimen does not need further description.

Fig. 39.

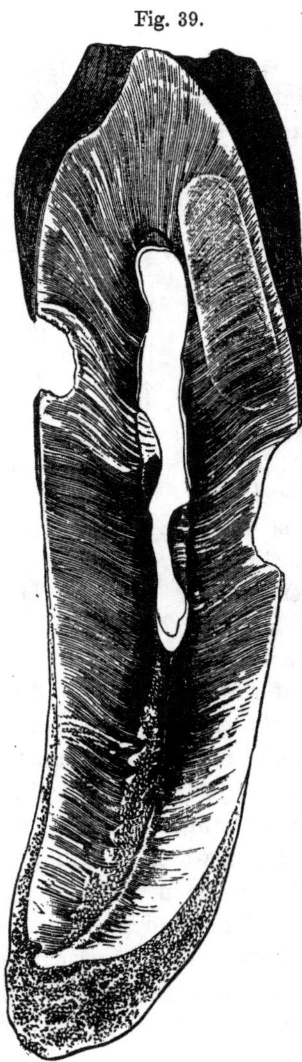

Osteo-dentine and *dentine excrescence* are not infrequently seen in teeth that are worn and exhibit dentine of repair; they are evidently associated, and have a similar exciting cause. *Dentine of repair, however, always forms upon that portion of the pulp-cavity next to the lesion, and is adherent, and in direct structural continuity with the primary dentine; whereas osteo-dentine and dentine excrescence occur almost always first towards the extremity of the fang, and the former is frequently quite detached from the remainder of the dentine. Moreover, in dentine of repair, the pulp is detached, and can easily be removed, whereas, in osteo-dentine it is bodily involved in the new tissue.* Where both forms exist, they usually increase till they become confluent and confounded together, and the origin of the different forms of secondary dentine, and their relation to one another, is then lost.

But the formation of secondary dentine, particularly disposed for tooth repair, is not the only phenomenon that occurs for that object.

The filling of the dentine tubes with a secondary deposit has long been recognised in the fangs of teeth, where it produces a condition called "horny dentine," the tissue being rendered more or less clear by the obliteration of the light-refracting tubes. This condition is found in the fangs of those teeth which have caused much irritation, and where there has been periosteal inflammation. The same thing occurs in those tubes of the primary dentine which pass from the secondary repair tissue to the injured surface; they become more or less filled up with deposit, and are clear in proportion. The amount in which the filling up of the dentinal tubes occurs is subject to great variety, and is irregular in its amount in various and contiguous tubes; there are frequently little pencils of tubes which are completely filled up, amidst others that are scarcely altered. And this secondary deposit in the primary dentine frequently extends laterally to tissue that has been uninjured. It must be observed, moreover, that the secondary dentine itself has almost all its tubes filled up, and is consequently very clear. It has been supposed that secondary dentine is destitute of tubes, or contains very few; but it will be found, upon careful examination with high powers, that the tubes are present in large numbers, but are so completely filled up with secondary deposit, that when seen with low powers, in thin section, they do not interfere with the almost perfect transmission of light. The limit, however, of this extreme clearness of the dentine of repair is not defined by the line where its junction with the primary dentine occurs, but it extends slightly into the original tissue.

It must also be observed, that dentine of repair follows a regular growth in proportion to the injury at any particular part, and it exhibits, in the form of laminated incremental lines, registers of its progressive formation. The dentine of repair is laminated according to the approaching injury and the receding pulp, in equal parallel laminæ.

The subject of tissue-repair, of compensation for injury and disease by the modification of existing structures, or the production of new ones, is of much interest, not only from its exhibition of a *vis medicatrix naturæ*, but also from the bearing which the whole phenomena have upon the vitality and organic susceptibility of the tissue in question. As bearing upon the tissues of the teeth, whose claims to vitality have so often been the subject of dispute, the question is particularly important.

Before entering further on these points, I would wish to state, as distinctly as possible, the circumstances under which repair by secondary dentine does, or does not, occur.

In Mr. Tomes's Lectures on the Teeth the following passage occurs, and I quote it as exhibiting the generally-received, but, as I believe, inaccurate expression of these circumstances.

Mr. Tomes observes: "In the teeth of old persons, or in teeth that have been much worn, the pulp cavity becomes greatly diminished in size, or wholly obliterated, by what may be called a secondary development of dentine."

Now, the circumstance of *age, per se*, is really not efficient for the production of secondary dentine; and the fact that the teeth which exhibit secondary dentine are usually from aged subjects is merely accidental, and dependent upon the fact that it is in them that the teeth are most worn. Again, *mere wear* is not a cause, for no wear of the enamel produces the condition in question.

From a numerous and extensive examination of specimens, I have satisfied myself that the true and only cause of the production of dentine of repair is a *lesion* of the *dentine* of the primary system, which may occur at *any age.** The enamel may wear indefinitely, but no compensation occurs: immediately, however, that the dentine is injured, the repair tissue begins to make its appearance, and progresses in proportion to the lesion.

It would seem that the enamel does not possess that sort of vitality which is capable of taking cognisance, so to speak, of the injury done to it; but that the dentine, when injured, does receive the impression, and conveys it to the pulp. It is out of the question to imagine that any mechanical influence can be conveyed from the outer surface of the dentine to the pulp; the hardness of the intervening medium, and its great thickness when the repair commences, render such an idea untenable. It is obvious, however, that the influence is conveyed according to the direction of the tissue; for where the tissue does not run in a direction at right angles from the surface, the resulting repair is also, in like proportion, remote. It is physiologically, but not mathematically, opposite.

The dentine is a living tissue, capable of receiving impressions, and of propagating them to a proximate organ, which legiti-

* Dentine of repair sometimes occurs in temporary teeth.

mately has the power and the office of restoring it, and repairing the lesions it has suffered. Such a view is quite in keeping with what we see elsewhere; it is not the tissue itself that is its own means of repair, but its formative organ.

But in this case how perfect is the repair; and with what clearness is carried out the idea of a *vis medicatrix naturæ.*

I have never taken an opportunity of examining the fresh pulp of a tooth exhibiting dentine of repair. One would expect to find it present an increased vascularity at the affected part—a condition analogous to plastic inflammation, or perhaps rather to hypertrophic hyperæmia. In the clear, horny fangs of inflamed teeth is seen a part of these phenomena—the filling up of the primary dentinal tubes by secondary deposit—here always associated with increased vascularity, increased nutrition.

DENTINE EXCRESCENCES are little nodules of secondary dentine, occasionally found attached to the interior of the pulp-cavities of teeth which may be otherwise healthy, unassociated with injury or other disease. They also occur in the fangs of teeth which, higher up in the crown, are injured, and are the subjects of dentine of repair. They seldom give evidence of their presence; but it appears that sometimes they are associated with neuralgia.

Dentine excrescence fairly comes under the head of "Odontomes," or tumours of the hard tissue of the teeth, to the chapter on which the reader is referred for the further consideration of the subject.

OSTEO-DENTINE, as its name implies, is a form of secondary dentine in which the tissue combines the characters both of bone and ivory. It is developed by the general conversion and intrinsic calcification of the several tissues of the pulp. It is usually vascular; it is frequently arranged in systems *around* vessels, like the Haversian systems in bone, and it sometimes contains true lacunæ.

All the tissues appear to be calcified promiscuously: the vessels, or many of them, are the last affected; still they are early reduced in number, as those which occupy the axis of the dentine-Haversian systems are far less numerous than those of the original pulp. I have, however, frequently seen them of quite healthy structure when almost every trace of the other tissues has been lost. Upon treating a tooth-pulp with rather dilute acetic acid, I have followed the vessels among the calcified masses for a considerable distance, their coats exhibiting the characteristic nuclei with unmistakeable clearness, and quite unaltered.

In tracing the development of osteo-dentine, the calcification islands* are at first easily separated by needle-points; they become more and more coherent, but it is not before they are fused together that an intelligible section can be made. Osteo-dentine may exist in any number of systems, and the amount of pulp involved does not appear to affect the maturity at which a local calcification may arrive. I have figured a section of a carious bicuspid tooth containing one and only one perfect system of secondary dentine within the pulp cavity, the rest of the pulp not being affected.†

Fig. 40.

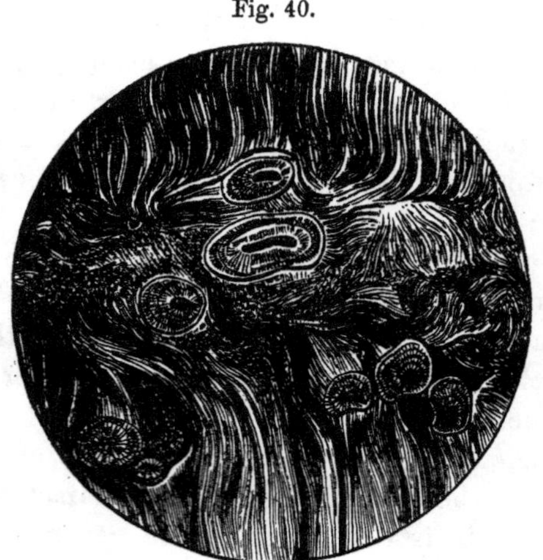

Usually, however, there are many systems of secondary dentine surrounded by and adherent to the primary dentine, as seen in the accompanying illustration (fig. 40).

Osteo-dentine has fewer tubes than any other form of dentine, and is usually very transparent: this does not altogether arise (as does the transparency of dentine of repair) from the filling up of the tubes with secondary deposit within them; many of

* These centres of calcification are particularly described in the chapter on "Diseases of the Pulp."

† *Guy's Hospital Reports,* vol. ix. pl. I. fig. 1.

the tubes are doubtless so filled up, as is the case with all dentine formed in states of tooth-irritation or inflammation; but they are nevertheless really less abundant. This circumstance is quite intelligible upon the idea that all the tissues of the pulp share alike in the common change; in this case doubtless the calcified nerves, blood-vessels, and connective tissue, would not develope tubes, but only those elements of the pulp which are similar to the cells constituting the membrana eboris.

The blood-vessel in the axis of a system of osteo-dentine usually remains open; but occasionally, and indeed not very infrequently, the central canal can no longer be seen. It is obliterated by the calcification of the blood-vessel and its contents, and its position is occupied by an indefinite

Fig. 41.

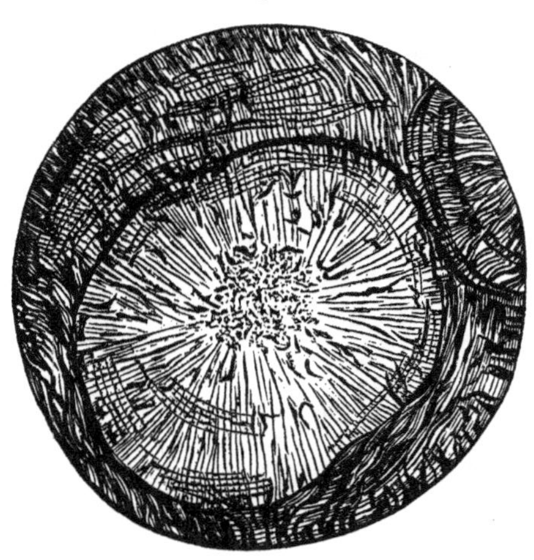

clearish structure. Such a condition is shown in the accompanying illustration (fig. 41). Here the last of the soft tissues of the pulp is swallowed up by the calcific change. But osteo-dentine may resemble bone other than by vascular Haversian systems. It may contain true bone lacunæ, especially resembling those of the crusta petrosa; and I have noticed this especially where there has been a preternaturally abundant communication between the pulp and the periosteum—the communication being large and short, so that the pulp and the periosteum are almost continuous.

I have several times found teeth, having short lateral canals passing from the periosteum to the pulp cavity of the fang,* in which the canal itself has been lined with a thin layer of crusta petrosa, and the same tissue has existed in the pulp cavity, either alone or mixed with secondary dentine. The same is seen in the pulps of temporary teeth, which are retained beyond the normal period of shedding. I have a remarkably good example of this from the mouth of a youth, eighteen years of age.† In this instance the fangs had been somewhat absorbed, especially on the inner surfaces, so as to lay open the pulp-cavities to near the main chamber of the tooth, and moreover the canals were considerably enlarged; by this means the pulp and the periosteum were almost as one. A section of this tooth shows the pulp converted into a mass of crusta petrosa and dentine confounded together.

* *Path. Trans.*, vol. v. p. 116, pl. IV. figs. 1, 2 and 3. 1854.

† *Guy's Hospital Reports*, vol. ix. pl. II, figs. 1 and 2.

CHAPTER VII.

CONGENITAL DEFECTS OF STRUCTURE AND FORM.

ENAMEL and dentine are both liable to defects of original structure, but this can scarcely be said of the late-forming and ever-changing tooth-bone.

The enamel rests on the surface of the dentine, and between its fibres the dentinal tubes project more or less. A continuation of the tubes by small contracting narrow points into the enamel is a natural condition; but occasionally these prolongations assume the form of elongated bulbous cells, still clearly connected with the ends of dentinal tubes. This often exists to an extent that is clearly abnormal, large and long-branched excavations passing a considerable way towards the exterior of thick enamel. I have shown* that these cavities are really prolongations of the dentinal tubes, and that they have the same definite walls as the tubes themselves. Presuming that the dentinal tubes are in some way the main vehicles of tooth-structure-sensibility, this condition would endow the enamel with an abnormal perception of external agencies; and this probably explains some of those cases of hypersensitive teeth which occur in persons of early age, where the enamel has not yet been sufficiently worn to reach the dentine.

The enamel itself is liable to defects of structure. The fibres, instead of being homogeneous, may be granular; or each fibre may have an axial cavity within it, instead of being solid; and again, contiguous fibres may be imperfectly united to each other.

But the most important defects in the enamel, as bearing on the life and health of the tooth, are "rocky" enamel, and defective

* Truman's *Archives of Dentistry*.

enamel formation at the bottom of the crypts between the cusps in molar and pre-molar teeth.

Rocky enamel is, I believe, always associated with imperfect formation of the immediately subjacent dentine; and it is a manifestation and permanent record of depressed nutrition at a period of tooth formation. In this condition the enamel is pitted or grooved, or both, and the surface is honeycombed and

Fig. 42.

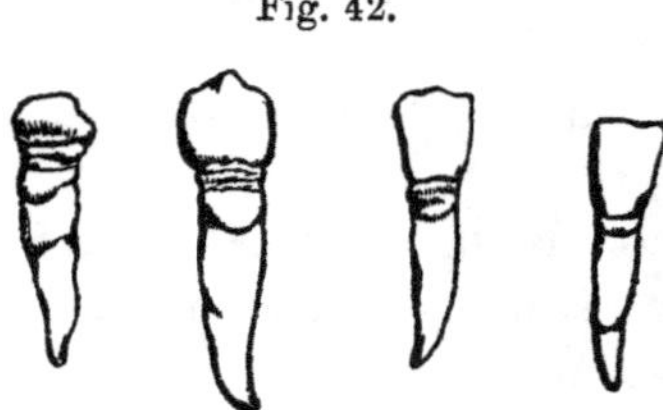

irregular. The tissue also is often discoloured, being brown or yellow, and opaque. In sections of such teeth the general arrangement of the enamel reminds one of what geologists know as *faults* in stratified rocks, and the tissue is often distinctly brown coloured.

Where one tooth is thus formed, its companion on the other side of the jaw will, as a rule, be found in exactly the same condition; and very often several teeth are affected, not at the same part of the crown, but at a point corresponding to the amount of development which each had attained at one particular date.

This defective enamel is thus shown in a series of teeth—central incisor, lateral, canine, and bicuspid—taken from one individual (fig. 42).

À priori, this honeycombed enamel would seem to indicate fragility of the tooth, and a speedy yielding to decay; but in effect it is not necessarily so. A large proportion of these teeth remains till late in life, and as useful and wearing as others. Here and there, where the enamel is defective down to the dentine surface, the result is very different, and decay rapidly ensues.

Defects in the enamel between the cusps of the molar teeth are very common and very fruitful of destructive disease. The fissures are frequently deep, and at the bottom there exists only a confused, ill-developed enamel that is cracked and porous, affording a most incomplete protection of the dentine from external influences.

Depressions in the enamel sometimes occur in unusual positions, giving rise to similar results. Perhaps the most common of these occurs at the back of the superior lateral incisor teeth, and is a pretty sure cause of decay in that situation.

The congenital defects of dentine may be divided into—

Imperfect calcification,
Vascularity, and
Replacement by modified bone.

Imperfect calcification of dentine is a common and serious defect in its structure. It, however, occupies a singular position as between that which is normal and abnormal. It is an incompletion—an arrest at a half stage—of that which is a normal process.

I need scarcely observe, in reference to the coarse anatomy of a developing tooth, that the dentine of the organ commences formation upon, or rather in the surface-structure of the formative pulp, and that the increase of growth is from above and without, downwards and inwards—the growth being strictly endogenous.

When a very small and thin layer of dentine (its organic element) is formed upon the upper outer surface of a tooth—and I would here use the term *layer* rather for convenience of expression than as implying a truly laminated structure, though a sort of latent lamination does really exist—when, then, a thin layer of dentine in a soft state is formed over the surface, its calcification rapidly follows the development, only a very minute thickness of animal substance anticipating this change.

The calcification consists not in an even, slow impregnation of the whole basis with earthy matter, nor in the interstitial deposit of earthy particles in a web of animal matter, nor a change having relation to the course of the tissue affected: it is an independent element of nutrition, affecting isolated points of the animal basis—points which become completely calcified, while the intermediate tissue remains unchanged. These points, gradually invading the contiguous tissue, evenly enlarge in each direction, becoming spheres; these still enlarge till they touch each other, and, progressing still further, gradually merge into one another; and, if the process continue to its complete issue, the fusion is so thorough that all indication of the calcification globules, and the intermediate uncalcified cartilage (if cartilage it may be called) is obliterated. The dentine is even, compact, and complete.

If, however, from a deficient nutrition, from an imperfect supply of calcareous matter, the animal basis of the dentine becomes only partially calcified, then the calcification globules remain distinct, or are unevenly fused, the intermediate cartilage being soft and unaltered; still the internal growth goes on, fresh layers of dentine being formed, thus separating the imperfectly developed layers from the nutritional influences of the receding pulp. A thin layer of dentine appears to be sufficient to effect this purpose, and this may itself be completely elaborated or not; but when once this separation has occurred, no change appears to take place subsequently in the imperfectly calcified layer, and that which should have been a temporary and transient condition becomes permanent, and therefore abnormal.

It must be remembered that during life, though there is this great difference in density between the calcified globules and the interglobular cartilage, there is no interruption in structural elements; the interglobular space is completely filled with uncalcified cartilage, and the dentinal tubes pass indifferently through the hard and the soft structures. When, however, such teeth are extracted and allowed to get dry, the tenuous animal substance shrinks and dries up to a mere film, while the calcified globules remain hard, sharp, and firm. These circumstances it is necessary to recollect, as they imply and explain certain optical appearances which would otherwise be unintelligible. The result of the drying up of the animal substance is, that interspaces filled with air occur between the globules, and have outlines exactly corresponding with the spherical bulgings of the hardened dentine. These interglobular spaces are opaque-black by transmitted light, and dead-white by reflected light; on the same principle, and for the same reasons, as such is the case in the tubes and loculi in dentine, and the lacunæ, canaliculi and interspaces in bone.

This condition of half-calcified dentine may exist in any

degree, from the slight indication known as the "contour-marking," in which thin alternate layers exhibit this state to a slight degree, to others in which the whole mass of dentine is a conglomerate mass of globules.

It *usually* happens that, when the dentine of the crown exhibits imperfect calcification, the enamel is imperfect at a spot corresponding with the external abutment of the imperfectly calcified layer, and exhibits the condition known as "rocky" enamel,—the converse of that is, I believe, *constant*, namely, that whenever a tooth exhibits rocky enamel, it will be found that the dentine beneath the grooves, irregularities, or pits, displays the condition I have been describing. This will be seen illustrated in fig. 43.

Fig. 43.

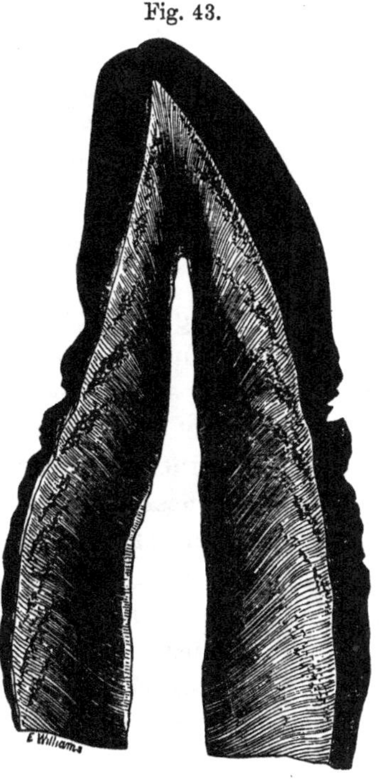

If a section of imperfectly calcified dentine be examined dry, or mounted in Canada balsam so rapidly as to prevent the fluid resin from running into and filling up the interspaces, the dentine globules are seen in various spherical and convex forms bounded by black, opaque interspaces (fig. 44). The dentine in the globules themselves is perfectly formed, and the tubes may be traced across the globules, and skipping the interspaces across succeeding globules as though in a continuous line. The globules are largest towards the centre of the tooth, and smaller and more numerous towards its surface, where, in the fang, they spread out beneath the crusta petrosa, forming what Mr. Tomes has called the "granular layer." The term "layer" is incorrectly used, for it is not continuous beneath the crusta petrosa, being interrupted, and consists only of the external abutment of the sheets of imperfectly calcified dentine.

If a specimen of globular dentine be mounted slowly, so that the Canada balsam can run in and fill the interspaces, the structure loses all its black opacity, and becomes very trans-

Fig. 44.

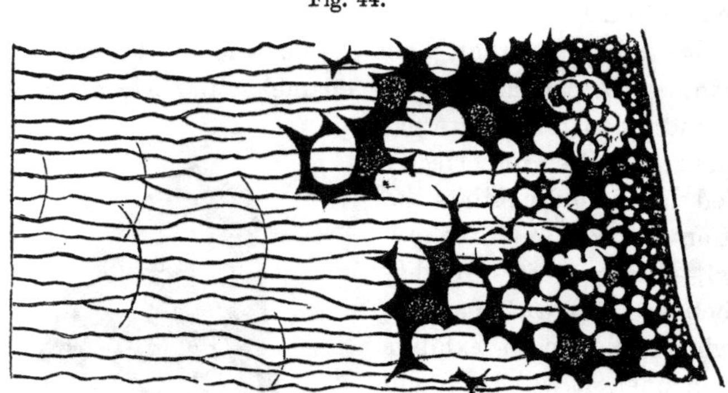

parent. The conglomerate nature of the mass is very distinct, and exhibits a curious appearance: some of the globules are seen sharp, clear, and in focus, while others are indistinct and looming obscurely out of focus; some isolated and spherical, others fused together in every variety of proportion.

The circumstances under which this condition is produced, all point to a depressed and imperfect nutrition at the time of development, as its cause:—

1. I believe it is almost universal in rickets: at least, as far as my own experience goes it is so: and it has been observed by others in that diseased condition.

2. It frequently happens that an illness in early childhood affects the layer of dentine that is formed during that period, and this is in the form very generally associated with rocky enamel. Where this is the case, all the teeth are affected—at least all that have commenced calcifying—not at the same part in each, but at a position which corresponds with the amount of development which each tooth had attained at that particular time.

3. This condition is not infrequent where the tegumentary organs generally are feebly developed. I have noticed this especially in young ladies with preternaturally thin and transparent skins, with short papillæ, whose eye-lashes and eyebrows are small and thin, hair of the head very fine and soft, papillæ of the tongue very short. There is a peculiar stamp of

complexion which is characteristic: and in these people the teeth are usually found very small, the cusps short, the fangs short, and the dentine exhibiting in a marked degree this condition of imperfect calcification—the teeth, in fact, as dermal organs, sharing in the general defect of the tegumentary system.

Vascularity of Dentine is an unnatural condition, but not altogether uncommon. It is, however, associated sometimes with the development of bone around the erratic vascular canals, and may thus lead to pathological changes which are inconsistent with normal dentine. Critical observations on dental pathology have not yet furnished sufficient data to generalise further on this subject. But what is known is sufficiently suggestive, especially if taken in conjunction with what follows.

The Replacement of Dentine by masses of bone. This condition involves a liability to some at least of the diseases to which skeleton bones are obnoxious. It is probably from insufficient and neglected opportunity that I must rest upon a single, but most remarkable specimen of abnormal structure to illustrate this subject.

The specimen in question is a molar tooth which was given me by Mr. Topping, the accomplished mounter of microscopical specimens. It had three canals piercing the neck just below the edge of the enamel, as seen in fig. 45. These canals were short and horizontal. Upon sawing the tooth vertically in half, it was found that the substance around these canals, extending considerably in the crown and down one of the fangs, was yellower and clearer than normal dentine, and it had a cancellated aspect.

Fig. 45.

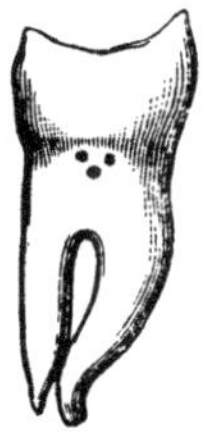

Upon examining this doubtful tissue with the microscope, it was seen to be bone, resembling very closely ordinary cancellated bone of the skeleton. This occupied about a fourth of the crown and neck of the tooth. Upon referring to the figure (fig. 46) it will be seen that the whole of the margin of the section is normal dentine: the bone is not merged by degrees into the dentine, but the limit between the two is defined and sharp, though irregular and jagged. The osseous tissue presents circular, oval, and irregular interspaces, like ordinary cancellated bone. Upon examining this structure with higher powers of the microscope, it is found to resemble skeleton bone more than crusta petrosa: the laminæ are smaller, more uniform both in size and arrangement, and the canaliculi are fewer and smaller, and altogether less conspicuous. The laminæ are even and regular, and are parallel with the outlines of the cancelli. Mixed up with these laminæ, and among them, are here and there to be seen some small isolated patches of dentine.

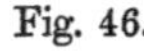
Fig. 46.

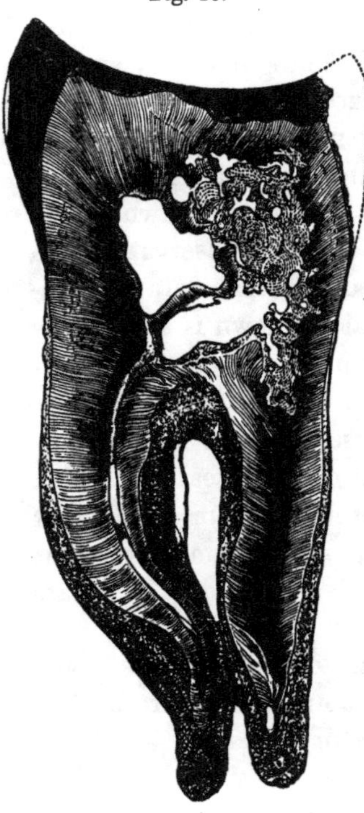

Here, then, we have true vascular bone occupying a considerable portion of the crown of a tooth. The specimen is, as far as I know, unique. But it is very unlikely that the morbid condition has not occurred many times before. Bone structure would be liable to bone diseases, and these occurring in teeth would, in such a situation, occasion anomalous and unexpected symptoms and results. It is probable that some such condition may have existed in the few reported cases of abscess in the hard substance of teeth, to be referred to hereafter.

Modifications of *form* and *size* of teeth are frequent; the latter, however, can scarcely be considered as coming within the limits of *disease;* though the disproportion in the size of the teeth and the jaw, especially when the former is in excess, often renders surgical interference necessary. The superior wisdom tooth and the lateral incisor are more frequently modified in form than other teeth.

I have a specimen of the former twice its natural size, with seven distinct cusps and seven fangs, the latter curved and thin. Another dens sapientiæ is similar in form and size to a single grain of wheat. The superior lateral incisor is sometimes reduced to a small compressed cone. The superior central incisor is occasionally nearly twice its natural breadth, and sometimes with a groove indicating an imperfect gemmation.

The incisors and canines may have conical cusps on the lingual surface; and I have seen both upper and lower bicuspids with a third cusp.

The fangs are liable to very great variety. The lower molars may have three or four fangs and the lower bicuspids and canines two. The upper molars may have four fangs, or two, or they may be fused into one. I have a singular modification of fang in a molar tooth; the implanted portion of the tooth consists of a single cylinder without any grooving or indication of separate fangs; the cylinder is slightly expanded at the extremity and hollow; around the edge, and not in the centre, are several minute foramina for the entry of the nerves and vessels.

A similar example of this rare condition is described in the "Transactions of the Odontological Society" for 1871.*

Occasionally fangs are unusually long, those of the upper molars very widely spread; and those of the lower molars much curved backwards. There are other modifications in the form and disposition of fangs which have an important practical bearing on the difficulties of tooth-extraction. These will be considered in the chapter on that subject.

Why many of the foregoing modifications in the form of teeth should arise is at present quite unknown. Some distortions of the fangs appear to be mechanical, the misplacement of other and contiguous teeth hindering the regular growth of the fang and pushing it aside. This is a gradual process, but sudden mechanical violence may shift a partially formed tooth from the soft immature pulp upon which it was growing, and this without preventing the continuation of development. This has been called "dilaceration" of the tooth. Such a specimen is shown in the accompanying figure, 47, of an incisor tooth, enlarged two diameters.

Fig. 47.

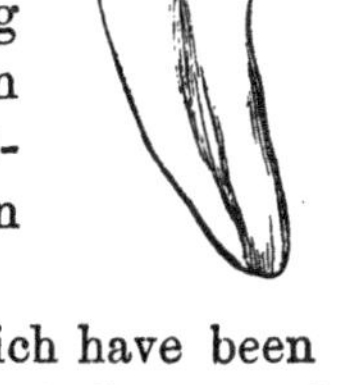

There is one other form, or series of forms, which have been clearly traced to a specific origin, namely, to the influence of inherited syphilis.

* New Series, vol. iii., p. 200.

Syphilitic Teeth. — We are indebted to Mr. Jonathan Hutchinson for pointing out one of the most interesting malformations of the teeth, and for establishing, by unanswerable evidence, its singular cause.

A certain number of children born of parents under the influence of constitutional syphilis have incisors and canine teeth exhibiting very characteristic peculiarities. The teeth are small, peg-like in shape, narrow at the free edge, and either excavated by a crescentic notch at the margin, or marked by a crescentic groove. The conical peggy condition is most marked in the lower teeth; the crescentic notch is most conspicuous in the upper incisors.

These conditions are usually, though not always, confined to the permanent teeth, which Mr. Hutchinson attributes to the fact that hereditary syphilis does not develop itself during intra-uterine life. Mr. Hutchinson supposes that attacks of syphilitic stomatitis are necessary to produce these malformed teeth; but I quite agree with Mr. Tomes, that such an idea is unnecessary as an explanation of the condition in question. Syphilis perverts the nutrition of many organs and structures; it acts with special virulence on the tegumentary system of which the teeth are part; and it seems to me that the malformation of the teeth is probably more the result of perverted nutrition than of inflammation.

CHAPTER VIII.

CARIES, OR DECAY—ABSCESS IN DENTINE—STAINING OF DENTINE.

The disease of the teeth known as Caries, or Decay, is the most common morbid change that occurs in the body. It is almost universal, to a less or greater degree, in persons who have reached adult age. As a result of its frequency and its great importance, much controversy has arisen in regard to its nature and causes.

The term caries is singularly inapplicable, as it has no relation whatever to those diseases of true bones which are so defined; but the name is so generally adopted that it is useless to attempt to disturb it or replace it by another. Decay is a far better expression, for it asserts the truth, without implying any incorrect theory.

Dental caries may be defined as a softening and disintegration of the tooth's surface, gradually penetrating towards its centre. It affects the enamel, the dentine, and the crusta petrosa, when the latter is exposed. It is essentially a superficial affection, dependent on external influences, though modified somewhat by vital action.

The most obvious commencement of caries takes place on the surface of dentine, immediately underlying faulty enamel; but it certainly in some instances commences in the enamel itself.

When the enamel is attacked it becomes opaque, whitish or grey, and then gradually stained of a brownish colour, and this is soon followed by still more obvious changes in the dentine. The latter tissue undergoes more rapid alteration than the enamel; it becomes brown and soft, and the change penetrates in the direction of the tubes towards the pulp, while it spreads laterally beneath the as-yet healthy enamel.

These changes occur in endless variety, one form passing into another: the extreme varieties have been described as distinct *species* of decay, without, however, sufficient justification.

Caries may affect a large area of enamel at once, and break it down into a chalky state: this is called "calcareous." In the dentine it may pass rapidly from the surface of the tooth to the pulp for a small and limited area: this is called "perforating" or "penetrating" caries. Sometimes the whole or a considerable portion of the dentinal surface of the crown of a tooth becomes rapidly carious: this is called "spreading" or "peeling" caries. At times the disease advances to a certain stage, and ceases to progress: this is called "arrested," "stationary," or "carbonised" decay. With the exception of the latter, the varieties are mere matters of degree. As regards colour it may vary from the slightest tinge of brown to nearly black, the enamel being always less affected than the dentine. The consistence of the carious dentine may be scarcely less than the healthy tissue, or it may be soft and almost diffluent. The superficial part of the decay is always the softest, and in cutting it the structure is found harder and harder as the subjacent healthy dentine is approached. The colour of caries is brown; it varies from the palest stain to nearly black, but it is pretty uniformly a modification of the same hue. Among pigments burnt sienna is the nearest approach to the colour. In a section of a slightly carious tooth, mounted in balsam and viewed under the microscope with low powers and a full, transmitted light, the appearance is very brilliant.

As a rule the colour is deepest in the slowest decay, and palest in that which is most rapid.

One of the most remarkable characteristics of dentinal caries is its smell, which is constant. It is quite distinct from any other odour that emanates from the body, and it is altogether different from that which is given off in the neighbourhood of dead bone.

I am only acquainted with one source of a similar smell. The species of the genus of neuropterous insects, *Chrysopa*, all have a precisely similar odour. This is intense in the exquisite little *Chrysopa septempunctata*.

The *chemistry* of caries is one of its most interesting points.

It consists in a process of decalcification, progressively going on, both as regards the area and depth of tissue invaded, and the degree of the change.

The process is best traced in the dentine. The decalcification may be very slight, and then the tissue remains proportionately hard; or it may be so considerable that the dentinal cartilage can be readily cut with a knife. When even a large amount of the earthy salts has been removed, the form of the dentine is still retained; but by degrees the animal matter of the surface is so robbed of its mineral support, that it breaks down and becomes decomposed and disintegrated. It is, however, never completely decalcified, as it may be by artificial processes.

I am indebted to my colleague, Dr. Stevenson, for an analysis of carious dentine. The material was obtained principally from molar and pre-molar teeth, and it may be accepted that it was of an average density.

When in a moist state, as it would be in the mouth and immediately after extraction, Dr. Stevenson found that 55·53 per cent. was lost by drying at a temperature of 212° F.; and of the remainder the animal matter rather exceeded the inorganic. The result of the analysis was this:—

Water	55·53
Organic matter	23·40
Ash	21·07
	100·00

The ash consisted mainly of phosphate of lime, with a little magnesia: there were carbonates in very small proportion, and a trace of alkaline salts. As I have before observed, the decalcification of the dentine in caries varies indefinitely; and the foregoing analysis merely represents an average condition. But there is always some residue of inorganic matter. By calcining the softest carious dentine in a platinum spoon with a blow-pipe I have always found an appreciable ash.

It may be broadly stated that the change, brought about by the chemical influences which occur in caries, consists in the withdrawal of the earthy constituents of the dentine and their replacement by water.

Carious dentine when moist gives an acid reaction with litmus-paper. If dried and re-moistened after a long time it is still acid. When immersed in water the liquid becomes acid; after two or three washings the carious dentine will be found neutral, and it will remain so, unless exposed to some further chemical or fermenting action.

Mr. Coleman, in his interesting and valuable paper on dental caries,* suggests, what is probably correct, that the acid reaction of carious dentine is due to superphosphate of lime. He has found that the dentine, but slightly softened and deep in the substance of the tooth, is quite as acid as that removed from the more superficial portions of softened dentine in the same tooth. It must be remembered that the phosphate of lime, as it exists in bone and ivory, can only be converted into superphosphate by the removal of a certain portion of the lime and its replacement with basic water—this changes the neutral insoluble salt into one that is acid and soluble. But to accomplish this a free acid must have removed a portion of the basic lime; and though, as Mr. Coleman suggests, the acid reaction probably depends on the soluble superphosphate of lime, especially where the dentine is not superficial, it involves the pre-existence of an acid from some extraneous source.

The microscopical characters of enamel caries are less distinct than those of dentine, as they are so closely associated with disintegration of the tissue. In the immediate neighbourhood of the carious enamel the prism structure is usually very distinctly marked; but where caries has actually set in this rapidly disappears, and an irregular highly pigmented molecular mass takes its place. The depth of colour and the disintegration of the enamel usually bear a direct proportion to each other.

In carious dentine the intertubular tissue is first and most powerfully acted upon, and its density is diminished, so as to be easily removed from the tubes, and at the same time its optical refraction is lowered, so as to be even less in proportion to that of the tubes than relatively exists in health. The result is that in transverse sections of carious dentine the peculiar appearance of a thick wall to each tube, produced by the diffraction of light by the cut end of the tube-wall, is generally strongly

* *Trans. Odont. Soc.*, vol. iii. p. 82.

marked; and the appearance has been very aptly likened to the ends of a number of tobacco-pipes. When, however, the same tubes are seen in a longitudinal section the illusion is manifest, and the tubes are observed much as in healthy dentine, with the exception of occasional varicosity. The tubes of carious dentine appear to me to be generally, if not always, occupied by solid material. It is not improbable that upon the first inroads of caries the contents of the tubes become calcified, as we see them in the clear limitary layer, and that they slowly undergo the partial decalcification which occurs in the whole tissue as the decay progresses.

When seen in longitudinal aspect, in very soft and diffluent caries, the tubes are occasionally found in a varicose and bulbous condition, and I have seen them quite moniliform; and in such specimens the tubes are not infrequently found projecting free, beyond the intertubular tissue. By treating carious dentine with strong hydrochloric acid, or what is even better, with caustic alkali, the intertubular substance is readily removed, and the tubes displayed standing free from the cut edges, in the form of short cylinders. These have been described by Mr. Tomes as fibrils and as tube-contents, but they are the tubes themselves. These cylindrical projections are very apt to break off; and if a specimen of carious dentine be steeped in caustic alkali and then thoroughly picked abroad with fine points, the field of the microscope is seen scattered with short lengths of these little cylinders.

With low powers the carious dentine is seen to show a marked tendency to crack and break up in two nearly opposite directions—in the line of the tubes; but still more in the course of calcification, that is, along the contours, or incremental lines.

But one of the most remarkable appearances displayed by carious dentine consists in the projection from its surface of enormous numbers of very minute threads of a truly vegetable character. These constitute a cyptogamic vegetable growth, known as *Leptothryx buccalis*, which, however, is probably an incorrect name, as the genus Leptothryx is one of the Oscillatoriaceæ, and the structure found upon dentine appears rather to be the mycelium of a true fungus. In the uncertainty, however, it would be undesirable to suggest an alteration of the name. This growth has a power of penetrating into the dentinal tissue.

Leber and Rottenstein * assert that the Leptothryx enters the carious tubes, and, where they are dilated, fills them with a molecular mass which is identical in nature with the other vegetable structure. I have myself found Leptothryx burrowing for great distances between the tubes, and in very soft caries completely occupying the intertubular spaces, and twining around the tubes.

The causes of caries may be divided into *predisposing* and *exciting*.

The predisposing causes are faults or deficiencies in the enamel, such as have been indicated in the chapter on defects of the tissues. These practically leave the surface of dentine open to the attacks of fluids in the mouth; and where the defects are only superficial the enamel itself may alone first suffer. Mechanical injury is a fertile source of caries, either by exposing the dentine, or by disintegrating the enamel and rendering it porous. The latter condition very often occurs where teeth are in close contact and in crowded jaws—the enamel at the points of contact becomes crushed and disintegrated, so that it no longer excludes the fluids of the mouth, but imbibes them.

Imperfect calcification of the dentine is, in one sense, a predisposing cause: teeth in which the calcification globules are imperfectly fused decay rapidly when once attacked; but, I believe, if the enamel remains sound, they do not show any exceptional disposition to caries.

Another but vague cause must be considered as tending to predispose to decay. I mean some hereditary condition of *quality*, which is passed from parents to children. The tendency to decay which runs through some families is so marked and unmistakable, and so independent of all other explainable cause, that it can only be supposed to result from some imperfection in the nature of the teeth, apart from or superadded to histological defect.

The exciting and immediate causes of caries have been very carefully worked out, and they may be stated without lengthened argument.

* *Recherches sur la Carie Dentaire.* Paris, 1868.

Nearly all the changes which occur in carious teeth have been imitated artificially, either by dead teeth being worn as substitutes, or by submitting teeth out of the body to certain agencies, which have been contrived to imitate the influences which are presumed to operate in the mouth.

The fact that dead teeth worn artificially undergo changes very similar to ordinary caries, shows how far the changes are dependent upon external and non-vital agencies.

One of the most manifest changes which teeth display in caries is decalcification—a removal of the previously insoluble earthy salts; and it has been found by experiment that the action of acids, such as may be supplied by the fluids of the mouth, or by the decomposition of articles of food, will produce results in dead teeth having a close resemblance to true tooth-decay.

It was long ago shown by Westcott, an American dentist, that even vegetable acids, though in weak solution, have the power of dissolving out the lime-salts from teeth; and these observations have been repeated by others. But the most interesting experiments are those of Magitot,* who found that neutral substances, moistened or in solution, in contact with teeth, would produce carious-like decay and an acid reaction. Thus solution of sugar acted, and its energy was increased, by the addition of animal matter, the fluid becoming acid; and that this arose from some catalytic process was proved by the fact that it was arrested by the antiseptic action of creosote, and by the boiling and hermetic sealing of the vessel in which the experiment was conducted.

Mr. Coleman † has shown that teeth placed in a solution of sugar in water, with saliva added, and in a mixture of bread-and-water with saliva, undergo decay, and the fluids become acid; and he has also proved that the presence of saliva is an active if not a necessary element in producing the result. The sources of acidity within the mouth are mucus, saliva, and acids produced by fermentive action of matters of food entangled with the teeth.

Buccal mucus is very commonly acid, and I find that the

* *Traité de la Carie Dentaire.* 1867.

† *Trans. Odon. Soc.*, vol. iii. p. 80.

oozy secretion around the necks of the teeth nearly always turns litmus-paper pink.

It is by no means uncommon to find the saliva giving an acid reaction, even temporarily, in healthy people, and I do not think that this has been sufficiently dwelt upon as a cause of decay.

But as regards the acidity both of the mucus and saliva, it must be remembered that, however slight, if efficient to cause the least amount of decalcification, it is accumulative, and any slight withdrawal of bone-earth from the tissues leaves them so far carious and the more prone to further mischief.

The acids produced by fermentation of food entangled by the teeth probably supply the largest amount of solvent material.

There is yet another agency which probably has a large share in the decay of dentine. I allude to the growth of the Leptothryx, already mentioned. I believe it pervades all carious dentine, pierces it, and perhaps grows at its expense.

What its precise action may be is mostly a matter of speculation. Its growth may be catalytic in its effect, as the growth of torula acts upon sweet-wort, determining an atomic arrangement, in which fresh chemical combinations arise; and thus insoluble matters may be rendered soluble; or its own nutrition may rob the tissue of a solidifying element; or again, its perforation of the dentine may (and no doubt does) weaken its cohesion, and help to disintegrate it. But whatever the mode of action, it seems to me that this vegetable growth cannot form on and in dentine without aiding its destruction. Conditions of ill-health must be looked upon as exciting causes of caries; and though the expression is vague and the mode of action at present uncertain, there is evidence, beyond dispute, that maladies, especially those deranging digestion and primary assimilation, are potent, immediate causes of tooth-decay. This is especially marked in those maladies which occur during pregnancy. It is not uncommon for each pregnancy, with some women, to be regularly attended by loss of teeth by decay; and that with persons who, before marriage, showed no tendency to caries; and in such cases the disease is usually attended with disproportionate suffering.

That ordinary decay of teeth is to a certain extent mimicked by the changes which occur in ivory and animal teeth used as artificial substitutes, cannot be questioned; but there are distinct and important differences between the two, which have not yet been imitated by any artificial process.

From accidental circumstances I have had peculiar opportunities of examining very numerous specimens of ivory masticating-blocks and human teeth, that have been worn as artificial substitutes. The general resemblance of these in a state of decay to true caries of dentine is very striking, and the miscroscopic changes in all are to a great extent the same. There are, however, several marked distinctions. In the ivory and artificial teeth there is (*a*) a want of limit to the change, (*b*) an absence of the calcified zone and clear pencils of tubes around the decay, and (*c*) an entire absence of the characteristic smell.

When artificial molars are made of ivory they become sodden and soft throughout; and the dentine of artificial human teeth becomes affected in the same way. The zones and the pencils of clear tubes with calcified contents are certainly absent in the ivory and dead teeth that have been worn in the mouth. I commit myself to this statement after very many investigations; and in this I entirely agree with Magitot,* in contradistinction to Wedl.†

I can only conclude that the latter observer has mistaken the pale deepest layer of decayed dentine for the condition in question. The innermost layers are the least coloured; when decalcified in the process of decay, they become, to a certain extent, translucent and horny upon drying. And I have seen the same appearance, the result of fatty matter imbibed from the food, and which yielded to the action of ether. This, however, is quite distinct from the transparent zone, and the pencils of clear tubes, which latter never appear, nor are imitated, in these specimens of artificial teeth.

The calcification of the tubes in the neighbourhood of caries, though it does not affect the question as to the chemical and extraneous influences which soften and remove the decaying dentine, does, however, affect the matter when considered as a whole. I quite agree with Magitot that it is a vital process,

* *Recherches sur la Caie de Dents.* Paris: 1871.

† *Pathologie der Zähne.*

curative in its tendency, or at all events preventive. We see the same in the crowns of teeth worn by attrition. Here we frequently find the tubes of the primary dentine sealed up by calcification of their contents, concurrently with the formation of dentine-of-repair. This whole process is obviously one of vital nutrition, the nutrient material being furnished by the dentinal pulp. We see the same changes occurring in the dentine of the fangs of teeth from young persons after inflammation, and, it may be assumed, hypernutrition, as well as in old people.

That this transparent dentine is the result of calcification of the tube-contents is to my mind beyond all question. The material ordinarily occupying the dentinal tubes is so thin, that when the tissue is dry scarcely any evidence of its existence is left, and the tube is filled with air. When once the dentine of a living tooth has become transparent, no amount of drying, even by artificially high temperature, will admit air to the tube. I have tried this repeatedly; and after such treatment a transverse section of such tubes shows them to have a solid axis. No uncalcified animal tissue could thus comport itself; it is physically impossible.

Smell is another circumstance which distinguishes true caries from any artificial attempt to imitate it. The smell is absolutely peculiar to carious dentine and it is constant. Offensive as decayed ivory and artificial teeth may be, they never have the characteristic odour. I have had exceptional opportunities of observing on this point. For the first ten years of practice (1851 to 1861) I was in the daily habit of seeing and handling artificial teeth in which ivory of some kind and human teeth were used; and unless the artificial piece came in contact with a carious tooth I never met with the particular smell. I was so struck with the similarity, in many respects, of caries of standing teeth and decay occurring in artificial ones, that I was always on the look-out for an example of this additional resemblance; but I never met with one. And I have found, moreover, that if a carious tooth be allowed to dry and remain till the characteristic smell has passed off, it does not come back if the decay is continued by artificial means.

It has been asserted that caries of dentine is associated with the death of that tissue, and indeed that its death is not only an absolute element in its production, but the essential first step in the changes which occur.

But certainly this is not the fact, for (*a*) the death of a tooth and its severance from vital nutrition derived from the tooth-pulp does not render it prone to caries; and (*b*) caries may attack the ivory of a tooth, and yet that very tissue, already carious, will retain extreme sensibility.

Teeth become carious on different parts of the crown and of the neck and fangs when exposed. When the crown is attacked there is, I believe, always some previous defect of enamel.

In the molar teeth the crypts between the cusps are usually first attacked. The necks of the molars near the outer gum are prone to decay, especially the back molars, where food often remains in contact with the teeth for a considerable time. This is especially the case with the upper wisdom-teeth.

The bicuspids, especially the upper, nearly always commence to decay where in contact with the next teeth. The same is the case with the upper canines and incisors. The latter sometimes decay at their backs, when by folding or pitting of the surface the enamel is imperfect, and irregularities exist, in which food may remain. The necks of the teeth when exposed will often decay. In the front of the mouth this condition is usually initiated by receding of the gum; in the back teeth by erosion, through absorption, of the enamel in contact with inflamed and spongy gum.

One curious fact is worthy of especial note: the fangs of teeth, when exposed after alveolar abscess, by absorption of socket around their apices, are never attacked by caries—a circumstance probably due to their being bathed with alkaline pus.

As caries progresses the pulp-cavity is approached and opened, giving rise to painful symptoms and a retrocession of the pulp, after which decay attacks the inner surface of the cavity and progresses outwards.

The teeth differ in a very remarkable degree as to their liability to decay.

In the temporary set the molars decay much more often than the incisors or canines. And it may here be mentioned that decay of the temporary teeth does not seem in any way to affect their successors.

As regards the relative frequency of decay in the permanent teeth many elaborate statistical tables have been drawn up, which are rather curious than instructive; and many of them give results which are hardly correct, according to my experience. The broad facts may be briefly stated as follows: The first permanent molar is much more apt to decay than any other tooth; next follow the second and third molars; the superior bicuspids succeed in order; the superior lateral incisors come next in frequency, followed immediately by the superior centrals. The superior canines are little prone to decay, and the same may be said of the lower bicuspids, especially the first. Caries is rare in the lower canines and incisors.

Taken as a whole, the upper teeth decay nearly twice as often as the lower; but the lower molars are more prone to caries than the uppers.

The extreme frequency of caries of the first molar is a most remarkable circumstance, and it has never been satisfactorily accounted for. It has been supposed by an eminent dentist to result from the constitutional disturbance occasioned by infantile vaccination; but this theory is certainly insufficient to meet all cases. It is true, however, that the first molar is undergoing development at that early period of life when children are liable to frequent disturbances of nutrition from the occurrence of the ordinary infantile maladies, and when their physical condition is extremely mobile and prone to diseased action. This may in some degree account for the peculiar frailty of the first molar in relation to caries.

Caries may occur at any time of life; but it usually happens that faulty teeth declare themselves before the twenty-fifth year of age, and that after that period there is comparative immunity from decay till long after middle life, when the majority of teeth are lost by loosening rather than by decay.

Caries of teeth is distinctly more common among women than among men; and this probably arises from those disturbances of health which are purely sexual.

It is much more common now than in past ages, and it

appears to have advanced with civilisation, and the use of soft and cooked foods.

As regards now-existing races tooth-decay is much more abundant among the highly civilised than among savages, though the scale of gradation is by no means even and unbroken. But what is remarkable is the fact that the poorer classes in highly civilised communities are those who suffer most of all. In this country the labouring classes in purely agricultural districts are afflicted with caries of their teeth beyond all others. I make this assertion after very considerable observation.

The *treatment* of caries consists in the removal of the decayed material, leaving behind a healthy surface, either polished and exposed, or covered in by some foreign material—a stopping, in fact.

Caries has a constant tendency to increase both by contact and continuity, and the removal of the decayed matter is a first step towards an arrest of the disease; and though this proceeding may leave dentine exposed and unprotected by enamel, decay will often be arrested so long as the surface is kept smooth and polished, and thus prevented from being the nidus of parasitic growth, or the seat of fermentine changes from the attachment of putrescent material.

When the caries is superficial it may be removed by filing and subsequent polishing with pumice-powder and chalk, care being taken in every case to retain as much of the front of the tooth as possible. The filed surface should, too, be left as flat as it can be, for a small concavity will occasion a lodgment of foreign material, and so start a renewal of the decay.

When the caries is deep and perforating, excavation with cutting instruments will be necessary, the hollow thus produced being stopped or plugged, so as to exclude all food and moisture.*

The removal of carious dentine is often attended with considerable pain, for, as has already been remarked, it retains its vitality, as manifested by sensitiveness, long after the decay has commenced. And it is necessary in some instances to prepare the surface with some benumbing application before

* The proceedings adopted in tooth-stopping are now so mechanical, and belong so entirely to 'Dentistry' proper, rather than to Dental Surgery, that they do not come within the scope of this work.

the filing or cutting can be borne. The late Mr. Arnold Rogers, many years since, recommended to me a strong solution of chloride of zinc for that purpose, and it is certainly most efficient.

Abscess in Dentine.—This is one of the very rarest diseases to which the teeth are liable. For a long time the evidence of its possible occurrence rested on a single case recorded by Mr. Bell; * since then another instance has been published by Mr. Spence Bate.†

Mr. Bell describes his case as follows:—

"Mr. S——, a medical gentleman, had long been suffering extreme pain in the right side of the lower jaw, apparently produced by the second molar tooth, which, however, had no external marks of disease. After a time inflammation took place in the periosteum of the root, and the tooth was in a measure loosened." The tooth was extracted; "and as no diseased appearance was found on the surface, I sawed it asunder at the crown, and found a cavity in the solid bony structure, perfectly circumscribed; the surrounding bone being white, and of a healthy and sound texture. Not the slightest appearance of disease existed in any other part of the tooth, excepting that from the inflammation which had so long existed. The pulp itself had begun to suppurate.

"In this case, then, it appears that inflammation had occurred from some local cause in the bone of the tooth; that the vessels of the bone had formed pus, and that absorption had taken place in consequence of its pressure, and formed a cavity for its reception."

In Mr. Bate's case a first upper molar was removed on account of abscess of the antrum. On examining the tooth the pulp was found in a state of complete suppuration. But external to the pulp-cavity, and having no connection with it, there was, in the palatal fang, a cavity containing pus—"abscess in the dentine," as Mr. Bate defines it. Though there was no communication with the pulp-cavity, there was a small orifice opening to the periosteal surface.

Mr. Tomes ‡ describes two interesting specimens of circum-

* *On the Teeth.* London: 1835, p. 173.

† *Trans. Odont. Soc.*, vol. iv. p. 97.

‡ *Lectures on Dental Surgery.* London: 1848, p. 245.

scribed cavities in the tusks of elephants, which were probably abscesses. Each contained some inspissated material, and in one there were numerous canals for vessels, visible to the naked eye, in the dentine around the cavity.

As regards Mr. Bell's case, it should be remembered that no microscopical examination of the tissue around the abscess took place, and any peculiarities that it may have exhibited are unrecorded. In Mr. Bate's case there was an external orifice, which probably gave admission to a slip of vascular periosteum; and in one of Mr. Tomes's specimens the dentine around the probable abscess was certainly vascular.

I cannot conceive that ordinary dentine, so unprone to change and nutritional action, could undergo suppuration; but where it is vascular, and especially where fibro-cellular tissue permeates it, the case is quite different; and there is no more reason why, in such a condition, suppuration should not occur in a tooth than in a bone.

I have shown (p. 79) that dentine is sometimes vascular; that the vascular condition may be attended with the development of bone in the vascular track. I have also shown that very rarely a portion of the ivory of the tooth may be replaced by cancellated bone. If it is conceded, as I think it must be, that fibro-vascular tissue may find its way into, or be entangled within the ivory of a tooth, conditions are present which may yield upon inflammation, an abscess-sac within the hard tissues of a tooth. And I venture to suggest that this is the explanation of the foregoing cases.

Red Inflammatory (?) Patches in Dentine.—It is not uncommon to find small portions of dentine exhibiting a red colour; and I am surprised that the circumstance has not attracted more attention. Ivory may be coloured artificially by the administration of madder during its formation, and probably such stains may occur by means of certain foods taken accidentally.

It was my opinion, when first studying the diseases of the teeth, that such colouration was mere dyeing of the tissue during its formation; but more extended observation has led me to believe that the red patches are frequently the result of inflammatory action.

Mr. Bell, while endeavouring to establish the idea that

dentine is a blood-circulating tissue, wrote the following passage; and though his inferences are not sustained, his facts cannot be denied:—

"I have, in many instances, on purposely breaking a tooth, immediately after extraction, where the pain and inflammation had been severe, found distinct red patches in the very substance of the bone." *

I have found these patches of red stain in two distinct forms, one radiating from the pulp-cavity towards the surface in the direction of the tubular tissue, the other in belts mostly parallel with the surface of the tooth, and concurrent with the incremental markings, that is, with the successive areas of calcification. Accepting the opinion that these marks in dentine may arise both from staining in development and from extreme inflammation of the pulp in disease, it would be presumed, *à priori*, that the radial patches were inflammatory and the contour bands were developmental. But I have not found this to be constantly the case. I believe it to be true of the former, but not always of the latter. I have found incremental bands of pink dentine in teeth violently inflamed, when I am satisfied the colour was occasioned by hematine in the tubes. The real distinction between the two conditions I believe to be, that in developmental colouring, the intertubular tissue shares the pigment; in inflammatory staining the colour is within the tubes. It is many years since I satisfied myself that hematic colour enters the dentinal tubes in destructive inflammation of the pulp, and in necrosis of teeth; and in 1863 I observed the appearances of tube-staining in pulp-inflammation, which have since been figured and described by Heider and Wedl.†

* *Loc. cit.* p. 12.

† *Atlas zur Pathologie du Zähue.* Leipzig: 1869. T. x. fig. 94.

CHAPTER IX.

MECHANICAL INJURIES TO THE TEETH:—SURFACE-WEAR (ABRASION AND EROSION)—FRACTURE.

The term *abrasion* has been applied to those lesions of a tooth's surface which have clearly arisen from friction-wear. Where a similar removal of the outer layers of a tooth occurs without an obvious mechanical cause it is customary to call the affection *erosion*. To the latter, Hunter applied the term "decay by denudation."

I believe that abrasion and erosion are essentially the same conditions, and that they are equally caused by friction, though perhaps not only by that influence, as it is possible that a solvent power of the fluids of the mouth may assist in the process. The anatomical conditions of the two are so precisely the same, and they are so very frequently associated in the same mouth and in the same tooth, that I cannot believe them to be essentially different.

In considering this question it must be recollected that when any spot on the surface of a tooth has suffered abrasion, the tissues are there at a disadvantage, and they will sustain loss of substance far more rapidly, and with a less amount of friction, than contiguous, uninjured, or slightly injured parts. Then, again, the hard enamel will protect the immediately contiguous dentine, and that more remote from it will suffer more loss of substance though the tissue is the same. A damaged point on a tooth will be worn into a cup, while the rest of the tooth's surface, being sound, shows no indication of wear.

Again, be it remembered, food and the act of mastication may occasion friction and consequent wear on *any* part of the crown of a tooth, and this will attack the part that is predisposed to it by frailty of structure or damage.

It is quite possible that a solvent power of the fluids of the mouth may assist in the process; but an acid that would act on the calcified tissues of a tooth would not, by itself, leave the denuded surface smooth, hard, and polished.

All these premises being granted, I do not see any difficulty in accepting the view that abrasion and erosion are essentially the same; and, indeed, I do not see how to escape from that conclusion.

I think both the terms abrasion and erosion ought to be merged in one phrase, such as *surface-wear*, which I have suggested at the head of this chapter.

The most frequent situations for surface-wear to appear is on the masticating surfaces of the teeth, and on the edges of the incisors, where they meet end to end in the two jaws. It frequently occurs as a horizontal groove along the necks of the teeth on their buccal and labial surfaces (figs. 37 and 39), and occasionally as irregular excavated patches on the front surfaces of the teeth, especially the upper incisors. Any part of the crown of a tooth may be thus affected, but it is comparatively rare on the lingual surface.

The loss of tissue may be superficial or deep, and in the case of horizontal grooving a tooth may be completely cut through; and, were it not for the development of *dentine of repair*, the pulp cavity would be opened.

Sometimes the whole surface of the teeth is slowly and evenly removed, appearing like a sort of atrophy, though of course the diminution is superficial (Tomes).

Cases have occurred, though rarely, in which certain individual teeth have become worn down and truncated rapidly while contiguous teeth have suffered little. A remarkable

Fig. 48.

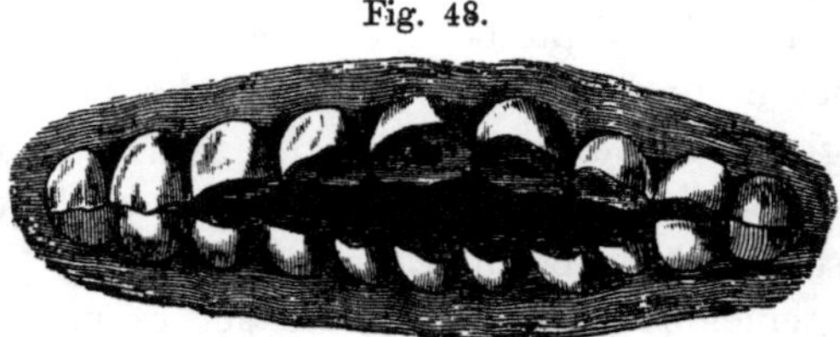

instance of this is described by Mr. Bell, and is illustrated in this figure, 48. Here the central incisors had first worn, then the laterals, then the canines, and ultimately the bicuspids: this occurred in both jaws, and the result was an elliptical separation of the front teeth as shown in the figure. I have little doubt that this was an example of syphilitic teeth, as I have seen a very similar example, which was undoubtedly syphilitic. In this condition the teeth, especially the incisors, are sometimes liable to very rapid wearing. Though the teeth had ceased to be themselves in contact, they would be rubbed by food in mastication, and this accounts for the polish of the surface, which existed in both cases.

The causes of surface-wear may be stated to be *predisposing*, consisting of an inherent softness of structure which certainly exists in some syphilitic teeth and probably in other conditions; and *exciting* causes, such as molar-mastication with incisor teeth, gritty food, a hard tooth-brush, certain tooth-powders, especially vegetable charcoal, which usually contains particles of silicates of lime and potash. The friction of artificial teeth will often remove the surface and polish the teeth where mastication would not easily account for it.

It is probable that in some cases the wearing is assisted by a solvent, or at least a softening action of the saliva, but the polish I believe is always occasioned by friction.

The consequences of surface-wear are interesting and important. When the dentine has become fairly exposed it assumes a yellowish colour, and more or less translucent from the calcification of the protoplasm in the dentinal tubes. The pulp takes on a renewed formative activity, dentine of repair is developed, and the pulp undergoes intrinsic calcification as already described (p. 69). When the wearing reaches the calcified pulp it is seen clear and yellow like amber. The dentine, when denuded of enamel, is more or less sensitive.

If the polishing friction is suspended, caries generally supervenes sooner or later.

In the grooving across the necks of the teeth, as it extends in breadth, the gum recedes, sometimes to a very remarkable extent. I have seen the fangs of teeth laid bare and polished by this process nearly to their apices on the buccal and labial surfaces, while on the lingual surface they were undisturbed. This is occasioned by hard brushing, and for a very long time does not disturb the firmness of the teeth.

In treating these cases it is desirable to smooth and round-off any sharp projections of enamel.

Any carious cavity should be carefully filled; and the extreme sensitiveness that often arises may be allayed by the application of camphorated chloroform, or a solution of chloride of zinc.

Fracture. Teeth are liable to fracture, both on account of the position they occupy and the functions they perform. Fracture may be occasioned by a blow, by hard substances in food, and even by the mere force of vigorous mastication. I have also known it occur from the spasmodic action of the muscles in tetanus.

Fracture may occur to any degree, and in any part of the tooth. A cusp of a molar or bicuspid may chip off, an incisor may be broken across the crown, or a tooth may be split more or less vertically. The most important question is between a simple and a compound fracture—one, that is, in which the hard tissues are alone fractured, or, on the other hand, where the pulp-chamber is opened and its contents exposed or lacerated.

A simple fracture is comparatively trifling, but a compound fracture is most serious, and usually leads to the loss of the tooth, when the fracture occurs in the crown so as to expose the pulp to external influences. When, however, the fracture is in the root, though the pulp chamber may be opened, the consequences are less threatening, the fracture may unite and the tooth be retained.

A simple fracture of the crown of a tooth only exposes the dentine to external influences; but being a sentient tissue, it is at first painfully affected by physical agencies—changes of temperature and friction. This usually subsides by degrees and the tooth is restored to its natural functions. In other cases, however, the irritation may be such as to set up inflammation, even to a destructive degree, of the pulp, leading to alveolar abscess, and such pain as to render extraction necessary. At first there is nearly always a certain amount of sympathetic inflammation within the alveolar cavity when a tooth is simply-fractured; there is tenderness of the whole tooth to the touch, and often some looseness, and when extracted, inflammatory deposit is found on the fang. But as a rule these conditions subside.

When the fracture is compound the pulp becomes the seat of intense inflammation and pain of a most distressing kind. These conditions are described in the chapter on Diseases of the Pulp (p. 157). The intensely sensitive exposed pulp may remain without much change for an indefinite time, or it may become the seat of sphacelus, attended or not with alveolar abscess.

When fracture of the fang occurs, I believe the pulp-cavity is always opened; but at the same time the pulp is not exposed to external influences unless the alveolus be also broken, and the gum lacerated. Circumstances are present, therefore, for union of the broken parts. And under these conditions union does really occur sometimes. Wedl mentions some fourteen specimens which have been described, in which fracture has been cured by re-union of the hard tissues.

From microscopic examination it appears that this union is brought about by a fresh growth both of the dentine* and crusta petrosa, the latter having a tendency to be in excess and encroach on the former.

The *Treatment* of tooth fracture depends on its nature and extent. In simple fracture of the crown, all rough edges and projections should be removed and smoothed down. Tenderness of exposed dentine may be greatly reduced by the application of chloride of zinc or nitrate of silver; and chloroform mixed with an alcoholic solution of tannin has the same effect more slowly. The alveolar inflammation, if it arise, may be reduced by leeching.

Where the fracture is compound it is desirable in the majority of cases to extract the tooth and its remains at once. There are, however, some exceptions to this rule. The fangs of the six front upper teeth, if not seriously injured, *may* be retained for pivoting-on new crowns; but if the irritation and inflammation consequent on the fracture are considerable, it will be preferable to extract the roots and supply artificial teeth in another manner. When either the canine or the

* It is very rare indeed that the pulp, when exposed, resumes a *dentine* development; but Tomes and Wedl both mention instances of its occurrence.

lateral incisor is broken in early life it may be removed in the hope that that first bicuspid will replace the former, and the canine come forward and close the small gap left by the latter. When, however, a compound fracture of a tooth occurs in childhood or adolescence, while yet teeth are coming, and the jaws are still undergoing growth and change of form, other considerations arise.

There is, however, one condition in which it is very desirable if possible to retain the fang of a tooth, even though broken to expose the pulp, and that at the cost of much suffering. I mean where a superior central incisor is broken in a young person. This is the most important "feature" tooth in the mouth. The extraction of its fang in childhood or youth will lead to the collapse of the contiguous teeth, leaving a space too small to pair with its fellow; or, if the space be obliterated, leaving an unsightly irregularity.

CHAPTER X.

NECROSIS OF TEETH.

THE term Necrosis is usually applied to teeth whose dentinal pulp has lost its nervous and vascular connection with the jaw, and in which that element of the tooth, together with a certain contingent portion of the dentine, has lost its vitality. The term, however, is not strictly correct as thus used, for such a tooth still retains a considerable degree of vitality from its connection with the periosteum, both as regards the cement and much of the dentine of the fang, and not improbably as regards also an outer indefinite layer of the dentine of the crown.

A tooth may be likewise partially necrosed as regards the periosteum, while the pulp retains its living connection with the nerves and vessels of the maxilla. Still the term necrosis, as applied to a tooth, relates to the death of its dentinal pulp. That form of tooth-death which is associated with the periosteum is dependent upon other causes, such as absorption of the socket and retrocession of the gum, or alveolar abscess. When a tooth becomes necrosed from death of its dentinal pulp it undergoes a change in its external appearance. It becomes discoloured; usually of a greyish dirty hue; and it is also more transparent than the contiguous teeth. The change of colour varies very considerably: it may be scarcely perceptible, or the tooth may become of a livid purple; and I have seen an instance in which, after an attack of scarlet fever in an adult, the two central incisors of the upper jaw, which were necrosed, were of a faded blood red; brighter, however, than the colour of venous blood.

When a tooth is necrosed, it may undergo a variety of changes. It may remain quite stationary in position, producing no apparent irritation; and be quite firm in the socket, the only alteration being that of colour. It may, however, immediately produce intense inflammation of the surrounding socket, leading to alveolar abscess, and even to necrosis of contiguous bone; or it may give rise to a chronic development of osseous tissue filling up the alveolus, and slowly dislocating the tooth.

The teeth which are most commonly affected by necrosis properly so called are the incisors, but particularly the central incisors of the upper jaw; and this arises from their being so much exposed to that which is the commonest cause of this condition, namely, mechanical violence.

The most frequent cause of tooth necrosis is a blow; but it may also arise from the poison of fever, destructive inflammation of the pulp, necrosis or fracture of the jaw, torsion of a tooth, or the pressure of an opponent or a contiguous tooth.

It, however, occasionally arises without being traceable to any distinct cause. An accidental tap with a tooth-brush upon an incisor tooth may rupture the vascular connection of the dentinal pulp at the foramen of the fang. A very common cause is the striking of an infant's head against its mother's front teeth.* As regards misdirected pressure, I have seen more than one instance in which the lateral incisor of the upper jaw has become necrosed by being shut back in a crowded jaw into the palate, and habitually struck by the lower teeth. Continued fever produces necrosis of teeth. I have had one patient who lost many teeth by necrosis immediately after an attack of typhus, and Mr. Bell tells me he has known many such cases in his own long-extended practice. I believe, as I have elsewhere stated, that the necrosis of tooth and bone which occurs in children after the eruptive fevers commences with necrosis of the teeth and their formative organs. As I have already mentioned, after scarlet fever in an adult I have seen the two central incisors of the upper jaw necrosed, and their structure rapidly pervaded by the colouring matter of the blood. Necrosed teeth are liable to absorption of their fang; and, especially where they are associated with alveolar abscess, the minute orifice at the apex of the fang is often enlarged by the

* This circumstance was mentioned to me by Mr. Bell many years ago, and it so happens that I have seen several instances in which this singular cause has unmistakably produced death of an incisor tooth.

removal of tissue. In the accompanying illustration (fig. 49) these two conditions are represented.

The tooth, a superior central incisor, had long been dead, and was slowly loosened and dislocated. A considerable patch of absorption will be observed on the side of the fang, and a marked dilatation of the foramen is also conspicuous.

Fig. 49.

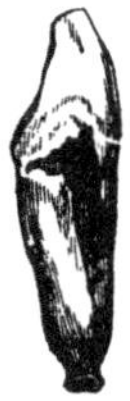

Upon the extraction of such teeth the fang is frequently found encrusted with minute grains of tartar, where a pus discharge has burrowed along the fang of the tooth. Upon opening the pulp-cavity it is found occupied by the dead and decomposed pulp, which may vary in condition according to the period which has elapsed since necrosis occurred. In an early state it is a dark, diffluent mass, which under the microscope exhibits a considerable amount of fat globules, whose nature is proved by their solubility in ether. Later on the pulp becomes dried up, and the contents of the cavity are small in amount, and comparatively dry. In this state there are a large number of extremely minute granules seen by high powers of the microscope. These are partly fatty, and partly the result of disintegration of the dentine. They are sufficiently minute to produce molecular motion when diffused through water. When a tooth has been so long necrosed as to produce a certain stain of colour and some transparency, the dentine itself and the dentinal tubes appear to be permeated by fatty material. If a section of such a tooth be boiled in ether, the original opacity of the ivory is restored.*

Treatment.—As regards the treatment of these cases, when first the necrosed condition of the tooth becomes apparent, especially if occasioned by a blow, it will be a relief freely to lance the gum, or to apply leeches. The acute inflammatory conditions which follow the accident may thus be staved off; and indeed, when the case has become more chronic, occasional leeching is very beneficial. If acute inflammation and alveolar abscess supervene, it may be necessary to remove the tooth at once, and at a later stage of the case extreme discolouration or

* Fatty Degeneration or Decomposition of the Tooth-pulp. *Transactions of the Pathological Society* for 1855; by S. James A. Salter.

dislocation of the tooth may render the same radical treatment necessary. It has been proposed to open the pulp-cavity, remove the decomposed pulp, and destroy the stain of the ivory by some bleaching reagent. I can scarcely think, however, that such a proceeding will yield results sufficiently marked to justify its adoption.

CHAPTER XI.

ODONTOMES.—TUMOURS OF THE HARD TISSUES OF THE TEETH.

In December, 1867, M. P. Broca read a paper before the Academy of Sciences of Paris, under the title "Recherches sur un nouveau groupe de Tumeurs désigné sous le nom d'Odontomes," in which he described some of the hard excrescences which hypertrophy and abnormal growth of the tooth-tissues produce. None of the abnormalities described by M. Broca were new, though the arrangement of them under the one head —tooth-tumours—had not been before adopted by authors.* Still, I think it must be conceded that to arrange all the tumours formed by the increased and perverted growth of the hard tissues of the teeth, under one head, is rational and expedient, and that the term "Odontome" is a convenient and legitimate expression.

It seems to me desirable to restrict the term odontome to tumours of the hard tissues of the teeth, and to include them all. Some, as, for example, enamel nodules on the fang, are small and trivial; still they are tumours, and the list would be incomplete without their consideration.

As regards the arrangement of Odontomes, I think that adopted by Broca both inaccurate and inconvenient; and I have thought the following logical and good:—

Congenital Odontomes—

- Warty teeth,
- Hernia of the fang,
- Enamel nodules on fangs.

Secondary or induced—

- Exostosis,
- Dentine excrescence.

* Professor Broca has since published a more complete history of Odontomes, *Traité des Tumeurs*, tome deuxieme, chapitre x. Paris, 1869.

WARTY TEETH.

THE morphological changes of membrane-surface which occur in the development of the teeth, would of themselves almost suggest to the mind of a physiologist the probable occurrence of the pathological condition which I am now considering. An exuberant growth, a contortion and folding of the superficies—and the circumstances are present by which a tooth-pulp eventuates in a warty tooth.

I was, I believe, the first * to apply the term "warty" to this condition of tooth; and indeed to demonstrate its histological nature. I cannot but think that the expression is apposite; and not only conveys an idea of the coarse appearance of the malformation, but implies a true anatomical analogy.

The warty condition may vary indefinitely from that in which the anatomical form of the tooth is utterly lost to that in which there is but a small puckering of the surface. Again, the wart may be a mass superadded to a tooth, otherwise perfectly well formed.

The few instances of warty teeth that have been recorded, sufficiently attest the rarity of this malformation. It is not mentioned by Hunter, or Fox, or Bell, or indeed by any of the English systematic writers on Dental Surgery up to recent times. I have been only able to discover two recorded instances prior to the publication of my own case in 1855—one by Oudet and one by Wedl.

The account of M. Oudet's case was published in Paris in 1821, † and the following is an abstract of it:—A man about 25 years of age, who was a patient at the Hôtel-Dieu, applied to M. Oudet on account of two hard bony tumours occupying, one on each side, the premolar region of the lower jaw. The hard masses were encrusted with tartar, and this M. Oudet supposed to be the real nature of the supposed tumours. But upon removing the salivary calculus, which was merely superficial, he came upon bright nodules of enamel, and these were scattered over the surface at many points. The masses were clearly

* "Description of a Warty Tooth:" in *Transactions of Pathological Society of London*, vol. vi. 1855.

† "Cas d'exostoses sur des dents devenues monstrueuses." Par M. Oudet. In *Nouveau Journal de Médecine*, p. 245. Paris, 1821.

modified teeth, and were formed by the fusion and irregular, formless development of the tooth germs in the region they occupied. These hard bodies were irregular in outline, but of a general oblong form. The eminences on the surface, which were enamel-covered, were some like the cusps of canine teeth, others like the edges of incisors; between these was a bony tissue like the roots of teeth. These growths had given some uneasiness, and occasionally, though rarely, pain. The right mass was removed, without much difficulty, by tooth-instruments; but the patient declined to have the other interfered with.

Wedl, in his "Pathological Histology,"* describes a specimen consisting of a molar tooth wholly transformed into a warty mass:—

"A remarkable new formation of tooth-substance came under our observation in a body removed by Dr. Jarisch, and which, after repeated and careful examination, we cannot but regard as a malformed tooth. It was situate in the region of the right wisdom tooth, and, after the considerable swelling of the surrounding parts had subsided, was removed without much difficulty by the forceps. After previous cleansing of the place, it was apparent that the body embraced the substance of the wisdom tooth."

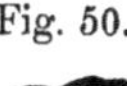

Fig. 50.

When extracted, the mass exhibited an irregular cubic form, about nine lines in diameter. It is displayed in the accompanying figure, 50, enlarged two diameters.

"The surface was nodular: on the attached or basal aspect could be seen an excavated depression, surrounded by a projecting ridge, the circumference of which corresponded with the borders of the crown of the wisdom tooth. Two kinds of substance could be perceived on the surface, even by the naked eye; the one towards the basal portion was whiter, smoother, and with a pearly lustre, especially on the circular ridge; whilst, on the surface of the other, larger and smaller holes could be

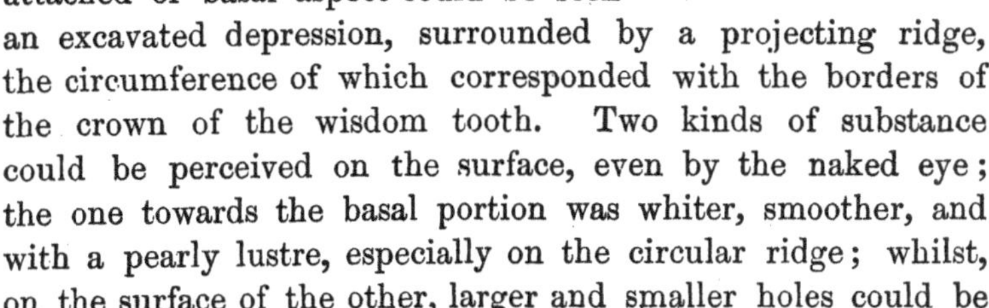

* Grundzüge der pathologischen Histologie. Von Carl Wedl, p. 626. Wien, 1854. A further description of this specimen is published in Heider and Wedl's *Atlas zur Pathologie der Zähne.* Part I. fig. 39. Leipzig, 1868.

perceived, which, when traced in section, were found to correspond with a number of fine white *striæ*. The consistence was compact.

"The examination of the section, which had been made perpendicular to the basal surface, at once showed the existence of radiating canals, running from the periphery towards the base, and filled with a material resembling fat-globules. No blood-vessels could be observed in the canals, nor did they give off any branches. These vacuities, which looked like medullary canals in a state of involution, evidently opened on the surface of the structure at the orifices, which were discernible by the naked eye."

Closer investigation showed that the bulk of this mass consisted of dentine: the tubules were irregular in distribution, and very much branched: they mostly originated around the medullary canals, curving not unfrequently at a right angle, and uniting occasionally from both sides into a single bundle. Entire fasciculi also of dentinal tubes, might be noticed arising from the cæcal ends of the medullary canals, whence they spread out in a fan-like manner. Between and among these systems of tubes were masses of globular dentine, with opaque interglobular spaces. Many of the tubes terminated upon the cuneiform masses of enamel, which penetrated the structure in all parts. The *enamel* was thickest at the circle around the base of the growth. The colour and disposition generally were those proper to enamel. The layers of enamel extended to a considerable depth in the upper half of the malformed tooth: they ramified in various directions, projecting into the dentine like sharply defined papillary structures, surrounded by clear concentric layers, and by the dentinal tubes running towards them. These enamel plates were in many places of a deep brownish yellow. Their texture could not be made out everywhere: in many situations, nothing was apparent beyond a brownish yellow substance, presenting no texture whatever; whilst in others, the enamel prisms were clearly displayed, divided either obliquely or transversely.

There was but a very small amount of true bone structure (*crusta petrosa*) involved in the complicated mass.

Interglobular spaces in the dentine were abundant throughout the structure, and often very voluminous.

I have myself had opportunities of seeing and examining more or less closely five examples of warty teeth.

The first was the most remarkable, and was similar in many respects to that described by Wedl. The case occurred in the practice of a distinguished surgeon many years ago.

A young man, about 20 years of age, was admitted into a metropolitan hospital, having a mass resembling bone within the mouth on the upper surface of the angle of the lower jaw on the right side. The mass had been gradually rising in the mouth for some time, and was, when the patient was admitted into the hospital, as big as a walnut; and by its continued projection, had gagged open the mouth. To all outward appearances, this mass very much resembled a piece of porous bone, denuded of periosteum; and this indeed it was considered to be.

For the purpose of extirpating the mass, a portion of the angle of the jaw in which it was implanted was removed; and, subsequently, to ascertain its anatomical structure, a vertical section was made through the whole. This at once disclosed the nature of the peculiar growth, and showed that it was in reality a malformed tooth in a state of warty complication.

The subsequent history of this case is very interesting in a surgical point of view. The error in diagnosis—the tooth being mistaken for an exostosis from the jaw bone—led to an operation—the excision of the angle of the lower jaw, which entirely destroyed the patient's mastication ever after. The loss of bone on the right side, and the suspension of antagonism of the muscles (especially the *pterygoids*) on the two sides, led to the permanent displacement of the horizontal portion of the jaw, and the teeth never met for mastication. The arch of the jaw was drawn to the right side by the left pterygoid muscles, so that the point of the left lower canine about corresponded with the interval between the two superior central incisors. The teeth could not be brought together: the jaw was bodily drawn over to the right side, and was incapable of masticating movements. An attempt was made to rectify this unfortunate condition, by fixing a false joint in the mouth fastened to an upper and lower molar tooth: the apparatus allowing an up-and-down action of the lower jaw, but rigidly resisting the lateral traction of the muscles which dislocated the arch. At the same time, the cicatrices from the operation were divided, under the idea that they were dislocating the jaw: this was a mistake, however, as the action was purely muscular. But the treatment was practically inoperative. The apparatus only partially restored the lower jaw to its position; the molars could not meet to crush the food; and soon the teeth to which it was attached became loose and painful, and its use had to be discontinued. Many months afterwards I saw the patient: he was then much emaciated, from total inability to masticate; and I subsequently learnt that he died from phthisis.

Considering that this tooth might have been extracted by a pair of forceps, it is distressing to contemplate the results of the mistaken diagnosis. I would venture to add further, that even supposing the mass had been a bony growth from the jaw, a division of the maxillary bone, with its inevitable injury to mastication, was not needed for its removal. And I cannot but think that the extreme importance of retaining the lower maxillary arch unbroken in all operations, where it is possible, has not been sufficiently appreciated.

M. Forget* has published two cases of warty teeth: in the one the whole parts of the teeth were concerned, and in the other the crowns only were malformed.

The former is perhaps the most serious case of this affection on record. In this instance, the patient, at twenty years of age, came to Paris, in 1855, to be operated on for the disease in his jaw. His sufferings commenced at five years of age—fifteen years before. At seven years of age, a small hard tumour, about the size of a nut, made its appearance on the outside of the lower jaw on the left side. It remained stationary for eight years, and then began to increase, and the whole of the left side of the jaw enlarged. The permanent molars were wanting on the left side: on the right they were normal.

"When the patient consulted M. Forget, his general health was still unaffected. Upon looking into his mouth, a round, smooth tumour, hard, unyielding to the touch, and about the size of a turkey's egg, was seen occupying the whole of the left side of the lower jaw; anteriorly it did not extend beyond the symphysis of the chin, while posteriorly it terminated at the

* *Des Anomalies dentaires et de leur Influence sur la Production des Maladies des Os maxillaires,* p. 25. Par M. Forget. Paris, 1859.

lower part of the ramus, the upper part of which, and the condyle, were free from disease. The alveoli were enlarged, and none of the teeth beyond the first bicuspids were present. The gum was of a dark red colour, unusually hard and thickened. At one spot there was a space, about the size of a sixpence, which was denuded of the soft parts, and left exposed a greyish coloured, rough, uneven surface. When this was struck with a metal instrument, it produced the same kind of sound as that which is caused by striking against a tooth placed in its socket. At the base of the tumour were several fistulous openings, and the submaxillary glands were enlarged and indurated." (Mr. Hulme's Translation of "Forget's Memoir" in *Dental Review*, vol. ii. p. 16. Lond. 1860.)

To remove this tumour, the greater part of the left horizontal ramus of the jaw was excised. Upon making a section of the jaw and tumour, the second bicuspis was found embedded in the jaw in front of the tumour: immediately beneath, and received into an excavation in the tumour itself, was the crown of a molar tooth. The tumour itself, which represented the two remaining molars, consisted of an irregular ivory-like structure, covered more or less with nodules of enamel. The microscope showed the mass to consist of dentine, enamel, and crusta petrosa folded together in an irregular and warty complication.

Another specimen, in which the entire tooth-structures were involved, was brought under the notice of the Odontological Society of London, Dec. 1, 1862, by Mr. Harrison. The specimen was obtained from the mouth of a pauper lunatic. It was first seen by the resident medical officer of the asylum, who * "found a large mass on the left side of the lower jaw, lying obliquely along the space which would ordinarily be occupied by the canine and two bicuspids: the gum around it was swollen, spongy, and inflamed, and discharged an offensive secretion. The hard mass was a little loose." The mass, after several weeks getting looser and looser, came away of itself, leaving a long deep groove on the top of the jaw, which discharged offensive pus: the surface of this granulated and healed, but left a deep depression on the alveolar border. This specimen appears to have represented the two bicuspids and the canine merged into one warty mass.

* *British Journal of Dental Science,* vol. v. p. 557. Lond. 1862.

The first specimen of warty tooth which I had an opportunity of examining histologically, was given me by Mr. H. Hamilton, of Poole. It was a right upper permanent lateral incisor. It is represented in the accompanying illustration (fig. 51), enlarged two diameters, so as to render its form and proportions more conspicuous. Upon consulting this figure, it will be seen that the tooth was bent upon itself from before backwards, and when viewed sideways, presented an outline like the letter S. The crown was well-formed, large, and somewhat compressed from before backwards: the root short and thick. In the front of the tooth, extending both above and below the neck, was an irregular lobulated mass, the size of a horse-bean, of a brown colour, and of a porous cancellated structure, and looking very like (especially when seen *in situ*) what one might imagine an exostosis from the edge of the alveolus denuded of periosteal covering. The surface was extremely irregular, exhibiting every species of complication—foldings, projections, pores, interspaces, and depressions. This abnormal growth evidently belonged to the tooth, and seemed intimately connected with, and to form a part of, the anterior inferior portion of the crown.

Fig. 51.

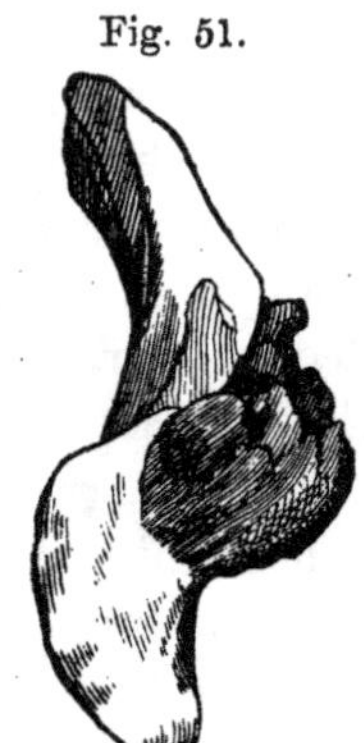

To ascertain the real nature of the mass, as well as to determine its precise relation to the tooth, I made a vertical section of it and the tooth from before backwards. The structure was extremely friable, and the section was made with much difficulty.

The accompanying figure (fig. 52) indicates the anatomical composition of this specimen, as seen during the progress of the section; and though rather diagrammatically expressed, it is, nevertheless, absolutely correct. There is necessarily much confusion in the appearances, as a section in any plane through a mass consisting of different tissues, moulded in every conceivable complication of surface and general arrangement, must obviously cut them in the most varied proportions and positions. In the progress of the section, I found that the pulp-cavity gave off at its neck anteriorly a large canal in a direction downwards and forwards. After a short passage, this divided into three or more smaller canals, some of which were soon lost in a confused mass of dentine and enamel; while another could be traced for a considerable distance in the centre of the outer layer of the warty mass. On tracing, in the illustration, the most

Fig. 52.

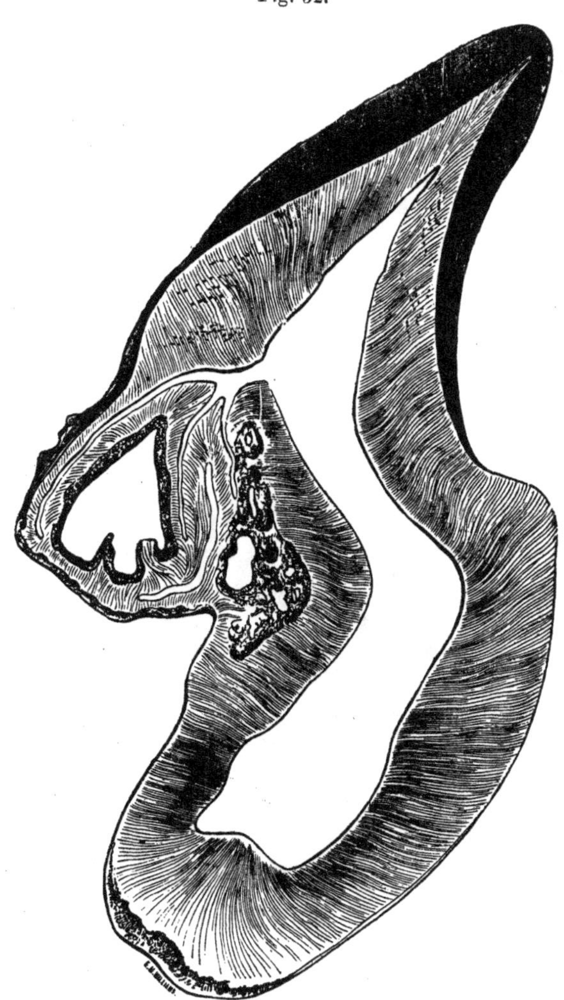

anterior of these canals, it is seen to pass forwards and downwards. The canal is of pretty equal diameter throughout; and the same is the case with the lamina itself. At the bottom, of the mass this canal ceases to be apparent within the lamina, from being ground out; but the lamina itself bends backwards, and from its upper surface project at this part two small papillæ of the same structure, and doubtless containing originally a vascular canal each. These latter project into a sort of heart-shaped cavity—an apparent cavity caused by the involution of the surface, which originally had within it many papillary and folded processes. This adventitious mass contains all the anatomical elements which are normally found in a tooth-crown,—pulp-cavities in the form of vascular canals, on each side of which are layers of dentine, and, beyond these again, coatings of enamel. The relation and proportion of these structures are very apparent in the lamina just described. On the outer surface is a layer of enamel, not only covering the exterior surface, but that (produced by the involution) of the heart-shaped cavity within it. The dentine is somewhat thinner than the enamel: it presents the ordinary arrangement of parallel tubes, diverging from the pulp-cavity, and passing in curves to the enamel base. This is displayed in figure 53,

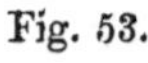

Fig. 53.

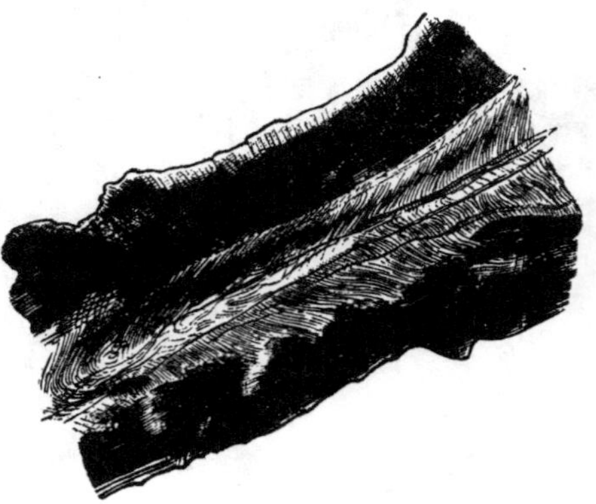

which is not a diagram, but an exact portrait of a portion of the lamina, magnified forty diameters.

In the more confused portions of the section, those parts nearest the tooth itself, the structure is less intelligible. Vascular canals are only seen for a short distance of their course. The dentine is irregularly distributed in small quantities; and thick opaque enamel is very abundant.

An example of "warty" tooth came under my notice and my

treatment in the summer of 1858, which was interesting in its history, and very instructive practically. A gentleman of about thirty-five years of age applied to me, complaining of great pain in the angle of the lower jaw on the right side, extending down to the shoulder: and there was swelling behind the wisdom tooth on that side. On examining the mouth, I found a small bone-like mass embedded in the mucous membrane immediately behind the *dens sapientiæ*, scarcely projecting above the surface, and surrounded by irritable bleeding granulations: it had much the aspect of a piece of necrosed bone.

By means of an elevator I removed the little mass; and then upon examination with a lens I found it to consist of dentine surmounted by irregular nodules of enamel. Some time afterwards the patient came back to me, complaining of the presence of another adventitious growth in the same region. This I also removed with the elevator. It was a thin plate of dentine, about half the size of one's little finger-nail, and on its upper surface were three projecting nodules of enamel.

Up to this point I considered the growths I had removed as two supernumerary teeth of malformed growth; but the subsequent history of the case disproved this conclusion. Some weeks after I had removed the last portion of the adventitious tooth substance, the patient again came to me, suffering much pain in the wisdom tooth itself, extending along the jaw on the same side and down to the shoulder. Upon examining the tooth I found that it was slightly loose, and raised above its fellows. By carefully passing the *searcher* over its surface, I detected on the posterior face of the neck an irregularity, and I suspected a small carious cavity. In a few days I found it necessary to extract the tooth; and then the nature of the original malformation, and the cause of the recent suffering, were at once apparent.

There had been a warty growth from the back of the wisdom tooth. On the posterior aspect of the tooth, near the neck, was an irregular jagged projection with a minute orifice in its centre, through which a fine bristle could be passed into the cavity of the tooth (fig. 54).

It was clear now that the warty mass, which I had considered as a separate tooth, had been attached to the *dens sapientiæ* at this spot, and had had, through the minute orifice, a pulp-cavity common with that of the tooth.

Upon making a section of this tooth, it was found that the pulp had entirely disappeared, and that the interior of the cavity, admitting the fluids of the mouth, was stained by early decay. The continuity of the pulp-cavity with that of the previously removed warty mass was now more clearly demonstrable, as the black bristle introduced into the small external orifice is seen to enter the pulp-cavity of the posterior fang (fig. 55).

The accompanying illustrations display (to the left) the entire tooth as seen on the posterior surface, and (to the right)

Fig. 54.

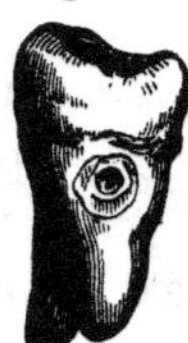

Fig. 55.

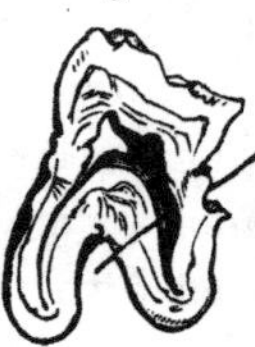

the section in which the bristle passes from the pulp-cavity through the external orifice. I am acquainted with two other specimens of warty teeth: they are preparations in the museum of Guy's Hospital.

One of the specimens is a superior *dens sapientiæ*, and the warty excrescence consists of a small conical mass attached to the side of the tooth: it is irregularly folded in surface, and the enamel which covers it is particularly white—more so than in either of the other specimens I have seen. The form and size of

Fig. 56.

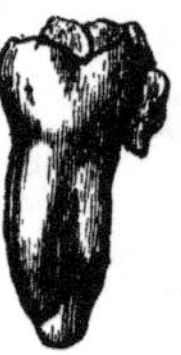

Fig. 57.

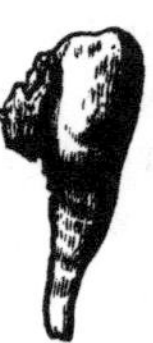

the little mass will be best understood by reference to the accompanying figure (fig. 56). The other specimen is also from the Guy's museum. It is a superior lateral incisor (fig. 57), with a considerable warty projection on its outer side and back part.

The mass is irregularly folded, and yellowish in colour. The front of the crown of the tooth is well formed; but on the back the outer half of the tooth is swollen out and forms part of the mass.

As these specimens belong to the hospital museum, I have not had an opportunity of examining the structure of the warts by microscopical sections: but their enamel is continuous with that of the crowns of the teeth, and it is quite obvious that they have the same relation to them as in the lateral incisor whose minute anatomy I have already described.

The history of these specimens is unknown; but the lateral incisor, from the large size of the pulp-cavity, clearly belonged to a child, and was probably removed from its unsightliness.

The morphological explanation of these warty teeth is obvious —indeed there can be but one way of accounting for them. Since we know that the superficies of a tooth is the part first formed, and that it corresponds in every particular in shape with the original formative pulp, so it follows that the pulp must in these cases have been of warty complication—must have borne the same relation to a normal pulp as a tegumentary wart does to normal papillary structure.

This complication of surface is a great departure from the true plan of human tooth-forms, which are essentially of the simplest kind. At the same time the aberration is only morphological.

This subject has its practical bearings, and those not un important.

It should be borne in mind by surgeons, that teeth occasionally exhibit such change of form and aspect that they can no longer be recognised as teeth, and that they may (as has happened) be mistaken for necrosed bone. It should be remembered too that, under such circumstances, the ungainly mass does not require the scalpel and the saw for its removal, but that its extraction may be accomplished by the same instruments as are employed for taking out ordinary teeth. I think the dental-surgeon should be on his guard lest he mistake one of these adventitious growths for a mass of tartar. Oudet made that mistake; and I am sure that in the cases I have seen the same error might readily be committed. Such a mistake, however, would be fatal to the tooth; at least it would involve a contingency as regards the retention of the affected tooth which the operator did not calculate upon; for the thin laminæ of the spongy mass would readily yield to the force of the scaling instrument, and the pulp-cavity would be opened. And this leads to the question, What treatment should be adopted in a case of warty tooth? Much must depend on the degree of the malformation and the particular tooth affected.

If the warty tooth or teeth constitute an ungainly mass, interfering with the proper use of the jaws, and the comfortable closure of the mouth, the structure should unquestionably be removed. Supposing the wart be an appendage to a front tooth, one visible to ordinary observers, the question arises, whether the tooth should be extracted and replaced by another; or the wart cut off, the pulp destroyed, and the tooth plugged. But these are points upon which it would be impossible to lay down an absolute rule: it is a matter of degree and of circumstance, which can be best adjudged by an intelligent practitioner to whom the whole particulars of the case are familiar.

Where the excrescence is small and out of sight, as in fig. 56, I think, without doubt, it should not be interfered with.

I suspect that these warty growths would, from their intrinsic nature, soon lead to caries, irregular as their surface is, retaining matters of decomposing food, and that in contact with a broken and imperfect enamel.

Hernia of the Fang.—I believe this title best expresses the nature of the odontome I am about to describe. The name applied to it by Broca, "Odontome radiculaire" is objectionable; it conveys no meaning beyond locality, and that is equally applicable to other tumours.

These odontomes are very rare, and I believe there are only four recorded examples.

They consist of an hypertrophy and expansion of the proper constituent tissues of the fang—an outer layer of crusta petrosa, a thin layer of dentine, and a large pulp, which may, or may not, be calcified.

The following are the examples in question:—

1st. One described by M. Forget.* It consisted of a large

* *Des Anomalies Dentaires, et de leur influence sur la Production des Maladies des Os Maxillaires,* par M. Forget, Paris, 1859. Obs. III. p. 27, pl. ii. figs. 1 and 2.

tumour, about the size of a bantam's egg, attached to the posterior surface of a lower molar tooth, adherent to the neck and a considerable portion of the fang. This specimen was taken from the mouth of a Frenchman, 40 years of age, who came to Paris to have the tumour removed on account of the annoyance it occasioned. The tumour occupied the left side of the lower jaw, expanding its sides, especially the outer, and disfiguring the face.

M. Maisonneuve, who attended the patient, determined to extract the tooth as a preliminary step to removing the tumour: the tooth, however, and the tumour came away together.

A section of the specimen through its entire length shows a complete continuity of tissue between the two, and the part in the illustration, where the tumour and tooth are united, is singularly like that seen in the specimen in the Museum of the College of Surgeons. Forget originally described his specimen of this odontome as consisting wholly of bone. At my request he has had the structure subjected to a further examination. This was conducted by M. Robin, who discovered a layer of dentine between the crusta-petrosa and the bone-like nucleus, as I predicted he would.

2nd. The second example was recorded by Mr. Tomes in a paper read by him before the Odontological Society of Great Britain, April 6th, 1863.* The specimen was presented to the Odontological Society by Mr. Hare of Limerick. "The tooth, a molar, was taken from the upper jaw of a countryman, 41 years old, who for some years previously had suffered severe pain in the jaw. The cheek was perforated by a canal through which matter constantly poured. After the removal of the tooth the pain in the jaw ceased, and the wound in the cheek healed." Connected with the fangs of the tooth is a large lobulated mass, four or five times as big as the tooth itself. "The number and relations of the roots of the tooth are obscured by the mass of cementum by which they are surrounded. The mass itself may be roughly described as built up of three coalescing flattened lobes, not very distinctly

* Description of a 'Remarkable case of Exostosis,' by J. Tomes, Esq., F.R.S., in *Transactions of the Odontological Society of Great Britain,* vol. iii. p. 335. London, 1863.

marked: one immediately investing the roots of the tooth, and composed of dense cementum; a second, continuous with the first, marked by abrasions produced by superficial absorption of the tissue, and presenting an appearance of less density than the preceding lobe. The third and terminal division is double the size of either of the preceding portions of the tumour." Though Mr. Tomes spoke of this tumour as an exostosis—as being composed wholly of crusta petrosa—no examination of its tissues had then been made with the microscope. The opinion was merely an inference. A subsequent examination of this specimen, made by Mr. Charles Tomes, showed that this tumour was not an exostosis, but of the same nature as the condition I am describing.*

3rd. Heider and Wedl † have figured with a brief description a specimen of this tumour, of typical structure in all essential respects like that which I examined and now proceed to describe.

The fourth specimen is that existing in the Museum of the College of Surgeons.‡ The only published reference to it with which I am acquainted occurs in Mr. Heath's admirable work on "Diseases and Injuries of the Jaws." § Mr. Heath, perceiving the similarity and the apparent identity of this tumour with those figured and described by Forget and Tomes, includes it in the same category, and describes it as a large exostosis.

This preparation consists of a rather small molar tooth, from the posterior fang and neck of which passes off a large lobulated tumour, flattened from without inwards, more than twice the size of the tooth itself. The continuity of the tissues of the two is complete: the tumour is adherent to the tooth for its entire thickness from side to side. The form of this adventitious growth and its relation to the tooth will be better understood by referring to the accompanying figure, 58, than by any lengthened description. The surface of the large distal lobe

* "Description of an Odontome," *Trans. Odont. Soc.*, new series, vol. iv. p. 81.

† *Atlas zur Pathologie der Zähne.* Leipzig, 1868.

‡ No. 1,022 of the Pathological Museum of the College. This specimen is supposed to have belonged to John Hunter.

§ *Injuries and Diseases of the Jaw,* the Jacksonian Prize Essay of the Royal College of Surgeons of England, 1867, by Christopher Heath, Esq., F.R.C.S. London, 1868.

is very white and polished: the structural continuity of the tumour and the tooth at their junction is very conspicuous.

Fig. 58.

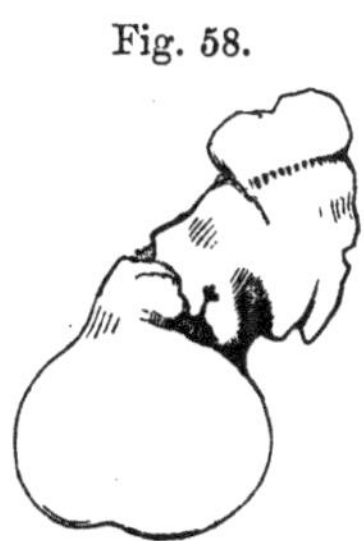

Molar tooth with hernia of fang.

Desirous of ascertaining the histological character of this tumour, I made a lengthwise section of it as nearly in its axis as possible. It was not strictly axial, as that would have involved the tooth, injury to which I was anxious to avoid: still the section was sufficiently near the centre to disclose the nature of the growth and its relation to the tooth to which it was attached.

In grinding down the specimen, a small portion of the thin layer broke away from the narrow extremity: this does not, however, interfere with the demonstration of its structure, as I had already proved, by repeated examinations with low magnifying powers, what were the histological elements constituting the section before it was sufficiently thin for permanent mounting.

Fig 59.

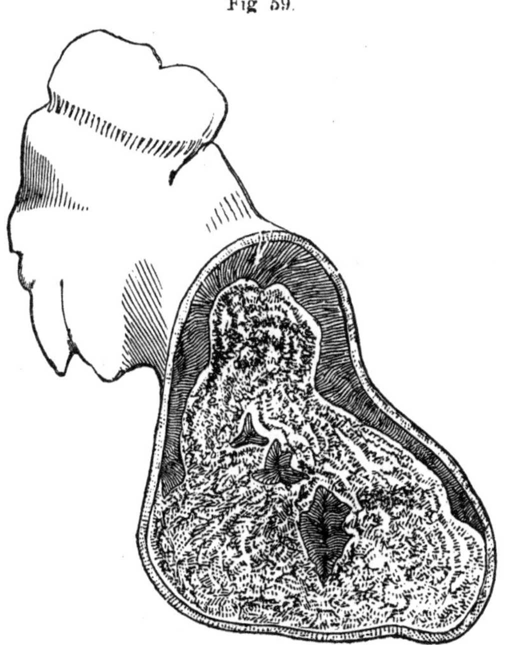

The illustration (fig. 59) shows what is the structure of this tumour. It is especially intended to display the relation of the parts of the growth to the tooth to which it is attached; and, though somewhat diagrammatic, is nevertheless strictly true.

A section of the tumour in the direction indicated in this figure shows the outer layer to be composed of a coat of crusta petrosa or tooth-bone: it is even, compact, and of the usual character seen on tooth-fangs. Within this is a layer of true dentine: this does not constitute the entire circle of the section, but for about two thirds of its circumference separates the external cemental layer from the *nucleus* of the growth, as it may well be styled. It is the two thirds towards the attachment of the tumour to the tooth. For the remaining third there is no limitary band of dentine separating the nucleus from the crusta petrosa; but the line of demarcation between the two is perfectly distinct.

Upon examining the tissues of this section with high microscopic powers, the nature, the meaning, and the relation of these several histological elements are quite clear, as is their source of developmental production.

The outer layer is one of ordinary crusta petrosa, such as is seen on healthy tooth-fangs: it is laminated, non-vascular, and with the usual scattering of lacunæ, parallel to the axis of the laminæ.

The layer of the dentine is equally conspicuous and unmistakable; and, as is usual, the tubes have a general direction at right angles to the pulp-cavity and to the external surface of the growth of which they form part.

The nucleus of this odontome, its structure as displayed by high magnifying powers, and the inference as to its nature and source, constitute the most important points of interest in the specimen: they involve its meaning—the question what it really is.

1st. The *structure* of the nucleus. It is highly vascular, and the arrangement of the vessels is like that of the tooth-pulp; they branch and unite, and diverge in every conceivable direction; and their average diameter is about that which is seen in an uncalcified dentinal pulp. As regards the minute elements of structure, lacunæ largely prevail, and frequently occupy the whole field of the microscope: they are, however, somewhat peculiar, being large, without axial definition, and surrounded by crowds of canaliculi, looking like patches of moss. From this extreme form there is every conceivable variety of shape, passing by degrees to distinct and unmistakable dentinal tubes. Again, in other parts of the nucleus, isolated patches of true dentine are to be found, and some of these remote from the dentinal band and close to the crusta petrosa which bounds the bulbous end of the tumour. Moreover, in many parts there are masses of those calcification globules characteristic of dentine. In fact, the nucleus is composed of a confused mass of bone-structure and dentine-structure, arranged around and separating an elaborate vascular network of the same character as that of a dentinal pulp.

2nd. As to what may be inferred regarding the nature and source of this structure. It must be observed that the nucleus is *embraced within* a belt of true dentine :—that for two thirds of its limit it is thus separated from true tooth-bone : that it is essentially different from the crusta petrosa hard by. It must be remembered further that whereas bone lacunæ may be found in a calcified dentinal pulp, dentine is never found in an exostosis—is never produced by the periodontal membrane.

In a paper which I published in the "Guy's Hospital Reports" (1855), "On the Intrinsic Calcification of the Tooth-Pulp," I showed that the dentine pulp, when it had undergone calcific impregnation of its whole structure, would often yield a mixture of bone tissue and dentine ; and I figured one specimen, that of a temporary molar long retained in the mouth, and whose pulp had become calcified, in which the axis of the tooth did present this mixture of dentine and bone. Now it would be impossible to distinguish the calcified pulp of this tooth from portions of the nucleus of the tumour I am now describing if they were placed under microscopes side by side.

This nucleus was produced by the intrinsic calcification of a large dentinal pulp, of the same size and form as the nucleus ; the belt of dentine was the primary and normal development of that pulp ; and the hypertrophied and abnormal pulp, ceasing to contract and prolong centripetally the dentinal tubes, underwent a confused bone and ivory genesis, retaining its then vascular condition. It is unnecessary to refute the idea of this being an exostosis. Dental exostosis is entirely external, superficial to the ivory of the tooth : it is an extraneous growth deposited outside the dentinal system and in no way affecting it.

A section of a tooth-fang, however incrusted with exostosis, has its dentinal elemental unaltered.

Exostosis is a secondary affection occurring in after life. This expanded cone of dentine necessarily involved an original development of the same form—as dentine growths from without inwards; while crusta petrosa forms from within outwards.

There is one point in reference to Forget's and Tomes's specimens of interest and of anatomical value: they both display hollows or cavities, and, in the latter, the bulbous extremity of the tumour was little more than a hollow calcified cyst. This is never seen in true exostosis; but it is quite consistent with the idea of an hypertrophied, expanded tooth-fang, whose pulp had not undergone calcification; it would be the equivalent of the specimen I have described, in which the tooth had been removed before the nucleus had passed from a soft pulp to a calcified mass.

Enamel Nodule, or Submerged Cusp on Tooth-Fang.

This little odontome is by no means uncommon. I have several examples of it in my collection. It occurs on teeth which are otherwise healthy and generally well formed, and I believe its presence is never indicated by any symptoms while the tooth remains implanted in the jaw. I have usually seen it on molars and not far from the neck of the tooth: it generally occupies the groove at the side between two fangs, and very frequently there is a conical process of enamel passing down from the crown of the tooth towards the nodule, the two resembling in form a note of exclamation, thus—!. At other times the nodule is quite alone and free, and may be at any distance from the crown of the tooth. I once saw an enamel nodule at the very apex of the fang of a pre-molar. The nodule is like a little white pearl stuck to the side of the tooth-fang. When the tooth is fresh extracted the enamel pulp is stretched over it and can be opened and folded back, just as can be done to the crown of a young tooth before it pierces the gum. It seems that, in the formation of this tumour, a little pocket of the enamel sac of the crown had to be shut off, as it were, from the main sac of the crown. The accompanying illustration is taken from an upper molar tooth. The nodule, in this case, was quite independent of the enamel of the crown. The structure of these nodules is not so simple as appears

Fig. 60.

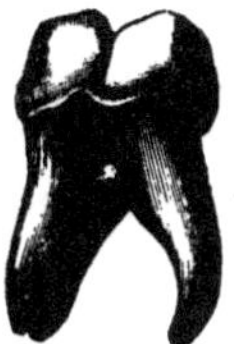

from mere external examination. They look, indeed, as if they consisted only of a grain of enamel adherent to the fang, just as is the case with a nodule of exostosis—a simple external addition without, and not affecting the dentinal system of the tooth. Such, however, is not the case. The nodule is in reality a minute tooth-cusp, consisting of a cone of dentine clothed upon by a thick tubercle of enamel: the structure is in every respect the same as that of an ordinary cusp on the crown of a tooth; the form rather rounder, perhaps, but essentially the same histologically.

I do not further dwell on this subject, as it is of very little practical importance. A description of the hard tumours of the teeth would, however, be imperfect without some reference to this, the least considerable of them.

Exostosis.

The crusta petrosa, or tooth-bone which forms the outer layer of the fang, is very liable to hypertrophy. The amount of this tissue which exists in health is variable, and it would be difficult in a slight case of exostosis to define the limit of health and disease. In other cases the increase of growth is very considerable.

The amount of tooth-bone on any particular tooth which is the seat of inflammation or irritation seems to be an ever-varying quantity; it undergoes perpetual absorption and redeposition.

The hypertrophy is usually a mere increase of the normal tissue, consisting of non-vascular laminæ with an abundance of lacunæ. Occasionally, however, a blood-vessel is involved in the new growth and becomes the axis of a "system" of tooth-bone; and more rarely still the exostosis is cancellated, porous, and very vascular.

Exostosis may occur at any part of the tooth-fang, but it is usually confined to the lower third, and in some cases it enters the pulp-cavity through the terminal foramen.

In exostosis, or layers of tooth-bone formed under hypertrophic action, the lamination is apt to be very marked, the lacunæ large and abundant, and the crescentic outlines, where absorption and redeposition have occurred, are usually distinct and numerous.

Fangs that have been retained long after the decay and break-up of the tooth crowns are nearly always the subjects of exostosis, and in such instances large masses on one side, where the periosteum remains, correspond with the living attachment of the tooth to the jaw. Where the periodontal membrane has been stripped from the fang, as by an abscess, no further development of tooth-bone occurs: but the growth may, and very often does, go on to considerable hypertrophy on the side where the attachment remains.

Exostoses differ very much in form. They may be even incrustations involving the lower third of the fang of the tooth and gradually diminishing upwards; or they may form an abruptly defined mass encircling the end of the tooth. In other cases they may form a globular termination to the fang, like the root of a turnip; or again, the exostosis may be a small isolated excrescence, with a lobulated surface, like chalcedony, and this form, as far as my experience goes, is that attended with the severest and most painful symptoms. The exostosis may consist of a general thickening of tooth-bone around contiguous fangs, increasing till they come in contact and then fusing them together in a common encasement of tooth-bone. In these cases the alveolar septa are absorbed before the progressive enlargement of the fangs. And this may occur not only as regards the fangs of the same tooth, but also with the fangs of contiguous teeth. See Chapter V. on United Teeth, and illustrations of this condition. And lastly, though very rarely, the bony growth may be porous and cancellated.

The general thickening of a tooth fang by an increased development of crusta petrosa is a change which must be considered in the least degree morbid. It is one of those simple excesses of growth which exuberant nutrition produces. And here I must venture to take exception to the stereotyped description of symptoms which exostosis is said to produce. They are sufficiently vague, and it would be interesting to examine prognostically more than one author who defines the symptoms of exostosis;—to place before them cases where certain indefinite and painful symptoms exist, and to require from them, before tooth-extraction, something approaching a definition of the morbid condition. A thickened, deep red-coloured gum, readily bleeding, with broad flat margins, accompanied by gnawing pains are conditions that constantly arise without exostosis; or, when the latter are present, are associated with other disease. Yet these are repeatedly enumerated as the characteristic symptoms of dental exostosis. They are common enough where dental caries happens to be associated with exostosis; but they equally occur where the exostosis is wanting.

There is, however, one form of exostosis which, I believe, produces severe symptoms, and those of a distinct neuralgic character.

These are examples of small isolated nodular exostosis, occurring on the fangs of otherwise healthy teeth in young persons, or at least before middle life.

I have not seen many of these. They are rare, or perhaps rather they are not readily traced. Still I have seen sufficient examples, and those sufficiently pronounced, to be satisfied that this is a distinct form of disease.

The accompanying illustrations are the results of such a case. A lady, twenty-three years of age, applied to me in 1858 on account of extreme neuralgic pain emanating from the left superior central incisor tooth; it was somewhat elongated, very slightly loose, and was particularly sensitive to changes of temperature. Every tooth in this patient's mouth was, to outward appearance, perfectly sound.

The patient, who was a very intelligent person, described the pain as intense and very peculiar in its character; it occurred spasmodically, and at irregular intervals, flashing over the left side of the head, *backwards*, as she described it, and like shocks otelectricity many times repeated; and it was accompanied by a great flow of saliva, and a taste as of salt. She particularly dwelt upon this latter circumstance.

Fig. 61. Fig. 62.

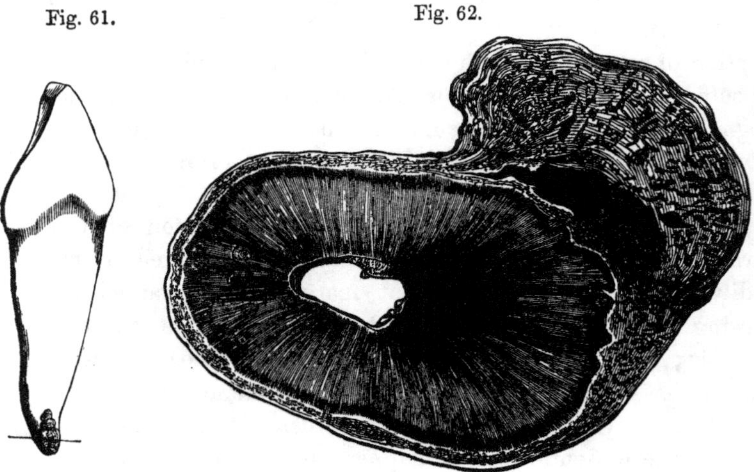

At my patient's urgent request, I took out the tooth, and the only morbid appearance I could discover was the exostosis on the fang depicted in the accompanying illustrations. The removal of the tooth was attended with extreme suffering, which, however, ceased soon after.

In figure 61, the incisor tooth is exhibited, enlarged two diameters, and the form and position of the exostosis are indicated. In figure 62, the section of the exostosis is shown; it was a dense, laminated, non-vascular mass, in many parts imperfectly calcified, and showing irregular hollows, having no histological meaning.

I did not see this patient again for some years; she had then lost two or three other teeth in the same way, and with the same sort of growth on the fangs.

And this I believe is a characteristic of this form of exostosis —that it affects many teeth in succession, and with a repetition of the same painful symptoms.*

Occasionally an exostosis forms a round root like a turnip. Many years ago a lady, who was wearing an entire set of teeth, came to me to have the root of a lower bicuspid removed. It

* See Chapter XX., p. 259.

was the only remains of a tooth in the mouth. The appearance was peculiar. The jaw was even and flat everywhere except around this stump, and here it exhibited a rounded swelling like half of a small marble, and was very hard; it had been increasing in size of late, and had injured the fit of the plate, which pressed upon it painfully. I did not contemplate any difficulty in extracting this root; but I failed to get it out after repeated trials both with forceps and elevator. The patient then declined to suffer more pain, saying she would call again. This she did, bringing the root in her hand. She had been to an eminent surgeon, who, after cutting the gum to the bone, chipped open the socket with a bone nipper, and so got out the fang. The bone was very compact and closely embraced the exostosis which could not have been removed by any other mode of procedure.

The exostosis was perfectly spherical, about twice the size of a pea. Upon making a section I found the dentine in the centre less than the tenth of the diameter of the whole.

I have two interesting specimens of exostosis found in an unusual situation. The tooth-bone which lines the fork between the fangs of molar teeth is usually thin, consisting of a transparent layer without lacunæ. In each of these specimens this region is occupied by a large exostosis. The teeth had decayed, the pulp-cavities were open, and caries had attacked the dentine in the middle of the floor of the cavity and just over the exostosis. The exostosis extended some way down the inner sides of the fangs, but was entirely confined to the fork. It looks almost like a repair against the approaching erosion.

Fig. 63.

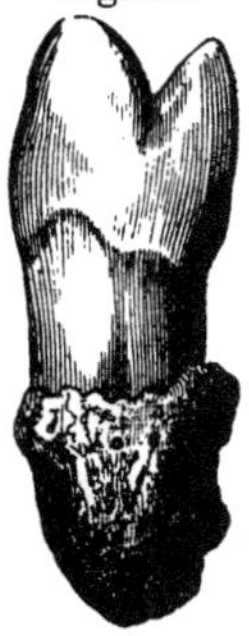

One of the most remarkable instances of exostosis with which I am acquainted occurred on the fang of an upper bicuspid tooth, given me by Mr. Walter Jones, of Worcester. The tooth was carious. On the lower half of the fang there was a considerable exostosis, commencing suddenly as a collar. It was a loose, porous, friable structure. In the accompanying figure, 63, of the tooth (enlarged two diameters) this porous surface is indicated. A section of the fang shows the tooth-bone to be cancellated and full of vascular canals. The condition is most manifest on the surface, for where the cement rests on the dentine it is as compact as usual.

The vascular canals are very irregular and erratic, and cannot be seen of any great length in a section; and their general character is shown in the annexed figure, 64.

Fig. 64.

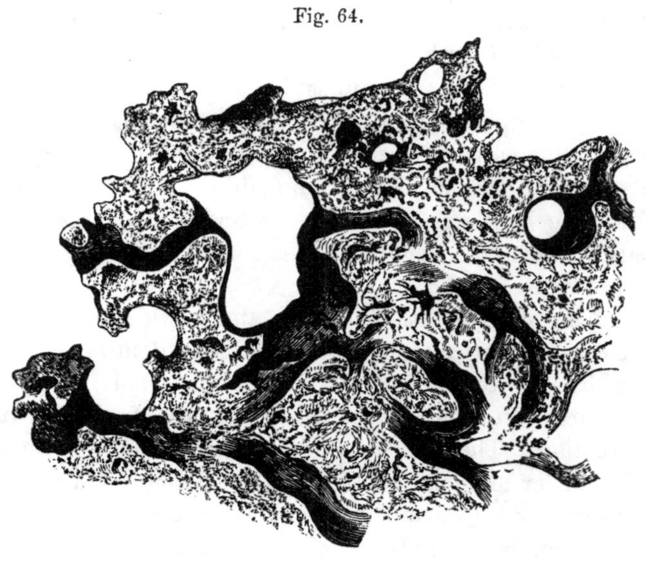

Seen with higher powers, numerous lacunæ are manifest: they are very irregularly scattered, and have no definite relation in axis and direction to the course of the canals near which they are situated—nothing, in fact, after the fashion of Haversian systems.

Dentine Excrescence.—I have thus defined the nodules of dentine, or osteo-dentine, which occasionally develope from the walls of the pulp cavity and press upon or grow into the substance of the pulp. They are not very uncommon, and though they must be considered pathological, they are not often traced as associated with painful symptoms. When I first described * these little tooth-tumours as an occasional cause of neuralgia, they had not been so recognised; a circumstance probably due rather to the imperfect investigation which the diseases of the teeth had received at the hands of pathologists than from the

* Before the Pathological Society, April, 1855.

infrequency of such cases. Since then, a few other instances have been recorded.

The form and number of these excrescences vary very much. I have usually seen them in the shape of a somewhat flattened nodule, with a constricted base of attachment.

Fig. 65.

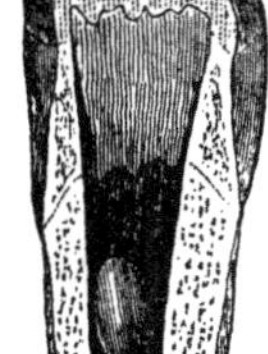

A very characteristic specimen is exhibited in the accompanying illustration (fig. 65), which displays a vertically cut upper incisor tooth (enlarged two diameters) with a nodule in the interior; and it is the more interesting as the excrescence was associated with severe neuralgia.

Upon making a section of the tooth (vertical from side to side) I found an oval pearl-like excrescence of dentine growing from the side of the pulp cavity, so as to encroach much upon it, and occupying, for a short space, more than half its diameter. It was of an oval form, its long axis corresponding with that of the tooth; in colour less opaque and yellower than the neighbouring tissue.

A section, as seen in the woodcut (fig. 66), shows the form of the excrescence and the general arrangement of the structure. It resembles the head of a mushroom, the central third being attached to the primary dentine. The dentinal tubes radiate by a somewhat tortuous course from the centre of the attachment, and these are crossed at right angles by a series of laminæ.

The dentinal tubes of the excrescence take their origin from the primary dentine at some little distance from the surface—the abnormal and irregular tubes radiating from that point, and the collateral tubes of the primary dentine being divergent. It is clear, therefore, that this abnormal growth commenced before the primary dentine was completed.

The tubular communication between the primary and secondary tissue is very circumscribed, for though the attachment of the excrescence occupies one-third of the basal surface, it has a far less extent of tubular continuity from the convergence of the tubes of the excrescence and the divergence of those of the primary dentine. They only anastomose deeply in the centre: and it would seem that from some local cause at that particular spot the growth took its origin.

The specimen, when seen with high powers, exhibits to a very marked degree those irregularities in the structure, course, and

Fig. 66.

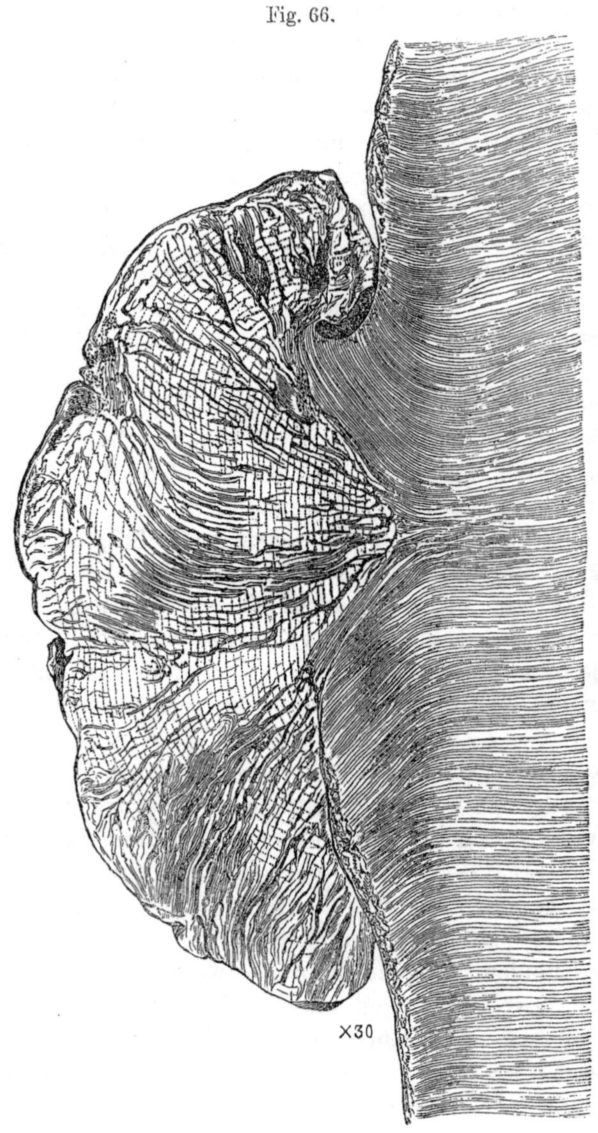

form of the dentinal tubes, which frequently occur in secondary dentine. The tubes are dilated, branched, and contorted in a remarkable manner, and there are many *dentinal loculi*, cavities with tubes radiating from them.

The patient from whom this specimen was obtained was a woman about thirty years of age. She applied to me at Guy's Hospital in 1854, on account of severe neuralgic pains obviously connected with one of the central incisors of the upper jaw The pain was described as of a gnawing character, abiding, but not constantly severe, frequently amounting to a mere consciousness of the presence of the tooth, and at other times sharp and darting. In the former condition it was confined to the region of the tooth; in the latter it flashed up the side of the face and through all the branches of the superior maxillary division of the fifth nerve on that side. Sudden pressure, or a tap upon the tooth, or a marked change of temperature produced a considerable augmentation of pain. The tooth itself was sound to all external appearance; it was somewhat elongated beyond its fellow, and was very slightly loose. The gum surrounding it was red at the edge, and a little swollen.

The tooth had not received a blow, nor was there any known cause for the symptoms which appeared associated with it.

The patient entreated me to extract it; which I did, expecting to find an exostosis. But there was none, and with the exception of some small patches of half organised lymph, the tooth appeared quite healthy.

The extraction of the tooth was attended by a violent paroxysm of neuralgic agony; but the pain never after returned.

That the symptoms from which this patient suffered were dependent on the condition found in the pulp-cavity there can be no doubt; and that the pain was occasioned by the pressure which this growth exercised on the nerves of the pulp seems the simplest explanation. Still it may be a question whether the pain and the growth may not have been both occasioned by some more remote cause, some local irritation of that region of the pulp.

Since the publication of this case, others of a similar nature have been recorded. Mr. Charles White, who is very assiduous in searching out interesting matters of dental pathology, has described two cases. In one a little boy eight years of age was suffering extreme pain from an apparently sound temporary canine. Mr. White extracted the tooth and the pain ceased. In the pulp cavity was found a lobulated calcified mass "filling nearly the whole cavity at the junction of its middle and lower thirds, and pressing the fasciculi of nerve fibres out of their course." The calcified mass appears to have been of the character of osteo-dentine.

In the second case a young lady, seventeen years of age, had suffered intolerable pain of a neuralgic character, which had emanated from a first lower bicuspid tooth. The tooth, however, was sound to external appearance; but upon extracting it and opening the pulp-cavity, Mr. White found "a large growing mass of nodular dentine pressing the sensitive pulp against the walls of its cavity." *

Mr. Coleman described at a meeting of the Odontological Society (January 9, 1871) a similar case; an upper biscupid being the tooth affected.

It is probable that unexplained cases of pain in the teeth may often arise from this condition. In all such instances, when the teeth are extracted, it is very desirable that a careful examination of the pulp-chamber should be made, and any intelligible results recorded, so that our knowledge of obscure tooth-pains may become more definite.

* *Trans. Odont. Soc.*, new series, vol. iii. p. 54.

CHAPTER XII.

DISEASES OF THE TOOTH-PULP.

THE pathological changes to which the tooth-pulp is liable are divers, and their importance is commensurate with that of the organ itself. They vary from those changes which may be considered in the lowest degree morbid, and even to some extent reparative, to those which entail the total destruction of the pulp and a corresponding injury to the nutrition and vitality of the surrounding dentine.

The diseases of the tooth-pulp may be classified under the following heads:—

1. Intrinsic calcification.
2. Suppuration and sphacelus.
3. Necrosis.
4. Polypus.
5. Sensitive sprouting.

Calcification of the Pulp.—This change in the pulp must be looked upon as morbid in the lowest degree, being to a great extent reparative and the result of trivial causes, though I believe it never occurs unless the tooth has been in some way the subject of injury or irritation.* The pulp of a young tooth that

* In estimating the sources of irritation which may lead to pulp calcification it is necessary to recollect how minute and superficial are the injuries to the surface of the dentine of which the pulp takes cognisance. The slightest external injury on the surface arouses morbid nutritive activity within.

Very large numbers of teeth, which would be declared to be sound by a superficial observer, have already been the subjects of diseased action or mechanical lesion. Being curious to test the extent of these earlier stages of disease, which give the first promptings to pulp calcification, I requested one of the Demonstrators of anatomy at Guy's Hospital to obtain for me a number of what he considered sound molar teeth. I selected molars, as they furnished one source of observation which single-cusped teeth would has been perfectly matured never exhibits this condition till after it has received some abnormal stimulation from morbid change or mechanical injury of the dentine. Its most potent cause is caries; but it may probably arise from any passing source of vascular excitement, and then become the register of a past event, when that itself has ceased to be.

The pathological change consists in the impregnation of the various tissues of the tooth-pulp with calcarious matter—their calcification, in fact—occurring in multitudes of isolated points; and by the multiplication and enlargement of these "islands of calcification," involving more and more of the structures of the pulp, and its ultimate *conversion*, under certain favourable circumstances, into *Osteodentine*.

The occurrence, to some extent, of islands of calcification in the pulps of carious teeth is universal. The complete issue of this process in the evolution of osteodentine is by no means common, and only occurs under certain favourable circumstances, when the process of calcification may continue for a long period, uninterrupted by the laying bare of the pulp-cavity.

The process of lime impregnation we are considering is, in important particulars, different from that which occurs in the formation of normal dentine and "dentine of repair." In these the calcification is superficial, and only involves those elements which constitute the animal basis of dentine—namely, the tubular prolongations from the peripheral cells and the hyaline intertubular substance. Their calcification, moreover, is "globular," as already explained.

not. He sent me thirty-four, from the mouths of adults in the Dissecting room. Not one of these had carious cavities, but none were free from the evidence of some injury or disease, past or present. I examined them all most carefully, making vertical sections of each crown, and transverse sections of all the fangs. The majority had suffered in more than one way.

Incipient caries between the bases of the cusps	existed in	28
Denudation of the dentine at the apices of the cusps from friction wear	"	15
The same from friction or absorption at the necks	"	11
Damaged enamel from pressure of contiguous teeth	"	15
Exostosis on fangs	"	12

Many of the fangs showed the horny transparency and the evidence of cemental absorption and redeposition which indicates periodontal irritation. All these teeth presented conditions which would explain pulp calcification in some degree.

In intrinsic calcification of the pulp the lime-impregnated islands are scattered diffusely through the several soft tissues, invading and ultimately solidifying them all.

In the early stages of pulp calcification no change is apparent to the unaided senses, but upon a deeper impregnation the pulp is found firmer and more coherent than usual; it does not shrivel up when dried, and is somewhat elastic when bent. It occasionally happens in extracting a carious tooth that it breaks across at the neck, the crown coming away, the pulps of the fangs slipping out of their canals and remaining stiffly bristling from the broken surface of the crown. Such a specimen is represented at fig. 67. In this instance the pulps were of the firmness and possessed the elasticity of whalebone.

Fig. 67.

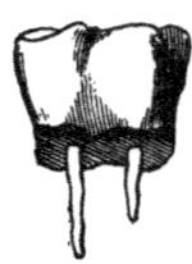

Fig. 68.

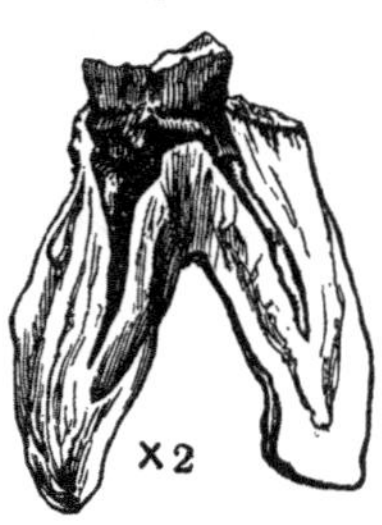

When the calcification is absolutely complete, as in the specimen, fig. 68, the whole is perfectly hard as ivory, but until this final stage it may be torn up with points of needles into fibres, which in the fangs are uniformly longitudinal. The axis of the pulp solidifies first and most completely, the exterior being more or less soft and pulpy till the osteodentine is fused and confounded with the dentine.

The colour is also modified by the change, according to the degree of calcification that has taken place; from pink and semitransparent it becomes whitish and opaque, and when the calcification is complete and the islands have fused together it is yellowish and horny-looking.

To investigate the changes that have occurred it is necessary to examine pulps with the miscroscope, assisted by chemical reagents.

As a rule, the more decayed a tooth is the more calcified will be the pulp. In some instances the calcification is very axial, with a broad, clear, soft external limit, as seen in fig. 69, taken from the specimen of which fig. 67 is an illustration. In

Fig. 69.

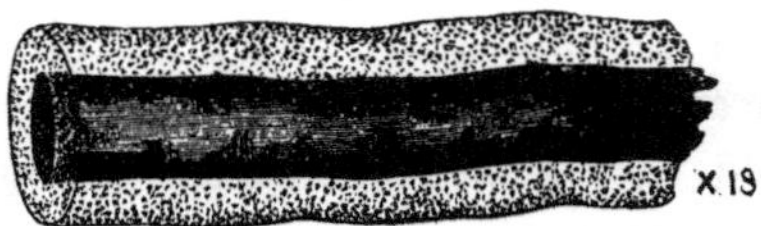

others, the outer limit is less thick and not so defined, but the soft outer layer is pretty constant up to the last stage.

In viewing a calcified pulp with higher powers—say forty diameters—it is best first to remove the general opacity by means of chemical reagents, and for this purpose caustic alkalis answer best. They render the whole very clear, exhibiting the calcific deposits and the nerves, the latter with much distinctness.

In fig. 70 is represented a portion of a tooth-pulp from the fang of a slightly carious molar tooth, treated with solu-

Fig. 70.

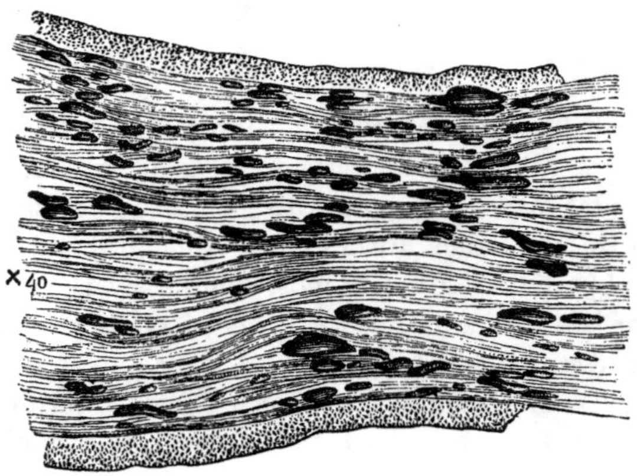

tion of caustic potash, and magnified 40 diameters. It displays the appearance characteristic of the calcific change in an early condition. Running along the pulp are numerous bundles of nerves with clear intervals, and scattered thoughout the whole promiscuously, except for a small space at the margin, are multitudes of small bodies, for the most part of a lenticular form, with very decided and dark boundary outline, lightening off to a brilliant centre, the long axis being that of the pulp. These are the "calcification islands." Upon examining pulps in which a very deep impregnation of calcarious matter has occurred with the same reagent, one finds traces of the original soft structures more and more obliterated, and the whole field of view is seen to be full of the calcification islands more or less fused together, giving an opaque, blackish or clouded appearance, in which little can be made out beyond a general longitudinal striation. The extreme of this condition is represented at fig. 71, taken from the fang of a very highly calcified pulp.

Fig. 71.

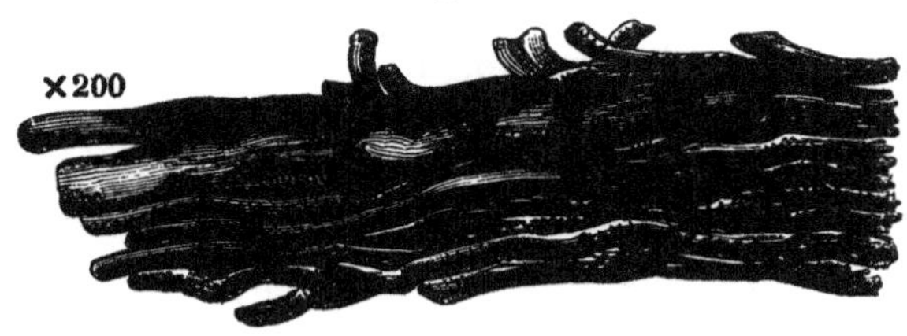

Here all residue of the previous tissue was lost, and the mass consisted of adherent calcification islands, in which the adhesion was closest in the longitudinal, serial direction, giving a coarse fibrous aspect.

The distribution of the calcification islands through the pulp is liable to some variety; but I have usually found them most abundant in those portions near the extremity of the fang, and in the central chamber of the molar teeth. At the necks of teeth, the summits of the cusps, and the outer surface of the pulp the change is latest.

The calcification islands, as closely examined with high powers, are found mostly lenticular in form, sometimes oval or club-shaped, rarely round. In the central chamber of molars they are sometimes branched, throwing out odd processes at different angles.

They very frequently exhibit evidence of being formed by the fusion of many smaller ones; and even where, with low powers, the islands appear like even ellipses, they are seen with higher powers to be formed of many elements, the union between which being still indicated. This is shown in the accompanying illustration (fig. 72).

When perfectly fused, the outlines are lost, and the whole,

retaining the original form of the pulp, becomes hard and semi-transparent, as in the specimen represented in fig. 68.

Fig. 72.

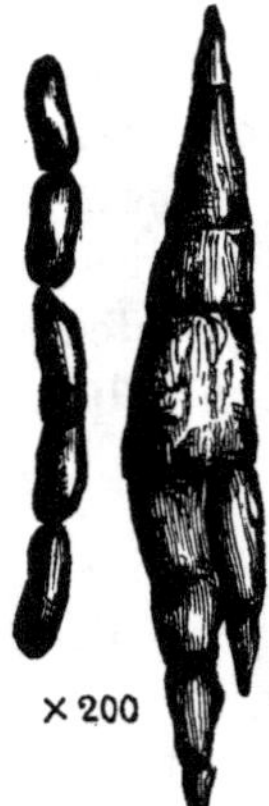

Chemically these calcification islands consist of an animal basis and earthy salts, soluble in muriatic acid, and they are probably analogous to ordinary dentine in these respects.

The relation of these calcified masses to the tissues among which they are found is very remarkable. The whole of the tissues, cells, nuclei, connective tissue, blood-vessels, and multitudes of nerves are swallowed up and obliterated by the calcification process. Hydrochloric acid removes the calcarious matter from the islands, leaving the animal matter of the same form.

The addition of caustic alkali to a specimen of pulp containing calcifications displays them conspicuously, and it shows their intimate relation to the nerves most remarkably from the fortuitous circumstance that the reagent, while it clarifies the mass generally, renders the nerve-structures only more distinctly visible. The calcification islands are very numerous among the nerves; the nerve-fibres do not seem in any way pushed aside by their presence, for we see them of considerable size in the axis of a compound nerve, without any bulging of its surface or edges. Such specimens are exhibited in figures 73 and 74.

The calcification is clearly not interstitial between the fibres, but swallows them up promiscuously with the other structures. This is sufficiently indicated by microscopical examination, and is confirmed by physiological evidence. The cells and nuclei, which are abundant in the adult pulp, share in the general change, and the former probably produce the dentinal tubes that are found in the osteodentine.

The blood-vessels are probably the last tissues to calcify, and this is certainly the case with the larger ones, some of which remain permanently patent and functional in the axis of Haversian systems of the matured osteodentine. Some, however, even of these become ultimately obliterated and calcified.*

The complete consequences of intrinsic calcification of the

* This subject is further illustrated in the Chapter on Secondary Dentine.

tooth-pulp are near obliteration of sensibility and greatly diminished vascularity, reducing the former to that of ordinary

Fig. 73.

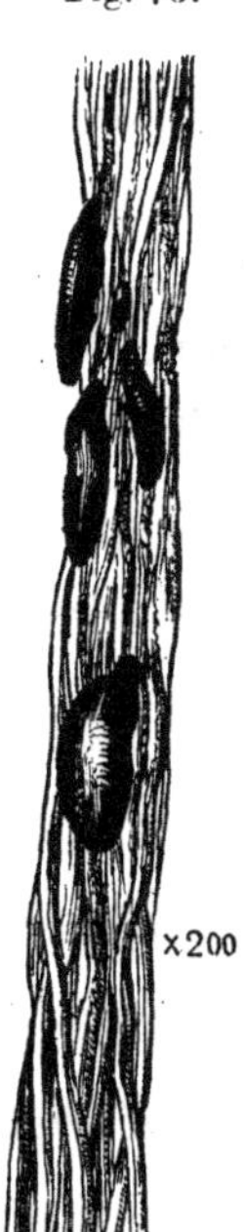

Fig. 74.

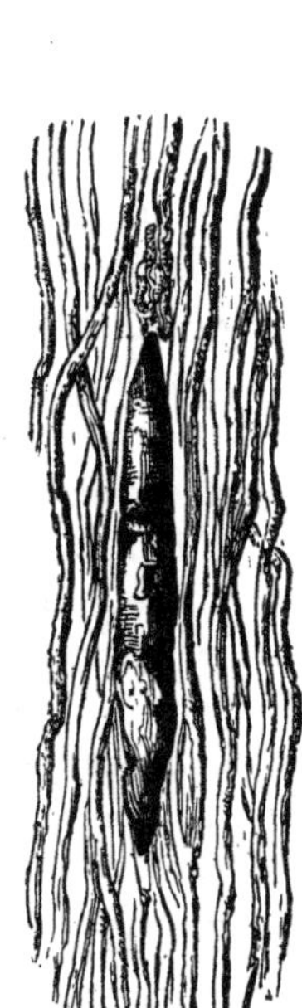

dentine, and the latter to less than that of bone. The change, however, is apt to be irregular; and while some parts of the pulp are converted into hard, insensitive dentine, other parts remain more or less soft and unchanged.

There are certain operations connected with the teeth in which we have to do with the pulp-cavity, and are influenced in our proceedings by the condition of the pulp itself, as, for instance, in tooth-filling or plugging, and in pivoting teeth.

In drilling the pulp-cavity for pivoting a tooth we have to deal with the pulp in every varied stage of calcification, and the vital phenomena which it exhibits are in accordance with the degree of change. Where the calcification is slight the pulp is exquisitely sensitive; the drill produces intense pain, and sometimes bleeding. As the calcification advances the sensibility and the tendency to bleed gradually decrease, till at length, in the completely formed osteodentine, these indications of vitality have practically ceased, and the calcified pulp may be drilled with as little inconvenience as attends the cutting of a hair or nail. Sometimes, however, small isolated spots of pulp will remain uncalcified and manifest their vitality.

The same phenomena are observed when the calcified pulp is reached in preparing carious teeth for stopping.

The calcification of the pulp, as I have already remarked, is a morbid process, though a reparative one. It falls under the category of those many processes which, evoked by injury or disease, are the means of averting results which would be fatal to the individual organ affected. The process has a close analogy to those many conditions in which irritation and increased vascularity, caused by disease in contiguous structures, issue in the deposition of adventitious matter; in this instance, as usually happens, the nature of the adventitious matter is determined by the normal nutritional affinities of the organ affected. There is a qualitative disturbance of nutrition, resulting from a vascular disturbance which would seem to be merely quantitative.

Suppuration and Sphacelus.—The formation of pus in the tooth-pulp is one of its commonest morbid changes, and happens much more frequently than is generally imagined. It may occur to any extent, from a minute development of matter in a circumscribed area of the pulp to the complete suppuration and sphacelus of the whole organ. This destructive purulent inflammation of the pulp is the usual commencement of alveolar abscess, and where the latter is associated with dental caries and an unopened pulp-chamber, I believe it thus arises always, or nearly so. But alveolar abscess *may* occur without suppuration of the pulp, and the pulp *may* suppurate without the discharge finding an exit.

The phenomena of tooth-pulp suppuration are parallel in all essential respects to suppuration in other organs, and the two conditions in which the matter is pent up, or freely discharged, have respectively the same distinctive and characteristic symptoms. A circumstance, however, which gives an especial exaltation to one of the symptoms, namely, *pain*, is that the pulp is peculiarly sensitive from its profuse supply of nerves, and that it is boxed up in a perfectly unyielding case—the tooth-walls. Suppuration of the tooth-pulp is usually of the same character as suppurations generally of internal structures: it is attended with a certain amount of destruction—sphacelus, of the structure itself. When the tooth-pulp, however, is exposed, especially if the exposure be gradual and effected without acute inflammation during its production, the pus-formation is superficial (as from granulating surfaces or mucous membranes), is unaccompanied by deep or general lesion of substance, or the attendant symptoms of such a change.

In many cases where there is no absolute proof of the existence of pus in the pulp, where the tooth has been retained and so could not be examined, one is nevertheless justified in inferring the presence of matter, by analogy.

I have so very frequently found pus in small quantities in the pulps of teeth only slightly diseased, and which have given rise to very moderate symptoms, that I am certain it is very frequently developed without being suspected, the tooth recovering from its painful condition, and being retained for a long series of years subsequently, as a useful and apparently a sound organ.

Thus, one person, who is impatient of pain, insists on having a tooth extracted, though apparently but little diseased. Pus is found in the pulp. In a similar case the patient prefers to attempt the saving of the tooth. The painful symptoms pass off by degrees, and although the anatomical condition cannot then be displayed, I am confident, in many such cases, that pus has existed. As will be shown hereafter, the subsequent examination of teeth, that have been thus affected before, corroborates such a view.

In considering the pathology of the teeth it must always be remembered that they have two sources of vitality—the periodontal membrane as well as the pulp, and that the latter may undergo the severest destructive changes without destroying the life of the tooth. This is conspicuously true as regards the plasmic circulation in the tubes of the tooth-fangs. I believe it is equally so in reference to the sensibility of the whole dentine. I am certain that, after the destruction of the pulp, portions of the crown of the dentine have been sensitive to mechanical violence.

I have been for many years in the habit of examining the pulps of a large proportion of the teeth I extract, and, having a microscope always set up and at hand, I have with great facility made a large number of such examinations.

The best way to get at the pulp is to crush the tooth in a vice. I first envelope it in a piece of calico, and then, placing it in a vice, slowly and carefully compress it till the walls give way. The calico keeps the parts sufficiently *in situ*, and one can examine the pulp and its relations to exterior disease quite satisfactorily.

When a tooth-pulp undergoes irritation, if of slight extent, the change which takes place in it consists of a general scattered calcification through its structure, the formation of numerous islands of dentine. When, however, the inflammation is more severe, pus readily forms in the substance of the pulp and its tissues rapidly liquefy, while (if the pulp-chamber be still closed externally) the matter frequently progresses rapidly to the apex of the fang, and finds its way to the surface, increasing in quantity, in the form of an "alveolar abscess." This process is attended by some interesting changes at the end of the fang, considerable absorption of bone around it, and the development of a mass of lymph, forming at first a sac, and, ultimately, as bone absorbs and the pus advances to the surface, a fibrous cylindrical canal, through which the matter escapes.

If a tooth be examined in which these morbid changes are fairly established, and while the pulp-chamber is still unopened by disease, a portion of the pulp-cavity, often considerable, will be found filled with liquid yellow pus—to the eye apparently pure and quite liquid, while another portion of the cavity is occupied by healthy pulp, perhaps a little extra-vascular, but exhibiting no other change. The point which separates the pus from the healthy pulp displays a very interesting condition.

The healthy tissue may be traced up to a certain point, where it ends, more or less suddenly, in a deep red demarcation or patch. This is succeeded by a mass of diffluent slough, of a dirty greenish colour, beyond which is the yellow liquid pus. The interval between the pus and the healthy tissue is often very narrow, and is occupied by but a small amount of structure.

The following descriptions and figures are taken from examples that I have recorded in my note-book at different times.

The first illustration (fig. 75) is a diagrammatic representation of a tooth in this condition, and as it was extracted from my own mouth I am the better qualified to describe its history. The tooth was carious on one side of the crown, but the pulp-cavity was still unopened, though the dentine was softened and discoloured to the interior. The tooth had been for some days slightly painful, a little loose, very tender, and susceptible to changes of temperature. Then occurred one day and night of acute suffering. On extracting the tooth it was found that the apex of one root was blood-pointed, marking a vascular orifice; the other was sealed up by a mass of half-organised lymph. Upon examining the pulp-chamber, about one-half of the pulp was found in a healthy condition (*a*), occupying one fang and nearly half the central chamber. The other fang and a small part of the central chamber were filled with a liquid pus (*d*); then occurred a mass of green diffluent slough (*c*), separated from the healthy tissue by a distinct band of a deep blood-red colour (*b*). The pus in the posterior fang was, as yet, quite shut in by the lymph around its apex.

Fig. 75.

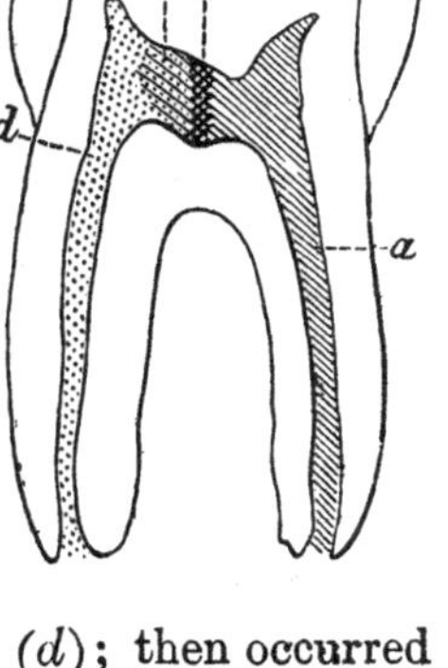

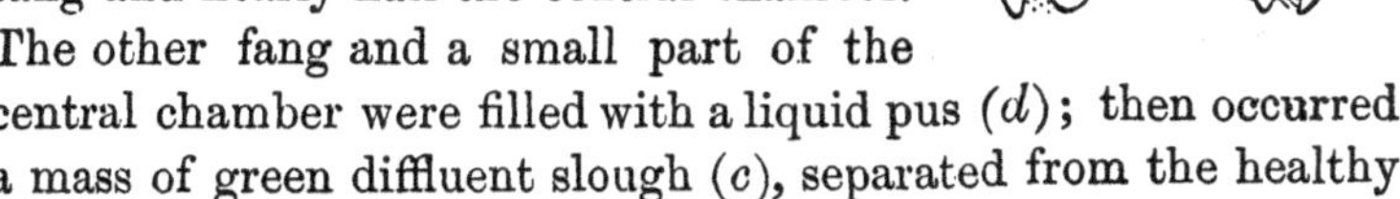

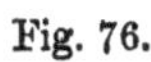

Fig. 76.

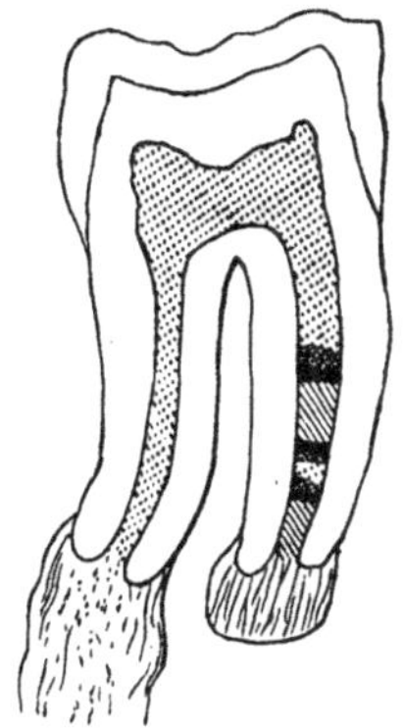

The second diagram (fig. 76) represents the condition of a lower molar. This tooth was carious on the posterior part of the crown, but the cavity had not opened the pulp-chamber. The posterior fang, the whole of the central chamber, and about half the anterior fang were filled with pus. In the anterior fang was a small, isolated collection of pus; above, below, and around this was some healthy pulp, but the structure in immediate contact with the matter was in a state of slough, as is always the case, and the healthy pulp was limited by a deep red outline, as is equally constant.

One other point, which is very general though not absolutely constant, is that the suppuration evidently commenced and was most advanced at that part of the pulp nearest to the dentinal caries. The extremity of the fang, which was wholly filled with pus, was surrounded by lymph, with a pus-canal in its centre, the matter being conducted by it and in progress to the surface, which, however, had not been reached. The extremity of the other fang was simply surrounded by half-organised lymph, in which suppuration had not yet commenced.

A third specimen examined was an inferior second temporary molar (fig. 77). There was a large carious cavity on the top of the crown; the central chamber was not opened, but the dentine above it was in an advanced state of caries. In the pulp of the central chamber were some minute drops of pus, isolated here and there, and surrounded by dark red walls, and an amount of sphacelus that was but just appreciable. This is a condition that I have frequently seen in carious temporary teeth, even where they have been but slightly painful, and I suspect it is very common indeed.

Fig. 77.

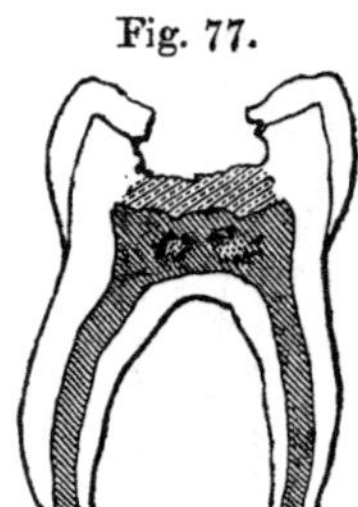

The examination of these suppurating and sloughing pulps with the microscope discloses a curious and interesting condition as regards the smaller blood-vessels where the healthy tissue is limited. The deep blood-red band which I have described is occasioned by the dilatation of the vessels into ampullæ filled with clots. They form the limit of the circulation, and the dilatations are doubtless produced by the lost vitality of the vessels upon the margin of the slough; the vital contractility has ceased, and the force of the blood-current dilates the thin walls, which passively yield, and the blood coagulates. Probably the same change occurs at all sloughing surfaces, but the minute size of the tooth-pulp, and the ease with which it can be isolated and examined with the morbid parts in undisturbed relation, afford exceptional opportunities for making the observation. In the accompanying illustrations specimens of this vascular dilatation are shown as they occur in the fang (fig. 78) and in the central chamber (fig. 79). In the former the general course of the vascular plexuses is longitudinal; in the latter the ves-

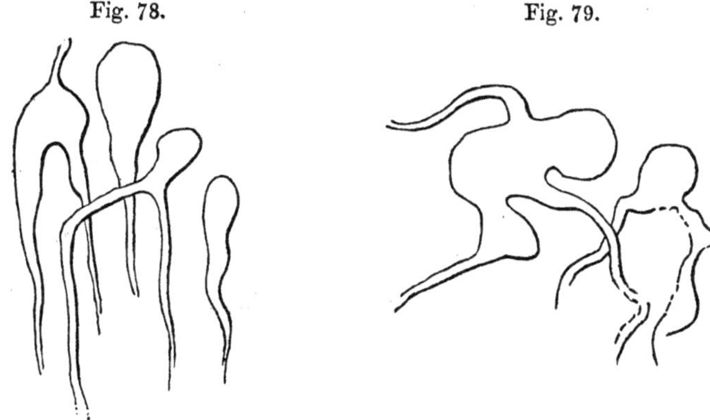

Fig. 78. Fig. 79.

sels are contorted and confused, and the dilated ampullæ vary accordingly.

The facility with which the tooth-pulp suppurates appears to be remarkable. This unquestionably varies much with different organs, and the persistence of the primitive cellular condition, which exists so largely in the tooth-pulp, probably leads to the rapid development of pus. It has appeared to me that the pus in the tooth-pulp is formed at the expense and by the multiplication of the cells (granules of Purkinje) which so largely pervade the pulp, by their direct conversion into pus-cells, just as Virchow has shown that the pus is formed in parenchymatous organs by the proliferation of the development cells of the connective tissue. Accompanying this rapid formation of pus there is a general softening and solution of the other tissues of the pulp. In the pus shreds of broken-up tissue are to be met with, and many "calcification islands" cast free; but often the pus is remarkably liquid and free from other elements in the canal which, but a short time before, had been occupied by healthy pulp.

As I have remarked, pus may be formed and long retained in the pulp-cavity without emission, and it may be found in such cases in all those stages of disintegration which Virchow has so ably described and so correctly figured—from the first fatty degeneration to the complete emulsion of the cells, and these changes probably always occur when suppuration of the pulp is unattended by a discharging alveolar abscess.

Suppuration of the tooth-pulp may and very often does occur with an opened pulp-chamber, and then the pathological changes are usually different. The exposed surface of the pulp is then constantly relieved by shedding of discharge from the surface in the form of pus or sero-pus, and the destruction of the parenchyma of the organ is far less liable to occur.

The regular progress of dentinal caries tends to open the pulp-chamber; and the pulp, though irritated by the advance of the disease, may remain without undergoing any destructive change till a communication is formed between the pulp-chamber and the exterior. This may lead to one of two conditions: either the pulp remains of nearly unaltered size, irritable, painful, with a suppurating surface; or, more rarely, it may grow into an insensitive tumour, polypus of the pulp. This latter condition I shall consider by itself hereafter.

Observations on the pathological condition and changes in pulps exposed by the progress of caries are very imperfect. There is usually much intrinsic calcification, of the axis especially, while certain portions remain soft and sensitive. The pulp in this condition may give very little uneasiness unless pressed upon by portions of food, when a sudden plunge of pain occurs; and this may rapidly pass off or continue as toothache. A tooth in this condition may at any time be the subject of acute odontalgia, with or without alveolar inflammation; and the latter may remain in a chronic and plastic form, or it may pass on to suppuration—alveolar abscess. This latter condition is, I believe, generally, though not necessarily always, attended by sphacelus of the pulp, extending to the apex of the fang (or in a molar it may be *one* fang of the tooth).

Necrosis.—The sudden death of a tooth-pulp is not an uncommon event, and is usually caused by some mechanical violence which severs the vessels of the pulp at the foramen of the fang. But it may arise from inflammation, from fever, and apparently spontaneously.

Necrosis of the pulp is attended with what is called necrosis of the tooth, though the death of the latter is not necessarily entire.

Tooth-necrosis is an interesting condition and is attended by phenomena and symptoms of particular importance. These are considered under the head of "Necrosis of Teeth" (see Chapter X.).

My present purpose is to describe the pathological changes of death of the pulp in relation to the pulp itself only.

Where the death of the pulp arises from inflammation and sphacelus with suppurative evacuation, the pulp disappears from either the whole or part of the cavity—from as much of it as is occupied by the affected pulp. The cavity of the tooth may be filled by the fluids of the mouth, and undergo caries on its inner surface.

When, however, the death of pulp is the result of mechanical violence, or of some disease which does not lead to suppuration, or an opening from the exterior to the pulp cavity—where, that is, the dead pulp remains boxed up in its impermeable prison—the changes which occur are essentially *fatty decomposition.* When the vital connection with the neighbouring tissues is severed destructive changes quickly occur; the pulp becomes dark coloured, soft, and diffluent. Under the microscope it displays countless multitudes of minute oil globules, among an unintelligible *débris*; and if the teeth are those of persons past adolescence, loose calcification islands are usually found. The oil globules, which are soluble in ether, are so minute that few reach the size of blood discs, and the majority are so small as to exhibit "molecular motion" like the base of chyle.* These, however, are not the only minute particles to be seen in dead pulps. In cases of longer standing I have found a considerable proportion of very minute granules which ether would not dissolve, but which were rendered either wholly or partially invisible by dilute hydrochloric acid. I take these bodies to be either disintegrated calcification islands or minute particles of broken-down dentine detached from the walls of the pulp cavity.

Polypus of the Pulp.—This consists of an expansion of the summit of the dentine pulp of a tooth in which caries has

* "Fatty Decomposition of the Tooth-Pulp," by S. I. A. Salter. *Path. Trans.* vol. vi. 1855.

exposed the pulp. It is not a very rare affection, but it was overlooked both by Hunter and Fox. I have almost always found that this condition, when present, occurs in young people, and in those in whom the teeth are imperfectly calcified, presenting that peculiar globular calcification in which the substance of the dentine becomes rapidly sodden with saliva and carious without limit from the enamel of the pulp. It has appeared to me probable that the pulp undergoes some influence or impression from the percolation of the saliva, before it is laid bare by the breaking away of the carious dentine, and that thus is lit up a series of changes which are widely different from those that usually occur as the result of ordinary caries. It seems not improbable that the sudden and complete saturation of the dentine with saliva might reach the pulp previous to its undergoing intrinsic calcification, while the crown still affords a protection from external violence. We may imagine an influence bearing on the pulp sufficient to alter its surface action, not of a nature to lead to the formation of dentine of repair, or intrinsic calcification; nor such as would produce abscess in the pulp, nor the painful inflammation which follows the fracture of a sound tooth.

This may be the reason why this character of tooth and this form of caries are so often associated with polypus of the pulp. If this be granted, it is obvious why it so constantly, when present, shows itself in early life; for teeth thus imperfectly calcified seldom long resist the chemical and physical influences to which they are exposed in the mouth, but early fall victims to general, soft, light-coloured caries. Whether the interpretation I have suggested be the correct one or not, the fact of such an association of character of tooth, and the youthful period of life with polypus of the pulp, is almost, if not quite, constant when the disease exists.

The physiological phenomena displayed by polypus of the pulp are remarkable as regards both the pulp itself and the tooth, and their oppositeness to the train of circumstances which attend the ordinary inflammation of the pulps dependent on caries—such as odontalgia, lymph deposit on fangs, alveolar abscess, &c.—does not appear to have been sufficiently appreciated or enforced.

The pulp grows into a mass, having very much the aspect and

about the same sensitiveness as the surrounding mucous membrane, the gum. The pulp does not undergo intrinsic calcification, nor is dentine of repair produced. True toothache does not arise; and alveolar abscess associated with these teeth is very rare, and does not necessarily involve the apex of the fang. Indeed, the phenomena of the two conditions are quite opposite to each other. They may perhaps be not inaptly compared to inflammatory action where it can, and where it cannot get rid of its results; as, for instance, to a granulating wound that sheds its pus without pain, distress, or irritation, and an unopened abscess with all the local and constitutional irritation and distress that accompany it. In the pulp polypus the swelling up of the tumour, unrestrained by compressing walls, and the free-shedding of its purulent or epithelial surface products, probably explain the absence of accompanying local pain and general irritation.

Fig. 80.

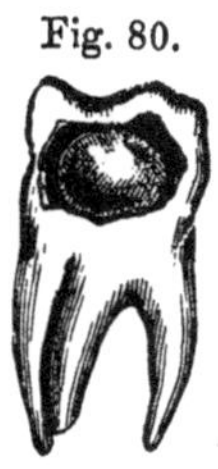

The polypus begins, as I have remarked, by the exposure of the pulp in a tooth that is imperfectly calcified, that does not ache and has not ached. The tooth is usually one of the second set, though occasionally, but very rarely, a temporary tooth may be thus affected. The tumour (fig. 80), generally fills the cavity, though not always, and is limited by it and the opposing tooth in the other jaw. There is usually an enlargement of the pulp in the fang or fangs of the tooth and a corresponding expansion of the fang-canals themselves. It is about as sensitive as the surrounding gum. With the exception of occasional and temporary variation in size—a sort of erection (often from cold or dyspepsia)—it seems to remain quite passive. It occurs, as I have observed, in young persons almost altogether, and more often in the molars, especially the first, than in other teeth. It has been my experience (perhaps an accidental coincidence) to have seen many more cases in young women than in young men. It frequently exists in many teeth in the same individual; and this is quite in keeping with the idea that it is dependent on an imperfect character of original tooth-structure. And I believe it is generally associated with soft complexion, fine hair, small teeth, and general tegumentary feebleness.

The examination of polypus of the pulp, in regard to its ultimate histological characters, has displayed two distinct conditions; which, however, appear to be mere stages of development.

In the great majority of specimens I have examined the polypus has had exactly the appearance of a mass of granulations, like those of a healing wound. The more superficial portions have consisted entirely of cells, about $\frac{1}{2000}$ of an inch in diameter, held together and at the same time separated by a nearly homogeneous blastema; some of the cells have seemed free *on* the surface, and others apparently detached and shed. Deep in the substance of the polypus the cells appear to have been developed into an immature fibrous tissue, and looping towards the surface are many capillary blood-vessels. I have never seen, on a pulp-polypus, any of the elongated or columnar cells, with their tube-forming processes, which constitute the membrana eboris.

The exposed pulp must be looked upon as a wound, and its surface in these polypi is in a condition of granulation. The cells of the granulations seem but slightly differentiated "granules" of Pinkinje. Occasionally, though not generally, the surface undergoes a higher degree of development into a more or less perfect mucous membrane.

I have found a very indistinct epithelium clothing a pulp-polypus, in which the nuclei appeared identical with the globular granulation cells, as though the latter had been clothed by an investing periplast, thus producing epithelium. In several specimens I discovered a folded film which appeared to be immature basement membrane covered by the pale epithelium. In others the papillary outlines were sharp and *prononcé*.

In a few examples I have found the surface of the polypus exactly like true gum, covered by a dense cuticular epithelium lying upon a regular system of papillæ. When a polypus has arrived at this structural condition it may be considered as having cicatrised.

The treatment of the polypus is to remove the tooth. The decay is usually so very far advanced that, apart from the presence of the polypus itself, the tooth is not worth saving. The polypus may be extirpated by the knife, but as far as my experience goes it sprouts again. I once attempted to save a tooth in which a polypus existed. I cut away the soft growth with a scalpel, and treated the cavity with an escarotic for some time, till I believed the growth had been entirely repressed. I then stopped the tooth. In a short time the polypus sprouted again and lifted the stopping bodily out of the cavity just as a growing agaric will lift a paving stone.

Sensitive Sprouting of the Pulp.—This condition, I believe, only occurs from the fracture, by mechanical violence, of a tooth the pulp of which had previously been in a healthy condition; or very little modified by calcification—practically a healthy pulp. It usually happens from an accident—a fall or a blow—but I have seen it occur by the breaking of a sound tooth whose removal was attempted for regulation of dentition; and also in extraction of slightly carious teeth.

When a tooth-pulp is thus exposed it exhibits intense sensitiveness to touch, to cold or heat, or indeed to any external influence; and it frequently sprouts into a small excrescence: this sometimes grows as large as a raspberry with nodular enlargements on the surface like the drupaceous elevations on that fruit, with the same semi-transparent aspect. When removed, like the other form of pulp-growth, it certainly returns, and of the same character as before.

In microscopic structure this sprouting of the pulp differs little from the insensitive polypus; it is, however, clearer and softer, and its vitality implies a more abundant nervous supply—vascular granulations appear to the observer to constitute its histological elements. This condition usually remains as a permanent torture to the patient, till the tooth is extracted, when it is of course completely removed. Sometimes, however, after much annoyance, it will slough away spontaneously.

I have known this state of tooth-pulp form a very distressing complication in a case of fracture of the lower jaw, in which a bicuspid tooth was broken and the pulp exposed: here the apparatus for fixing the displaced bone, and the introduction into the mouth of food, were attended with agonising pain, which continued till its source, a fractured tooth with a quick pulp, was discovered and extracted. Afterwards the treatment of this fracture was successfully and painlessly prosecuted. The possibility—indeed, occasional probability—of such a complication, in treating fractures of the maxillæ, should be borne in mind by surgeons; and it should be especially remembered that when extreme sensitiveness and pain manifest themselves in such cases, a fractured tooth ought to be sought for.

In treating these cases the effort should be to remove the tooth * which encases the sensitive pulp. The cure then is immediate and complete.

A singular and unintentional method of cure occurred to me, which I find thus recorded in my note-book:—

"A medical student from Guy's Hospital applied to me this day (November 8, 1864) on account of a fractured first upper molar, which had been broken off in an attempt to extract it. The large pulp of the tooth's central chamber was exposed and intensely sensitive. I attempted the extraction with the elevator, and lifted the tooth from the socket, when the patient plunged away, declaring he would stand no more torture. The tooth returned to its alveolar cavities; but the pain was cured. The exposed pulp had ceased to feel. In prizing up the fangs, the connection of the pulp-nerves with the maxillary nerve had been severed, and the case was so far cured. The tooth remained, and the periosteal union was re-established. The pulp sloughed away."

* Excepting where such a proceeding would endanger the development of the maxillary arch, as may occur in young people in regard to the superior central incisors.

CHAPTER XIII.

TUMOURS, AND OTHER AFFECTIONS OF THE GUMS.

These are certain small tumours connected with the gums, which frequently come under the observation of dental surgeons; and though their treatment may not be carried out by some, their diagnosis should not be in doubt.

These tumours may be enumerated as follows:—

Epulis.
Polypus of the gum.
Vascular tumours.
Warty tumours of the gum.

Epulis.—The term "Epulis" has been vaguely applied to various tumours that are formed in and upon the gums. The etymological meaning of the word (ἐπὶ, upon, οὖλα, the gums), entirely referring to position and not to structure, is likely to have caused and to continue this confusion. Where, however, distinction has been drawn, it has been applied to those hard and densely fibrous tumours that arise from the surface of the alveolar processes, involving the periosteum, and by their expanded growth stretching the otherwise healthy gum over them. These are essentially different in origin, history and structure, from those loose flaps and often pendulous masses of gum that are not unfrequently seen in the neighbourhood of decayed teeth, more properly called polypus of the gum.

An epulis tumour consists of a hard dense mass growing slowly and evenly from the edge of the alveolar process usually between two standing teeth, and more commonly on the labial or buccal aspect than the lingual. The point at which this growth generally makes its first appearance is beneath and involving the little tongue of gum which exists between the necks of two contiguous teeth: as it progresses in size, it displaces the neighbouring teeth, one usually more than the other: it has for the most part a broad base, and increases in basal area more than in projecting growth. The situation in which an epulis commences is liable to a good deal of variety: though usually at the free edge of the alveolar process, it may form at a distance from it; but I believe it is always associated with porous vascular bone, nearly connected with the periodontal membrane, and does not spring from the compact tissue limiting the outline of the bone. The growth sometimes commences *in* the tooth-socket. As I have remarked, the *endosteal* membrane shares in the genesis of an epulis tumour, and the fibrous growth appears to burrow, so to speak, into the substance of the bone, producing a general expansion of the whole structure. The surface of the tumour is like that of the surrounding gum; it is, however, sometimes mottled, and not infrequently slightly but broadly and flatly lobulated. It is as insensitive as the gum, and is not liable to bleed: when manipulated, it is tense and elastic. The tumour varies in size indefinitely—from the size of a pea to that of a walnut, or larger. It is generally stated that epulis tumours are more common in the upper than the lower jaw: this coincides with my own experience. I happen to have met with them in the proportion exactly of two of the former to one of the latter. The epulis tumour appears to have a certain relation to the teeth in whose neighbourhood it forms. It almost always makes its appearance where there *are* teeth: it usually invades one in a very marked degree more than any other near which it may be situated, by dislocating it and pushing it out of place: it has nothing to do apparently with caries of the tooth: the removal of the particular tooth, with excision of the tumour, is almost always accompanied by immediate and complete cure of the disease.

Occasionally these tumours appear where teeth have been removed and the gum seems to be edentulous: it will, however, generally be found in these instances that a fang of one of the teeth has been left behind, and is associated with the irritation that has caused the morbid growth. One of the most severe examples of this malady which I have seen consisted of a bi-lobular mass, the size of a large walnut, extending, on the left side of the lower jaw, from the dens sapientiæ to the canine tooth, the four intermediate teeth having been removed. The excision of the tumour had been repeatedly performed, but it always returned. Its removal on this occasion disclosed the remains of one fang of the first molar tooth in its very axis: this was extracted, and the disease did not again make its appearance. I believe this will generally be found the case where the tumour forms upon an apparently edentulous region of the jaw.

The accompanying illustration (fig. 81) is that of a characteristic example which occurred in my own practice many years ago, and which I described in the "Transactions" of the Pathological Society.*

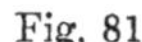
Fig. 81.

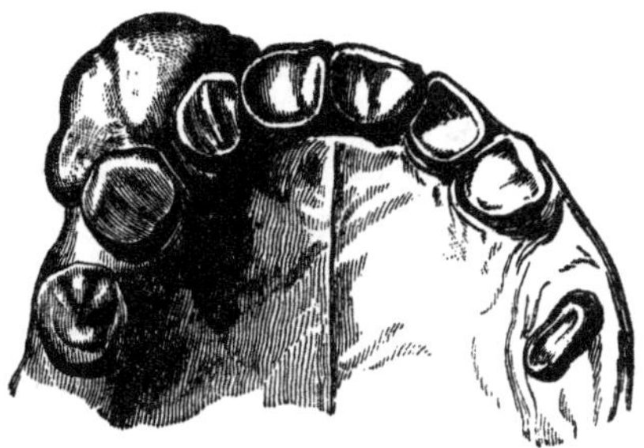

Epulis has its origin in the osteal membrane of the alveolus. The bone of the alveolar processes is very vascular, and almost cancellated in its loose open structure. The endosteal membrane which lines this cancellated bone, the periosteum which covers it, and which lines the tooth-sockets and the fibrous tissue of the gum, are all continuous, and alike share in the development of an epulis tumour. The bulk of the tumour consists of a dense web of fibrous tissue; and from its basal attachment, and passing into its substance, are usually small growths of bone. The fibrous tissue interlaces pretty regularly—some fibres being parallel to the surface, and others radiating from the base, intersecting the former at right angles. The bone-growths may be thin needle-like spicula or little flakes; at the point whence these bony processes arise the tumour receives its main vascular supply, and the subjacent bone is very porous. Mr. Cæsar Hawkins mentions an instance of an epulis attached only by a pedicle to the gum, in which there was a nucleus of

* "Specimens of Epulis," in *Trans. Path. Soc.* 1854.

bone. This could not at any time have had bony union with the jaw; but the circumstance indicates, in a physiological sense, the osteal character of these fibroid developments. Epulis tumours are perfectly innocent; nor do they, I believe, ever pass into a malignant character. Sometimes, though rarely, they ulcerate on the surface; but this is only under the influence of external agencies, such as produce ulceration of any portion of the gum; they may then become painful.

The histology of epulis tumours is consistent with their history—locally recurrent as long as the circumstances under which they occurred are maintained, destroyed by the removal of their local nidus, and never impregnating the system. Epulis tumours are always, I believe, a form of "fibro-plastic;" a combination of fibrous tissue and myeloid cells, the proportion of the two constituents varying indefinitely. In general, the main bulk of the tumour consists of fibrous tissue; but sometimes the myeloid-cell element preponderates, and may form the major portion of the growth.*

The *treatment* of epulis is very simple; it requires early and complete extirpation with the knife, and according to the extent and inveteracy of the case it may also need the removal of contiguous teeth and subjacent bone. These latter circumstances refer to an important circumstance in the *pathological history* of the disease: it is this, that as long as the alveolar process remains upon which the tumour grew, and which must necessarily be as long as the teeth which are implanted in it are not removed, so long will the tumour be inveterate, so often will it return, however accurately and carefully it may have been removed. Such, at least, is the very general rule. But when the alveolar process is gone, it shows no tendency to return. And it is a remarkable circumstance, that the spontaneous absorption of the alveoli that follows the extraction of the teeth is of itself, *in many instances*, where the disease is confined only to these processes, enough to prevent its recurrence. That is to say, if the tumour be removed to a level with the gum, and the contiguous teeth be extracted, the alveolar process vanishes by absorption, and the disease no more returns; though the same operation, without the removal of the teeth, may have

* "Myeloid Epulis of Lower Jaw," by J. Hutchinson, *Trans. Path. Soc.* vol. viii.

been performed unsuccessfully any number of times previously. In a first operation, when the disease is of limited extent, it will be well to try the result of its simple removal by the scalpel without the extraction of teeth or the cutting away of more bone than can be accomplished with the knife. The bone about the base and axis of the tumour being vascular and spongy, the knife readily cuts away small portions. Any subsequent sprouting of granulations in an undue or threatening degree should be checked and repressed by some caustic, and for this purpose nitric acid has been especially recommended. If the disease recurs, as it too often does, the same operation should be repeated, and accompanied by the extraction of a tooth or teeth whose socket or sockets have been implicated. Unless the disease have a deep hold on the bony substance of the jaw, it will seldom be necessary to cut away any large amount of bone; sometimes, however, this is the case; or the growth may have started deep in the socket of a tooth. In such an instance it may be necessary to extirpate a considerable amount of bone. A V-shaped portion or a cubical mass may be readily cut out by means of a Hey's saw and bone-nippers, according to the form and extent of the particular tumour. It will never, I believe, be necessary to go far below the limit of the alveolar process; for it is with the alveolar bone that the disease is essentially connected. In the lower jaw I would urge the necessity of never cutting through the entire bone, as the breaking of the maxillary arch most seriously interferes with the position of the remaining portions of the bone, and thus disturbs the normal opposition of the teeth in the two jaws relatively.

Polypus of the gum.—The gum is liable to a simple hypertrophy, the increase of growth—a sort of mucous tubercle—being confined to the gum structure alone, and not involving the osteal membrane, nor complicated with a growth of bone. The little tongues of gum between the necks of the teeth are liable to this affection, especially towards the front of the mouth; and they sometimes grow to such an extent, being confluent with those on either side, as to cover a considerable portion of the crowns of the teeth. This condition is usually associated with uncleanly habits, and may be generally cured and prevented hereafter by simple and easy means. The teeth should be thoroughly cleansed from tartar; the gums may be scarified: for the future the teeth should be abundantly brushed with a stiff brush, and the mouth washed with an astringent lotion, of which solution of permanganate of potass may form an ingredient.

An unusually large example of polypus of the gum came under my notice in 1863. A gentleman, 21 years of age, consulted me respecting a considerable growth which had formed on the alveolar border of the upper jaw just behind the second bicuspid tooth. It looked like an epulis, but its history and subsequent examination proved it to be a mere gum-polypus. The tumour was the size and form shown in the accompanying figure. The first permanent molar decayed very early, the crown disappeared, and the decay progressed till the fangs were isolated: the gum in the centre between them slowly expanded, separating the fangs, and then protruded in the form of a pedunculated tumour. The growth continued to advance till the patient consulted me. At that time the tumour did not

Fig. 82.

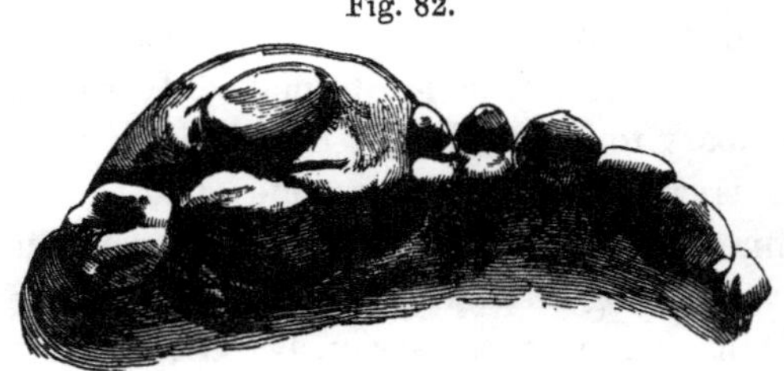

appear pedunculated, but broad based. It was a lobulated mass, as big as half a chestnut, with a small additional lobule on the surface the size and shape of a horse bean. It was of the consistence of ordinary gum. Upon examining with a bent probe I found it was attached by a very short stalk, less than half the diameter of the whole mass. I removed the tumour and then the tooth stumps, and the growth did not recur.

Hypertrophy of the gum of a truly polypus-like form not infrequently occurs in the immediate neighbourhood of teeth which are carious at their sides, and when the caries reaches the neck of the tooth: the irritation of the contiguous dentinal disease seems to stimulate this unwonted growth, and the mucous membrane bulges into the cavity and fills it up. The cavities of two teeth carious on their contiguous surfaces are apt to be associated with this condition, the little polypus of gum between them rising to their masticating surfaces. Such tumours are more or less pedunculated; they have a red fleshy look, and are very liable to bleed when roughly touched. The structure of these growths is in consonance with their aspect and the ease with which they bleed; they consist principally of hypertrophy of the true mucous-membrane element of the gum, especially the papillary structure: the epithelial covering is rather diminished in proportional amount, while the papillæ themselves become enormously elongated and increased in diameter, and some of the conical papillæ develop into the compound fungiform variety. These changes are accompanied by great dilatation of the capillaries which loop into the papillæ.

Polypus growths of the gum are so often dependent on the state of the contiguous teeth, that their treatment involves that of the teeth also. If the polypus, growing into a carious tooth, is extirpated, it will most probably return till the tooth itself is removed, or the condition of the tooth which had irritated the gum has been remedied. The caries should be cut away; ragged or sharp edges of tooth-substance should be smoothed and blunted, and the remaining cavity should be filled. The gum may still show some tendency to renewed sprouting, and this may be kept down for a time by the repeated application of a strong solution of nitrate of silver, sulphate of copper, or alum, when it will probably assume a healthy aspect. If the removal of the polypus is accompanied by the extraction of the offending tooth, I believe it never returns.

Vascular tumours.—The tissues about the necks of the teeth are obnoxious to the growth of vascular tumours, which vary from passive *nævus-like* swelling to those other forms of more arterial character—*aneurisms by anastomosis.* I have met with both these forms of the disease. The most common posi tion in which it develops itself is in the front of the upper jaw, between the incisors, or canines and lateral incisors. A rather severe instance which occurred recently under my care manifested itself in the region that should have been occupied by the left lateral incisor of the upper jaw; but as the laterals were wanting in this person, the tumour formed between the canine and central incisor. It had been about six months in reaching its then size, the dimensions of a large marble flattened on the surface. It was of a purplish colour, streaked with many vessels on the surface; it was easily compressed, but was elastic, and when pressed it became pale, exsanguine, and much reduced in size; upon removing the pressure it resumed its previous aspect in a pulse or two. The surface of the growth was tolerably smooth; the base somewhat constricted, being about one-third less than the head of the tumour. The whole of the gums were very red, turgid, and swollen, and the little tongues of gum between the necks of the teeth generally were enlarged and spongy. The patient had suffered no pain, but was conscious of a constant throbbing and pulsation. The most important symptom, however, was the hæmorrhage, which had latterly become a serious source of trouble and distress; it usually occurred at night; it would ooze from the mouth and stain the pillow and sheets, and sometimes trickle into the glottis and cause momentary suffocation.

The treatment which I first adopted in this case was determined by the very *arterial* character of the tumour. I attempted to destroy it by ligature: a needle armed with a double thread was passed through its base, and each portion of the thread was tied so as to strangulate half of its attachment. The ligatures were tied tight, but did not cut through the substance of the growth. Their effect was for the time to produce complete strangulation: the tumour was tense; and the blood could not be squeezed out of it by pressure. This plan did not ultimately succeed, for the size was not permanently diminished and the circulation was re-established. I next removed the tumour by a very tight ligature, cutting it clean off; after this it returned as before, and I finally extirpated it with a scalpel, cutting freely inwards so as to remove a portion of the spongy vascular bone which seemed to form its basal axis. The bone at the base of these growths appears always to be very vascular and open in its texture. Considerable hæmorrhage followed the operation, which ceased under cold and pressure. For a few weeks the cicatrix furnished freely-sprouting granulations: these were abundantly cauterised twice a week, and ultimately yielded a healthy scar. In structure this little mass, when removed, displayed a complicated vascular network, which, under the action of acetic acid, with the microscope, exhibited little else than an elaborate aggregation of the nuclei of blood-vessel muscle-cells. The surface was clothed with epithelium and papillæ, like the gum. I believe that no danger can arise in these cases from the use of the knife in at once extirpating the tumour: the bleeding may be profuse for a minute or two, but it soon ceases.

I have seen a vascular tumour, connected apparently with the periosteum of a loose molar tooth, in which the hæmorrhage was very severe, occurring at night to an extent that was really alarming: the patient was frequently awoke by blood trickling into the glottis, her person and pillow being saturated with blood. The tumour was a tense, pedunculated mass, the size and colour of a morello cherry, attached to the side of an upper molar tooth, half the fangs of which were naked. The extraction of the tooth brought away the tumour with it still attached. The growth immediately shrivelled up to half its previous size, and became soft and flabby.

The accompanying illustration (fig. 83) represents the tumour and tooth as they were after extraction. *l* indicates the neck of the tooth, and *n* the point to which the gum had receded. The stalk of the tumour was connected with the tooth just under the gum.*

Fig. 83.

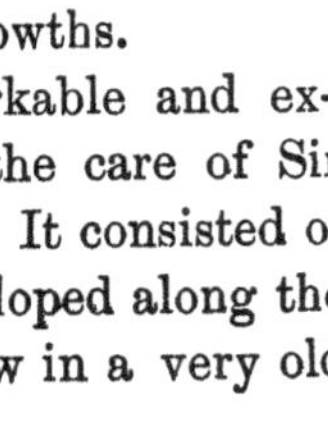

These tumours, as far as I have observed, occur in adult and middle life: they are perfectly innocent, and show no tendency to return when carefully eradicated.

Warty Tumours.—The papillæ of the gum occasionally become hypertrophied into warty growths.

During the summer of 1862 a very remarkable and extremely rare form of this disease came under the care of Sir William Fergusson, at King's College Hospital. It consisted of an exuberant papillary growth, which was developed along the alveolar border on the right side of the lower jaw in a very old man.

In this case the early history and the ultimate result are unfortunately both imperfectly known; and the only record

* "Vascular Tumour, connected with the Dental Periosteum," by S. J. A. Salter. *Trans. Path. Soc.*, vol. v., 1854.

of it which I have been able to obtain consists in a brief and crudely reported *clinique* delivered by Sir William Fergusson when he operated on the patient: this was published in the "Lancet." As, however, the pathological anatomy of the disease is so singular and exceptional, I have thought it well to quote this report *in extenso,* more especially as it is not long.

"Familiar as he, Mr. Fergusson, was with diseases of the jaw—and he had seen as many examples as most surgeons—here was an instance, Mr. Fergusson remarked, of disease he had never seen before or read of. About the middle of June the patient had called upon him with a letter from a friend. He noticed something wrong with his jaw, and, on looking into his mouth, he asked if he had a bit of potato in it. To his astonishment, he found it was a growth upon the jaw. Some surgeons would call it fibrous; but it was a form of disease which he had never met with previously in this or any other part of the body. It looked like vegetable matter or greatly elongated papillæ. He could not undertake to give it a name. It was something like malignant disease; and a question arose as to what ought to be done.

"The friend who wrote to him (Mr. Fergusson) had operated several times. It would, perhaps, have been better to have removed the whole jaw, but he did not like to submit so old a patient to such an operation, for his age was eighty years. He selected a milder method, that of cutting the disease out, instead of making a large wound in the cheek. He removed on this occasion (June 21st) probably the greater part of it, together with its base. It certainly was not unlike medullary disease. He thought he had succeeded in taking away the whole of it. If there should be any left, he expected to remove or destroy it by means of chloride of zinc. We shall see, Mr. Fergusson observed in conclusion, when the granulations spring up, the process the disease may take; and we must look upon the present case more as an instance of the curiosities of pathology than of surgery.

"It may be remarked that the disease was confined to the right side of the lower jaw, and looked like meat that had been macerated for a long time, and had become bleached of a pinkish-white colour.

"On the 12th of July it became necessary to repeat the operation; for although but three weeks had elapsed since the last occasion of removal, the tumour had grown very rapidly, and in general characters resembled its predecessor. It was cut away chiefly by means of curved forceps, and portions of it were scraped from the bone. With regard to the last, very little of it was left, and Mr. Fergusson mentioned that it was necessary to proceed with caution in such an old patient.

"After remaining about another fortnight in the hospital, the patient left for the country. Up to this time there has been no further recurrence. The cicatrix was, however touched with chloride of zinc." ("Lancet," Sept. 6th, 1862, p. 255.)

On applying at King's College Hospital some months afterwards, I was unable to obtain any clinical note, or, indeed, any record of this curious case. The gentleman, however, who had been Mr. Fergusson's dresser while the patient had been in the house, gave me this important information—that the disease of the jaw was unaccompanied by any enlargement of lymphatic glands in its neighbourhood; he also told me that the tumour did not appear to be connected with the bony substance of the jaw. The patient was eighty years of age, and he died shortly after leaving the hospital, apparently from old age and natural decay.

Through the kindness of Mr. Partridge, who secured a portion of the growth when removed, I had an opportunity of examining its structure. It was a curious white mass, consisting of sparse detached fibres, pointed and free at one extremity and attached at the other; in fact, it was a mass of papillæ, many of them nearly an inch long, and similar in shape to the "filiform" papillæ of the tongue; their surface was shreddy and broken; among these elongated processes were a few rounded eminences like "fungiform" papillæ, and these had a smooth unbroken surface. This is represented in fig. 84.

Fig. 84.

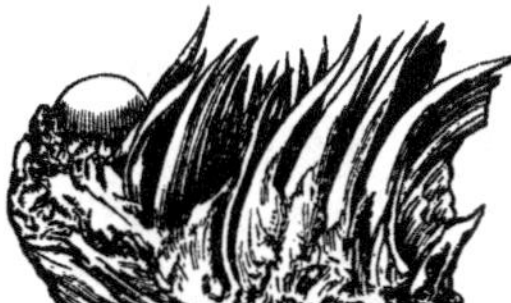

In microscopical structure I found the mass to consist almost entirely of epithelium, principally squamous and flattened; but in other parts the cells were aggregated together in groups, reminding one of the "bird's-nest" arrangement, considered by some pathologists to be diagnostic of epithelial cancer. The long filiform papillæ were striated or fluted in their long direction, and readily broke up into smaller hair-like processes; the centres of these processes consisted of very compact cells, not altogether characteristic of epithelium, but the more superficial were distinctly epithelial. The cells comported themselves as epithelium under the action of chemical reagents.

I did not succeed in making out the deeper structures of the papillæ, neither a limitary membrane nor a vascular loop. The base of the mass which was removed consists of fibrous tissue and a small piece of bone.

In the month of March 1866 a patient was sent up to Guy's Hospital from Dorsetshire to the care of Mr. Cock. In the upper jaw of this patient a growth had developed itself apparently having the same ultimate anatomical structure as the tumour in the previous case.

George Marsh, æt. 57, a butcher and small farmer, resided at Wool, near Wareham, in Dorsetshire. He was under the medical care of Mr. W. S. Granger.

In April 1865, the first upper bicuspid tooth of the right side was observed to be loose, and was removed; it was a sound tooth; the gum around it was supposed to be healthy.

Early in the following August the patient first noticed a slight roughness and swelling on the side of the palate, extending from the inner alveolar border of the gum, where the bicuspid had been removed, towards the vault of the palate; the area thus affected was then about the size of a finger-nail. Smoking made the place smart, but beyond that it was not painful.

The patient now applied to his medical attendant, who burnt the surface with lunar caustic repeatedly. Still the growth advanced; it increased in area, and the roughness became greater by the development of distinct papillæ; these were only partially repressed by the caustic from time to time.

There had never been any discharge, or pain, or general swelling connected with the growth.

At the time of the patient's arrival at the hospital (March

20th, 1866) the growth was the size of a split chesnut, the attached base being rather smaller than the extreme circumference of the tumour; it rested on the side of the hard palate, extending from the edge of the alveolar border to near the summit of the vault. The position, form, and general aspect of the growth, are displayed in the accompanying illustration (fig. 85). One very striking peculiarity cannot, however, be thus exhibited; it is the contrast of the colour of the tumour and that of the surrounding gum; the tumour was creamy white, and the surrounding gum the usual dark purple-red; the contrast was extreme, and the limit quite definite. The growth had much the appearance of a large, flattened, tegumentary wart with unusually long papillæ.

Fig. 85.

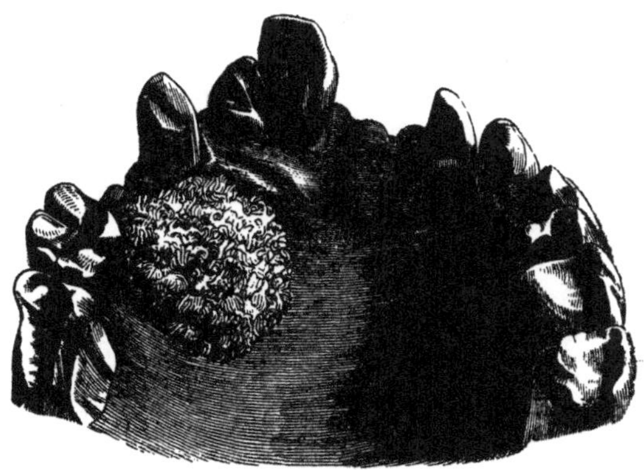

The illustration is drawn from a plaster-of-Paris cast of the upper jaw, which I took previous to the operation. The tumour looks a little smaller than it really was, from the pressure of the wax in taking the model.

On the 23rd of March Mr. Cock extirpated the growth. It was firmly attached to the periosteum of the hard palate, and in its removal the periosteum was stripped from the bone, which was left bare and quite healthy. There was much hæmorrhage and a good deal of difficulty in stopping the bleeding from one artery. As it became necessary to use the cautery, Mr. Cock took the opportunity of destroying by that means the entire circumference of the wound. The patient returned to the country, and was again under the care of Mr. Granger. On the 6th of July following (rather more than three months after the operation) that gentleman kindly reported to me the then condition of his patient.

The wound had healed with a healthy cicatrix; there were no glandular enlargements, and there was no return of the growth. Two small pieces of bone had exfoliated, most probably from the removal of the periosteum and the application of the cautery, as the bone was quite healthy at the time of the operation.

In microscopical structure the tumour consists of a hard mass of fibrous tissue, surmounted by papillæ, and the latter are mainly composed of dense coherent epithelium.

Fig. 86.

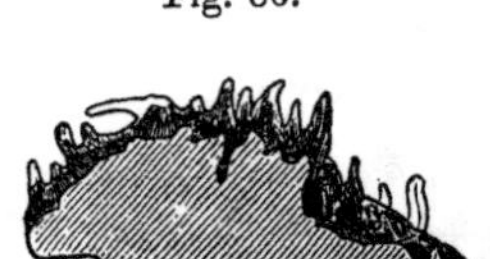

Fig. 87.

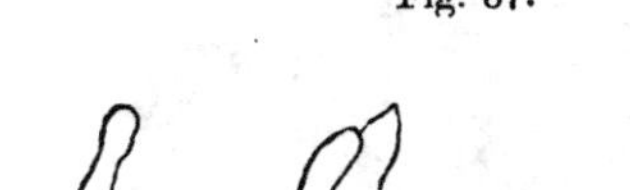

The accompanying figures represent a section of the growth the natural size (fig. 86), and outlines of some of the papillæ enlarged six diameters (fig. 87).

This patient enjoyed complete immunity from discomfort after the operation for nearly three years, excepting that on two or three occasions small pieces of bone were exfoliated. In February 1869 he first noticed that the cicatrix was rough and painful, and about this time the second upper molar on the right side became loose and tender. This was extracted, and about a week afterwards the jaws became firmly closed and fixed. The pain from this time increased and became erratic, wandering all over the side of the head, and the roughness of the cicatrix increased and extended so that the palate on the right side became covered in patches by small warty excrescences. In July 1870 the patient came to London to consult Mr. Cock and myself. The case had now evidently assumed a malignant character. The side of the face and the angle of the jaws were swollen by infiltration, and were hard and red: glands under the jaw were enlarged and indurated: the jaw was firmly closed. There were superficial warty growths all over the upper jaw within the mouth on the right side, and a patch of the same character had grown beneath the middle of the upper lip. The growths were pinkish, and covered with white sodden papillæ. The patient complained of constant and severe suffering over the whole side of the head. From the diffuse nature of the disease operative interference was not urged on the patient; and indeed he preferred to return to the country and allow the malady to take its own course. The poor man lingered on for two years, and died in September 1872, exhausted, starved, and unable to swallow.

The following is another instance of warty tumours on the gums that has occurred in my practice.

Mr. M., a gentleman, twenty-one years of age, came to me in September 1867. At that time nearly all the teeth in the upper jaw, except the canines, were carious, and all the lower molars were in a similar condition. But the most remarkable feature in the case was the state of the gums: the edges of the gums were fringed with wart-like growths, and where the carious cavities reached the necks of the teeth masses of these warts grew into and filled them. These were not the polypus-like excrescences of gum, which one often finds protruding into a carious tooth-cavity, but they were just like tegumentary warts with a cauliflower surface.

The patient informed me that when a little boy he had large numbers of warts on his hands and at the back of his neck. These were destroyed by burning sulphur. About fifteen years of age warts appeared on his face and nose, especially on the *alæ nasi*, and these have continued more or less ever since.

I extracted the whole of the carious teeth, with the view of supplying artificial substitutes, and at the same time pared away all the warty growths: this was in September 1867. In the following January, when the artificial teeth were made, some few small warts had again formed, and these were removed by the knife.

On the 26th of February 1869, the patient again came to me. The gums were covered with a profusion of warts, most of them small, but some as large as a pea: they had no relation to the remaining teeth, but grew principally along the cicatrices where the teeth had been removed. I again pared them away with a scalpel, and the accompanying illustrations (figs. 88, 89) represent the form and character of two of them, enlarged three

Fig. 88.

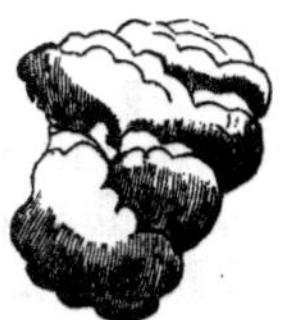

Fig. 89.

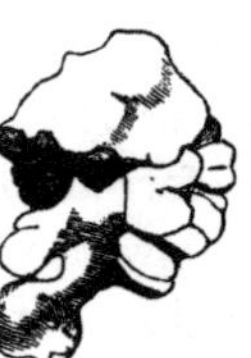

diameters. These figures were drawn from the specimens by my late brother, Dr. Hyde Salter. In structure they partook much of the nature of gum, folded into small tubercular elevations, looking like the head of a cauliflower. The ultimate elements, as seen by high magnifying power, were the same as gum-structure.

I directed the patient in future to brush the gums from time to time, as occasion seemed to require, with a solution of nitrate of silver, with a view to the repression of further warty development.

The histories of these three cases are very different. The histology of the morbid growths is apparently very similar.

In Sir William Fergusson's case the disease did not come to its legitimate issue, as the patient died from another cause, and the question of *malignancy* could not be fairly tested. There was no ulceration, there was no lymphatic-gland enlargement, though the disease had existed a long time. The fact that some of the groups of epithelium were rather bird's-nest-like is not a *proof* of epithelial cancer. I have often seen similar appearances from perfectly healthy gum, especially after maceration, where a cluster of epithelium, coherent together, has "shelled" from the end of a papilla.

The second case ultimately proved to be malignant. In the

third instance the growths were perfectly innocent, and they had, too, a much nearer resemblance, in physical characters, to the gum than in either of the other cases: indeed the warts were clearly of the same nature as those that commonly form on the skin.

I have seen several instances of warts appearing in the mouths of young people, generally where the membrane is dense and skin-like, as in the palate. Such growths I look upon as inno cent, and of the nature of common tegumentary warts. It is difficult to define in an early stage what is malignant and what is innocent; but I should have very little anxiety about one of these warty growths in the mouth of a young patient.

Other Affections of the Gums.

I propose now to consider other morbid affections to which the gums are liable. Some of these are not often submitted to the care or diagnosis of dental surgeons, and in works on our special branch of surgery are omitted, or are imperfectly considered. For convenience I may enumerate these maladies as follows:

Scrofulous ulceration,
Syphilitic affections,
True scurvy,
False scurvy or spongy gums,
Transparent hypertrophy,
Stomatitis in children.

Scrofulous Ulceration.—The structure of the gum is in so many respects similar to that of the skin, that we might naturally expect their morbid changes would be somewhat alike. I have already pointed out the entire similarity of common tegumentary warts and those which occur on the palate, and their occasional concurrence in the same person. I now proceed to describe a singular and interesting case in which scrofulous ulceration occurred on the skin and the gums of a patient at the same time.

John M., a native of Chatham, aged 19, was admitted into Guy's Hospital in July, 1853. He was suffering from phthisical symptoms; he had lost one of his parents from consumption, and other members of the family had shown marked indications of scrofula.

The patient himself was the very embodiment of struma. In early adolescence he was attacked with scrofulous ulceration of the skin and with suppuration of the lymphatic glands. His arms and legs were covered with the scars of the previous ulcerations, and these were of that dark livid hue which is so characteristic of the cicatrices of these strumous sores. His limbs were quite covered with these scars, and they gave the surface a most peculiar aspect. One sore on the arm was still open. The existence of these evidences of strumous ulceration gave a clue to the nature of the affection of the mouth, which would otherwise have been scarcely intelligible; at least it would have been difficult to decide on the nature of the ulcerative process.

There was no history whatever of syphilis. Three years before the date of my notes of the case a sore occurred on the palate, which soon perforated to the nose; so that when he drank some of the fluid came away through the nostrils. This ulcer was about half an inch behind the left canine tooth: it was small, and soon healed on the application of lunar caustic; and the orifice into the nose had completely closed in six months after its first appearance. It is to be remarked that this process was simply one of ulceration; there was no abscess, no exfoliation of bone; and the perforation into the nose was ulcerative.

About eighteen months after the first attack ulceration of a similar character occurred around the gums in the neighbourhood of the upper incisors, and increased until the patient's admission into the hospital; that is, for another period of eighteen months. The ulcerations were superficial and granulating: they were not attended by burrowing, or exfoliation of bone. There was a discharge of pus, but this was from the ulcerating surface.

The ulceration was confined principally to the gum around the four incisors, and it was attended with absorption of the alveoli and a consequent loosening and loss of the teeth. This became conspicuous twelve months from the date of this report and progressively increased.

On admission into the hospital (July, 1853) the condition of the patient's mouth was as follows:—There was a large irregular ulceration in the front of the upper jaw around the four upper incisors and extending backwards about half an inch. The ulceration was irregular and granulating and looking exceedingly like the scrofulous sore still discharging on the arm. There were no sinuses or appearances of dead bone and the alveoli appeared to have vanished by mere absorption. Three of the incisors were hanging quite loose, merely attached to the jaw by their apices and surrounded by pouting granular masses. The fangs of these teeth were quite naked, and the canines were affected in the same way to a less degree.

I extracted the three incisors, much to the patient's relief.

A week afterwards I saw him again: there was no attempt at a healing process. The accompanying illustration is from a model taken on that occasion.

Fig. 90.

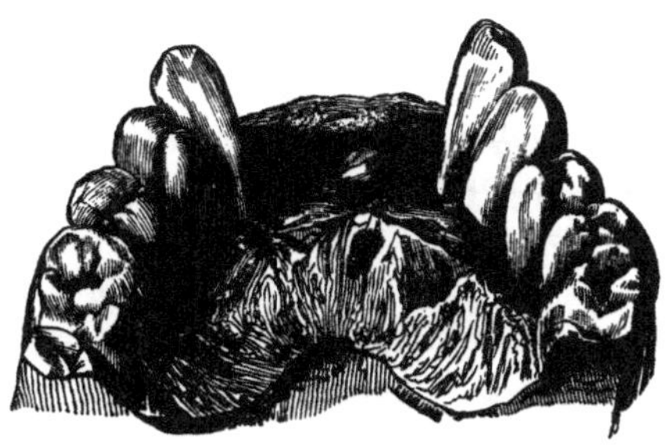

How far this ulceration and tooth-shedding would have proceeded cannot be said, for death terminated the case a few days after the taking of the model.

That similar cases have occurred is most probable, though I am not acquainted with recorded examples. They may have been unintelligible or misunderstood, as would doubtless have happened in this instance but for the very obvious interpretation which the surroundings of the malady indicated.

II. *Syphilitic affections.*—Syphilis is very apt to make its mark on the mucous membrane of the mouth. Probably the tongue most often suffers, and many an instance of ulceration, rhagides, and "glossy-tubercle" upon it, caused by syphilis, meets the eye of the tooth-doctor. Often is a sore of the tongue attributed to the irritation of a tooth, when the tooth's presence has only localised the outbreak of constitutional syphilis. The syphilitic affections, attacking the mucous membrane immediately surrounding the teeth, which I have seen, have been—

Psoriasis,
Ulceration, and
Condyloma.

An interesting example of the first has just occurred to me.

A. G—, a monthly nurse about 60 years of age, applied to me, May, 1873, at Guy's Hospital on account of a singular affection of the gums which existed around the two wisdom teeth of the upper jaw and extended to the soft palate. She had been seen by a general practitioner who was attending at the house where the woman was nursing, and he, considering that the complaint arose from the irritation of the wisdom teeth, sent her to me. Having seen a somewhat similar case before, with a clear syphilitic history, I suspected strongly that this was also syphilitic; but I could, on the patient's first visit, make out no history to tally with my suspicions. The malady had existed about a month, and was regularly and slowly getting worse. The appearances in the mouth were these—At the back of the upper jaw on each side the mucous membrane and gum were swollen, thickened and red, with here and there white patches. There was a great increase of epithelial growth, which was in parts soft and sodden, and in other parts hanging in shreds from contiguous red, raw-looking patches. It suggested to me a condition such as psoriasis palmaria would exhibit if constantly immersed in fluid. The affection was most marked immediately around the wisdom teeth, but it extended in a less degree to near the mesial line of the mouth. The patient complained of much heat and itching of the part; and she stated that taking her meals was a misery to her, on account of the pain which all condiments and even contact of food occasioned. The wisdom teeth were both useless—one carious, the other loose, and neither had opponents in the lower jaw. So I removed them, as a preliminary for treatment and diagnosis.

Seven days afterwards the patient again came to me, with the local symptoms entirely unrelieved by the removal of the teeth; indeed, the psoriasis had spread, and the whole of the soft palate, with much in the anterior part of the mouth, was involved in the disease.

I was now entirely satisfied that the malady was of a constitutional and not of a mere local character; but the explanation was still problematical. Here was a respectable woman past sixty years of age (and I know enough of the family to be satisfied of her respectability), whose husband had been dead for more than ten years, suddenly attacked with symptoms which I felt sure were syphilitic. She, an old woman, was leading a virtuous and industrious life as a monthly nurse in the family of a gentleman of fortune. The history of the family and the surrounding circumstances brought out the truth, and the mystery was solved.

At my patient's second visit I learnt the following facts.

Mrs. ——, whom she nursed, was duly confined, but the child was cachectic, its nates and genitals were covered with eruption, in fact it was afflicted with inherited syphilis. While attending to the child my patient cut her finger, and the wound instead of healing became an obstinate sore. Ultimately it did cicatrise, and then came the psoriasis of the gums and palate. Acting upon these indications, I ordered the patient to take three grains of iodide of potassium thrice daily, and to apply to the affected part a solution of nitrate of silver (eight grains to an ounce of water) with a camel's-hair brush night and morning.

This treatment completed the diagnosis by curing the patient. She rapidly got well: in three weeks every vestige of the malady had disappeared, and the patient's general health was much improved.

Ulceration is probably the most common of the secondary syphilitic affections which attack the gums. I have seen several unmistakable cases; but the narration of one will probably be more interesting than generalisations upon many.

F. T——, a medical student, had inoculated his finger attending a midwifery case. The chancre on the finger and many weeks of secondary symptoms followed, when he was attacked with ulceration of the gums. The ulcers occurred on each side of the lower jaw, on the lingual aspect; that on the right side was small and oval, on the left there was a long narrow ulceration about three-eighths of an inch in width, extending from beneath the wisdom tooth, about one inch forward. The surface of the ulcers was red, and the edges were grey and ragged; they were very painful, and excited a large secretion of saliva. The patient was taking iodide of potassium at the time of their appearance.

The ulcers rapidly healed under the application of a solution of nitrate of silver, eight grains in an ounce of water, as indeed most non-malignant ulcerations of the mucous membrane of the mouth usually do.

Condylomata of the gums are very rare. I can only call to mind a single instance: in this one there were rounded eminences on or rather in the gum, on the outer side of the lower jaw, apparently circumscribed plastic exudations. They were associated with glossy tubercle of the tongue, which is probably of the same essential nature, and ordinary condylomata in certain other regions of the body. The patient was a woman of more than doubtful character, and the case was certainly syphilitic.

III. *True Scurvy.*—Few dentists, I imagine, have seen or are likely to see cases of genuine scurvy, and few indeed are likely to have the treatment of such cases. Still it is possible that some members of the profession, residing in a seaport town, may be consulted as to the nature of the disease, where the gum element of the affection may be the only, or the most marked symptom of this peculiar form of purpura.

Many years ago, when in my pupilage, articled to a surgeon in a seaport, which had a large trade with Canada and Newfoundland, I saw not a few cases of scurvy, and I well remember that the very able and intelligent gentleman, whose pupil I was, pointed out to me the condition of the gums as one of the most characteristic symptoms. I was not, however, then sufficiently informed to appreciate the pathological instruction which these cases gave.

Since I have devoted my attention to the diseases of the teeth and their contiguous structures I have seen but one case of genuine scurvy. Indeed, the disease has of late years become very rare. Its cause is so well understood and its prevention is so readily effected, that ships are seldom sent to sea so ill-found as to render scurvy possible, if the ordinary daily diet is adopted; and the laws affecting maritime hygiene are such as to render those liable to severe penalties, who subject their mariners to a diet so defective as to induce scurvy.

Scurvy is a form of purpura in which the gums suffer with extreme and characteristic severity. The malady is brought on by the prolonged abstinence from vegetables, especially uncooked vegetables.

Dr. Budd, who was formerly physician to the hospital ship "Dreadnought," had peculiar opportunities of studying this disease, and he has contributed an exhaustive article on the subject to the pages of the "Library of Medicine" (vol. v., pp. 58–95.)

The affection of the gums in this malady he thus describes:—

"The gums soon become sore, and apt to bleed on the slightest touch. On examination they are found to be swelled and spongy, and of livid redness. Lividity of the gums first appears, and is always deepest at their free edges, diminishing gradually towards the roots of the teeth; while the lining membrane of the lips does not exhibit it in the slightest degree, but, on the contrary, is unusually pale.

"As the disease advances the gums become more swelled and more livid, forming, in some cases, a black spongy mass, which completely conceals the teeth; and they frequently slough, especially at their edges, leaving the crowns of the teeth exposed; the teeth themselves become loose, and often drop out, without having suffered decay; and the breath is remarkably offensive."

The case of scurvy which I have referred to as coming under my observation occurred in the practice of my late colleague, Dr. Hughes, and it displayed all the characteristics described by Dr. Budd. The gums alone were affected of the parts within the mouth; and the changes which they, the teeth, and the alveoli underwent were very interesting. The ecchymosis of the gums was complete; they were large thick fringes infiltrated with blood. These fringes of bloody tissue seemed so totally devitalised by the large amount of extravasated blood which pervaded them, that sphacelus followed, and considerable sloughing of the substance of the gum resulted, leaving the necks of the teeth bare. But the effects of the malady did not cease here; the alveolar socket-walls became absorbed, and the teeth were very loose, so much so that I thought their loss by falling out would inevitably follow at no distant date.

I should mention that this patient had many other symptoms of scurvy, among them various forms and characters of ecchymosis and blood extravasation in different parts of the body. Appropriate treatment was adopted, especially in diet—an abundant supply of succulent vegetables. The result was marvellous, almost magical; the escape of blood from the vessels ceased, and rapid repair of previous lesion concurred. That which struck me most remarkably was the complete restoration to a normal condition of the gums, and the rapid tightening of the teeth. The sloughing edges of the gums not only healed, but drew up around the necks of the teeth in a surprising manner. And the teeth themselves, especially the incisors (upper and lower), which one would, in any chronic case, have condemned as to be shed by looseness within a few months, tightened again completely.

The case, though acute, was not of long standing, and the patient was a vigorous young man; otherwise the issue as regards the teeth might probably have been otherwise.

I cannot take a better opportunity than this of narrating the following interesting case which occurred in the hospital practice of my late brother, Dr. Hyde Salter. It was a form of purpura most severely attacking the gums, and perhaps allied to scurvy. Dr. Salter sent me the particulars as I now give them in his own words, accompanied by a sketch of the little mechanical apparatus which he devised, and which so successfully accomplished its intended purpose. The patient suffered from a constitutional diathesis of a marked hæmorrhagic character, and had several attacks of general bleeding, of which the most severe is here recorded:—

"Catherine C——, aged about forty-five, of florid complexion, had been liable for many years to bruise visibly on the slightest blow or pressure, and to have black-and-blue patches of various sizes come out without any apparent reason on different parts of her body. On some occasions these patches and spots were so numerous as to be thickly scattered all over her person. They were of two kinds—small spots and specks of a red or purple colour, having all the characteristics of true purpura, and larger blue patches, from the size of a pea to that of a hen's egg, less defined than the others, and considerably raised above the surface. After remaining for a few days these patches would undergo a change, becoming green and then tawny, and so fading away. On the occasions of these purpurous eruptions spontaneous hæmorrhages would occur from the tongue, gums, fauces, lungs, bowels, &c. On some of these occasions she nearly bled to death.

"On one occasion the bleeding had continued so long and was so unmanageable that I admitted her into the hospital (Charing Cross), fearing that she would not survive above a day or two. The principal bleeding on this occasion, which all efforts had failed to control, was from the gum between the two inferior bicuspid teeth, on the right side, where the blood welled up without cessation, and had done so day and night for upwards of a month. I discovered that lateral pressure on the gum, applied with the finger and thumb on the inside and outside of the jaw at this situation, arrested the bleeding as long as the pressure was applied, though the blood immediately flowed again when the pressure was removed. I conceived therefore the idea of producing sustained pressure for an unlimited time by means of a spring, which should take the place of the finger and thumb, which the patient might wear in the mouth, and which might arrest the hæmorrhage for so long a time that it might ultimately be removed without its recurrence. This was easily managed by placing over the teeth at the seat of the hæmorrhage a little steel spring bent in a horse-shoe shape, the opening between the extremities of which was a little narrower than the distance between the inner and outer aspects of the gum. When applied it was found to exercise considerable pressure and completely to arrest the bleeding. It was put on about five o'clock in the evening, and the patient wore it all night, but in the morning the pressure it produced caused such pain and swelling of the gum that it could no longer be borne. When removed, however, no bleeding returned, the explanation of which I have no doubt was, that the little clip had left its equivalent behind it in the tension of the swollen gum—the extrinsic pressure of the spring had been succeeded by the intrinsic pressure of the swelling. The cure was final and complete. The poor woman is living at the present time, and has never had so alarming a return of the hæmorrhage since."

The accompanying illustrations, drawn by my late brother, show the apparatus and its application. Fig. 91 represents the steel spring itself, and fig. 92 is a diagram showing its action *in sitû*.

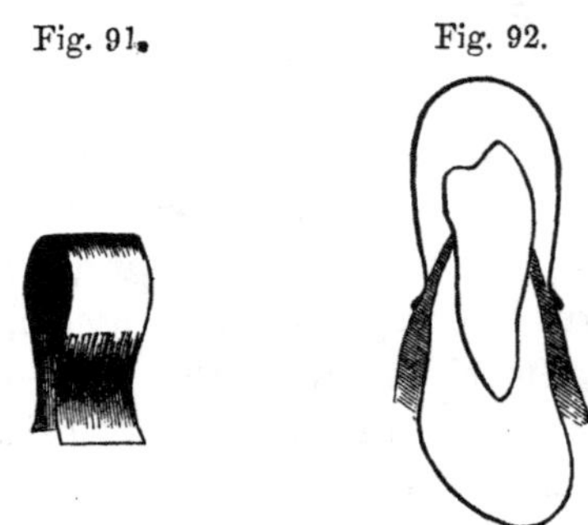

Fig. 91. Fig. 92.

This case occurred about five years since. A little more than a year ago I saw Mrs. C——, the patient, and I heard from her own lips a graphic account of her case, and of the efficacy of the device which Dr. Salter adopted to arrest the bleeding of the gum. The woman is now in very fair health, and though the hæmorrhagic diathesis remains, and ever will remain, she has long ceased to suffer from any acute symptoms.

False Scurvy, or Spongy Gums.—This malady has no relation whatever to scurvy properly so called. It is, I believe, generally more or less the manifestation of constitutional vice; but whereas, in true scurvy, there is sanguineous extravasation in the gums, in false scurvy there is vascular dilatation of the papillary and other capillaries,* with a general thickening of the gum itself.

In this malady there is a thickening and protrusion of the gums generally, especially along the edge. In young persons and in early cases the tongues of gum between the necks of

* Many years ago my friend, Mr. John Henry Roberts, of St. John's Wood, showed me a beautiful specimen of injected gum, obtained from a monkey suffering from chronic congestion of the gum. Since then Mr. Tomes has figured this identical specimen. To be properly appreciated it should be seen in contrast with healthy gum magnified to the same extent. As Mr. Roberts pointed out to me, the change consists of great enlargement of the capillaries, without increase of number or alteration of arrangement.

the teeth become elongated and enlarged, but in older persons and in cases of long standing these projections are lost, and the gum has a thick even edge. The gums are very vascular, and liable to bleed from very slight friction. Tartar is apt to accumulate, especially in rings and ridges out of sight, beneath the edge of the gum.

The gum, the subjacent fibrous tissue, and the periosteum of the alveoli are so continuous in structure, that they suffer together in this condition, and where the malady has been of long duration the sockets become less rigid around the tooth-fangs, the edges of the bone become absorbed, and the teeth loosened. It is attended by a considerable increase of the ooze which is secreted immediately around the teeth, and in some cases which are acute this secretion is certainly purulent. Pus is readily formed on the surface of certain mucous membranes; but in the gum there is a special structure from which it appears to emanate.

As I have stated in my introductory remarks, there is a special structure around the necks of the teeth which yields a secretion capable of rapid transformation into pus, and it is probably from this source that the purulent matter in spurious scurvy emanates.

The causes of this malady are neither constant nor always intelligible. It is frequently associated with chronic dyspepsia and general ill-health. It also occurs very often in females who have had frequent pregnancies, and in both sexes it frequently seems to depend upon irregularities of the teeth, in some instances where they are crowded, and in others where they are much separated. Another frequent cause is mercurial action at some previous time of life. Patients may have taken mercury even to a slight degree, and the gums may have apparently entirely recovered themselves, when at a distant period, sometimes many years afterwards, spurious scurvy will arise and produce rapid absorption of the alveolar processes and loosen the teeth. Other drugs besides mercury have the power of producing this condition, both as a temporary and evanescent state, and one of more permanent duration. This is particularly the case with iodide of potassium.

The *treatment* of this disease consists in endeavouring to restore general health, and extreme cleanliness of the mouth.

Patients are apt to shrink from the use of the tooth-brush, and the result is the necks of the teeth become uncleanly, and increase the congestion of the gums which already exists. In the first place, all the tartar should be removed from the teeth, and the bleeding which occurs during the operation will itself have a salutary effect. The patient should be enjoined to clean the teeth most assiduously, and a tolerably hard brush which will produce a certain amount of bleeding on each occasion will do good. At the same time an astringent wash should also be used, and this may well consist of a solution of alum in a decoction of cinchona. I am in the habit of applying this lotion with much benefit.

Transparent hypertrophy of the gums is one of the most singular morbid appearances I have ever seen. It is very rare. It is not described in books, as far as I know, and with the exception of one case which was under my own care, all that I have heard respecting it has been from my relative, Mr. Bell, who saw a few cases during the half-century he was in practice.

The change consists in the slow and gradual hypertrophy of the extreme edge of the gum, at first like a cord, and very sharply marked from the immediately contiguous healthy-looking structure; but the most remarkable circumstance is the singular colour of the hypertrophied part: it is pale pink and semi-transparent. It is very callous and insensitive, and scarcely bleeds when cut. As the disease progresses the hypertrophy of the gum-edge increases, but it does not alter its character or lose its sharply-defined limit. The teeth, where the affection exists, become slowly dislocated and pushed into irregular positions; they ultimately become very loose: when extracted scarcely any blood flows. Where the tooth is removed the gum heals very slowly indeed, and the edge of the wound long continues of the same pale transparent aspect.

Mr. Bell has furnished me with the following notes:—

"The most remarkable case of this form of gum-hypertrophy which ever occurred in my practice was that of a young woman, aged 22, who was under my care at Guy's Hospital for a considerable period.

"The whole of the gum in both jaws was greatly thickened,

and had a semi-transparent appearance, of a pale pink colour. The substance of the enlarged gum was very firm, and about a quarter of an inch thick at the edge; in extent it was abruptly limited to the gum itself, the integument beyond this limit not having any unusual structure. No pain was produced by cutting the growth, and so slight was the supply of blood that scarcely any flowed from the incision or upon extracting a tooth.

"The alveolar process gradually became absorbed, and every tooth, one after another, was lost. During this period there was not the slightest inflammation, nor did she suffer any pain; in fact, the looseness of the teeth produced no other trouble than the mere mechanical loss of power.

"As the teeth came out, or were extracted, the gums very slowly healed. Some months after the last was removed she was able to wear an entire set of teeth.

"During the whole period she was in tolerable health, with the exception of continued amenorrhœa.

"I should add that in the early treatment of the case I employed free scarification and strong astringent lotions, but they produced no effect. I kept the patient in the hospital for a very long time, for the purpose of watching the whole progress and termination of the case.

"I have seen this same condition in a less degree in a few instances. In each the patient was a woman, and suffering (I believe also in each) from amenorrhœa."

The patient whom I attended had been under Mr. Bell's care before I saw her. The malady was precisely the same as he describes, but it affected the teeth in succession.

Miss S——, a maiden lady about sixty years of age, of very unhealthy appearance, applied to me at Christmas 1861 to have a tooth extracted. Upon inspecting her mouth I found that only four teeth remained; all the others, she told me, had been extracted by Mr. Bell under the same circumstances as the bicuspid she now wished removed. This tooth was loose and slightly painful, and around it was hypertrophied gum, which looked like a ring of clear, pale pink glass, sharply defined, and about the thickness of a goose-quill. She informed me that for many years—more than twenty—she had been afflicted with this disease of the gums, attacking in succession the neighbourhood of one or more teeth in an indiscriminate manner at different parts of the mouth. When once the gum became thus affected the contiguous tooth was doomed. It was only a matter of time; the hypertrophy increased, the tooth first loosened and then became painful, and its extraction was soon necessary.

I noticed that the gum around another tooth had already commenced to exhibit the same change; and about a year afterwards I extracted this tooth also. Though so long a period had elapsed, the clear tissue around the cicatrix, where the last tooth was removed, had not all disappeared.

Since then I have extracted the last two teeth under precisely similar circumstances; the last of all was the left lower wisdom tooth. Being very ill and nervous, Miss S—— postponed the operation till the tooth was nearly buried in the glassy mass.

In this patient, as described before, the growth was insensitive and nearly bloodless.

In extracting the second tooth a small portion of the gum came away with it. I found that the epithelial covering was very thin, and the papillæ were short and seemed expanded; so that instead of being like the fingers of a glove they looked like a series of half-circles.

One of the most remarkable points in this malady is the stagnation which follows the extraction of the teeth. Instead of the wound closing and the gum becoming healthy and healing, it goes on for months with the least apparent change.

What the etiology of this condition may be I cannot suggest. It is altogether different from anything else I have ever seen.

Stomatitis in Children.—I have frequently had in hospital practice a peculiar form of ulcerated inflammation of the mouth occurring in children, not uncommonly though by no means always associated with caries of the temporary molar teeth. It affects the gum on the outer side of the jaw and usually the inner surface of the cheek, corresponding to the interval between the upper and lower teeth. It is accompanied with considerable induration of the sub-mucous tissue, and the surface is usually irregularly ulcerated. Children who are thus affected are more or less feverish, and the odour of the breath is most offensive. What is remarkable is that it occurs in children apparently in previous good health, and the malady is certainly either contagious or infectious, or at all events depends upon some generally prevalent influence, as it will attack several children in the same family or in the same immediate locality. In treating these cases I have always removed any teeth which might be supposed to produce irritation, and have treated the ulcerated surface with a weak solution of nitrate of silver, about two grains to an ounce of water, applied with a camel's hair pencil, at the same time treating the child's febrile condition with general remedies. I have had a large number of these cases among the out-patients of Guy's Hospital; and with the exception of considerable contraction of the cicatrices of the cheek in some instances, my patients have done well.

CHAPTER XIV.

CONGENITAL HYPERTROPHY OF THE GUM AND ALVEOLAR BORDERS OF THE MAXILLÆ.

THE diseased condition which I propose to treat in this chapter is very rare: it occurs in very young children, and in the recorded examples of it, has been noticed so early in infancy that it has in all probability been co-existent with birth. The first published example of this condition occurred in the practice of Dr. Gross, of Philadelphia, from whose elaborate* "System of Surgery" the following account is drawn:—

"The only case of the kind that I have ever seen came under my observation in 1855, in a lad of ten years old, remarkable for his stunted development, ill-shaped head, and large abdomen. The morbid growth affected the gums of both jaws, and was of a dense fibroid structure. It first began to attract attention at the age of nine months, but there can be no doubt, from its history, that it had existed from birth.

"The gums of the upper jaw formed a tumour of a pale colour, inelastic, perfectly insensible, and of a firm consistence, presenting very much the appearance of the snout of a hog. It stood off very obliquely, and received but a very partial covering from the corresponding lip. It was rough on the surface, and was about an inch and a quarter in its antero-posterior diameter, its width having been about one inch and a half. At its free margin, which was quite irregular, was seen the tip of the left central incisor. Extending back from this tumour, on each side of the whole length of the jaw, was the enlarged jaw, forming a thick, broad ridge, completely imbedding the teeth. At several points, particularly behind, the morbid growth was more than nine lines in width; in front and at the middle it

* *A System of Surgery, &c.*, by S. D. Gross, M.D. Philadelphia, 1862. Second edition, vol. ii. p. 534.

was less. It was of a more florid colour than the main tumour, but of about the same degree of consistence. Opposite the bicuspid teeth, on each side, it exhibited a remarkable granulated appearance, the excrescences having a pediculated form, and being folded upon each other. Projecting towards the roof of the mouth, it greatly encroached upon its cavity, lessening its capacity, and thus interfering with its functions, as well as with speech and respiration.

"The lower gum was in the same condition as the upper, being equally hard and insensible, but less developed. It was of a bluish florid complexion, and larger in front and behind than at the intermediate points; its surface was uneven, and so prominent as to hide all the teeth, except the central incisors, the point of the right cuspid, and the cusps of each deciduous and first permanent molars." In this case there was hypertrophy of the papillæ of the tongue.

Another example of this disease occurred in the practice of Mr. George Pollock, of St. George's Hospital, in the year 1859, and through the kindness of Mr. Pollock I had an opportunity of examining the case.* This patient was a little girl, and at the time of her admission into the hospital was eight years of age. At birth the only thing observed as unusual about the child was a very large quantity of coarse hair on the head, and also much on the arms and legs. At a fortnight old a tooth was cut, and by the fifth week six had come through the gum. It was then remarked that the gums were full, thick and puffy: they continued to increase in bulk; and at two years of age they were cauterised, and all the temporary teeth, which had appeared, were extracted. When admitted into the hospital (at eight years of age) the child's appearance was very strange: her head was covered thick with coarse, rank, auburn hair, which grew very low on the forehead and in front of the ears on to the cheeks; the arms and legs were also covered thick with hair. Her growth was short and heavy, and the expression stolid, stupid and dull. The patient was epileptic. But the mouth presented the most strange deformity. A large mass, pink and smooth, protruded between the lips, which they did not and could not cover; it was slightly corrugated and indistinctly lobed; the

* An account of this case has been published by the author in Holmes's *System of Surgery*. London, 1863, vol. iv. p. 18.

structure was very dense, inelastic and insensitive, and appeared skin-like on the surface. The greater bulk proceeded from the upper jaw, and was most developed in the front of the mouth; but the same condition appeared along the whole edge of both jaws, that of the lower jaw being less, and covered and overlapped by the upper.

The growth of this large mass was principally external as regards the alveolar border, and forwards as regards the oral cavity; still it encroached both on the front and sides of the palatal arch in the upper jaw, and somewhat upon the region of the tongue in the lower.

Fig. 93.

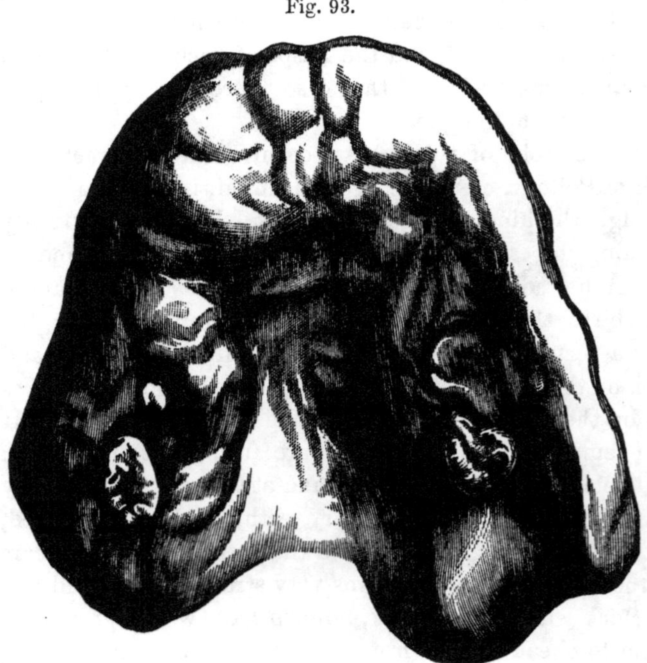

The accompanying illustration is taken from the plaster cast of the upper jaw: it is inverted—the edge of the jaw and the palatal surface being presented to view. The first permanent molars, and the posterior cusps of the second temporary molars, are seen to have pierced the gum—the rest of the teeth being hidden by the thick cushion of hypertrophied fibro-mucous membrane. In structure this hypertrophied mass consisted of an expanded and prolonged development of the alveolar borders of the maxillæ and an immense thickening of the fibrous tissue of the gum, with a proportionately exuberant growth of the papillary surface. The removal of portions of the mass by surgical operation gave opportunities of examining its precise nature. The edges of the maxillary bones had much increased in vertical growth and had extended laterally, while the buccal and labial plates of the alveoli were separated by a wide interval from the palatal: there was a general out-growth and expansion of the oral edges of the jaw bones. In the front of the upper jaw, where the development was greatest, the fibrous mass extended in some places more than three-quarters of an inch beyond the alveolar edge, which it thus covered in with a dense cushion. Those of the temporary teeth, which had not been extracted, were deeply embedded in the mass; the crowns of the second temporary molars in the lower jaw, and the posterior cusps of the same teeth in the upper jaw, being all that were now visible. The crowns of all four first permanent molars had appeared: the amount of the hypertrophy had been slight towards the back of the mouth, and their extrusion through the gum had been scarcely impeded.

Portions of the hypertrophied growth that were removed displayed in section the remaining temporary teeth completely clothed with the thick fibrous growth, the fangs embedded in sockets, but the crowns free of bone, and each closely surrounded by a serous-like chamber without any communication with the surface. One of the superior central incisors was overlaid by fibrous tissue and gum by a thickness measuring nearly an inch. The fangs of the permanent teeth were developed in accordance with the age of the patient: not so, however, was the relation of the bony covering of the crowns of the teeth. In many cases (as regards the incisors and first premolars) the bony loculi surrounding the crowns should have been removed by absorption; such, however, was not the case: the teeth were still surrounded by bone. In the socket of the first temporary incisors a small absorbed orifice existed leading into the loculus of the permanent tooth, such as is usually found about five years old: this patient was eight. But the most remarkable point of structure in this growth was the great development of papillæ.

The accompanying figure, 94, displaying a section (vertical to the surface) of a portion of the mass, shows how largely the papillary structure was hypertrophied. The epithelium had changed into a very thick and hard epidermis, beneath which were enormously long papillæ. In some parts these were evenly covered in by the epiderm; in other places, the exuberant epithelium was insufficient and bundles of papillæ stood up with clefts and fissures between similar contiguous growths: such masses were like warts. In the middle of the figure is seen the crown of the right temporary central incisor tooth.

Fig. 94.

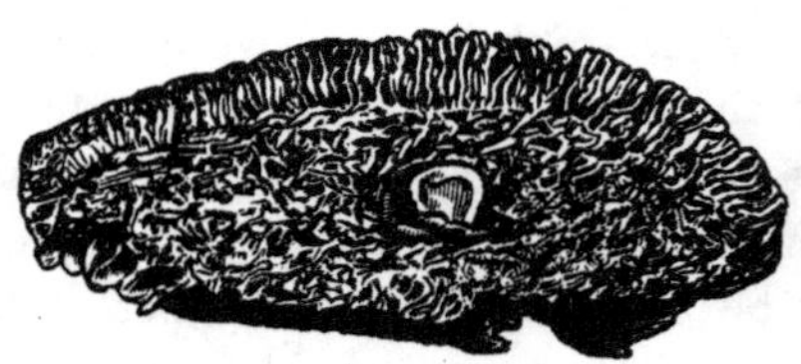

In natural, healthy gum the papillæ vary from about $\frac{1}{75}$ to $\frac{1}{35}$ of an inch in length; but in this morbid growth they appeared from the $\frac{1}{6}$ to $\frac{1}{4}$ of an inch long, and when by maceration the outer epiderm has been removed the papillæ stand up like the pile of plush or velvet and may be brushed from side to side by the finger. In the mouths of old people destitute of teeth, whose bare gums are exposed to the rough attrition of food, the papillæ become much elongated and enlarged, attaining sometimes the $\frac{1}{16}$ of an inch in length. In this case the exposure to rough external influences may in some degree perhaps account for the hypertrophy of the papillæ; but I apprehend that this anatomical condition has also another meaning, and that it is an essential part of the disease; it is quite in keeping with the rugged and thick skin which this patient exhibited, with the singular coarseness of the hair upon the head, and its abundant distribution over the body, and also the enormous teeth which were found embedded in the jaws. The permanent teeth, which were removed by the operations adopted for the relief of this deformity, are excessively large, especially the superior central incisors; they are larger than any others I have seen from a female mouth.

I need not here descant on the morphological relations which subsist between the teeth, the hair, and the papillæ: their exuberant development in these cases seems to imply a general tegumentary and papillary hypertrophy as the essence of the disease—this hypertrophy manifesting itself with especial stress upon those papillary structures the teeth and gums, which are formed on the free edges of the maxillary bones. The redundant growth of the alveolar processes, and the edges of the maxillæ are not at all inconsistent with this interpretation. In the evolution of the teeth the production of their sockets and the growth of the contiguous bone is altogether secondary and proportional; and this osteal expansion vanishes when the teeth are removed. An excessive developmental activity arising in the teeth and gums would of necessity involve exalted nutrition in those portions of the jaws which are contiguous, and in a certain sense *contingent* as far as the teeth are concerned.

The *treatment* in both Mr. Pollock's and Dr. Gross's cases was the same. It consisted in the removal of the projecting masses by means of the knife and bone-nippers. The operation was not performed at once, but in detail as the patient could bear it, and thus the alveolar borders were curtailed to within moderate limits. There has been a slight tendency in both cases to a return of the growth; it has, however, been but slight, and has not progressed: after a few months, in Mr. Pollock's case, it grew no more. Unfortunately the treatment employed entailed the loss of the teeth in the front of the mouth; but there was no alternative: to remove the tumour involved the teeth also, and had the growth not been cut away, the teeth, though retained, would have been useless—permanently embedded in the mass.*

* Two similar cases of later date have also been recorded. One occurred in University College Hospital under the care of Mr. Erichsen, and is described by Mr. Heath (*Injuries and Diseases of the Jaw*, p. 189. London, 1868). The other is published by Mr. Waterman, an American surgeon, in the *Boston Medical and Surgical Journal*, April 8, 1869, p. 167.

CHAPTER XV.

THE IMPACTION OF PERMANENT TEETH IN THE SUBSTANCE OF THE MAXILLARY BONES.

It not unfrequently happens that certain of the temporary teeth are found present and firm in the adult mouth, whilst the corresponding permanent teeth—those which should have succeeded and replaced them—have not made their appearance. This condition is most often seen in reference to the temporary molars of the lower jaw, and the canines of the upper. These teeth are sometimes retained to a very advanced period of life; and I have once seen the lower temporary molars firmly implanted and useful for mastication in a man at the age of sixty-five. In these cases the presence of the temporary tooth is almost always associated, not with the total suppression and absence of the corresponding permanent one, but with its presence in an abnormal position.

The permanent teeth may be thus locked up in the substance of the jaws in several ways. The teeth themselves may be perfectly developed, and placed in a normal direction, but too deeply embedded in the maxillæ; in other instances there may be an abnormal direction of growth, while the position as regards proximity to the alveolar edge is natural, in each case presenting circumstances which are efficient to bring about impaction in the jaw, and incompatible with the extrusion and replacement of the temporary teeth by the permanent. There is yet a third condition in which, though the tooth grow in a right direction, and is originally in a right position, it still remains impacted in the substance of the jaw, the temporary tooth retaining its original site; this circumstance being dependent upon the non-development of the fang of the permanent tooth.

The forces in operation which cause the impaction of teeth

are in some cases beyond our ken, but in others are obvious and easily recognised. In the former there are doubtless disturbed vital processes of development which we do not recognise, but which determine that one or more teeth should range out of normal order. In the latter the burying of the tooth in the jaw is simply accommodation for want of space, as for example an embedded *dens sapientiæ* in a short lower jaw: so the upper canine tooth, in a narrow jaw, where the lateral incisor and first bicuspid have long preceded it, and have come in contact, may find refuge obliquely buried in the substance of the jaw, nearly as readily as when it pierces backwards in the palate. I have known a lower bicuspid driven deep into the jaw, though not absolutely impacted, by a regulation plate worn on a temporary molar, the latter tooth having forced down and kept down the bicuspid by the pressure far below its neighbours.

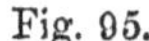

Fig. 95.

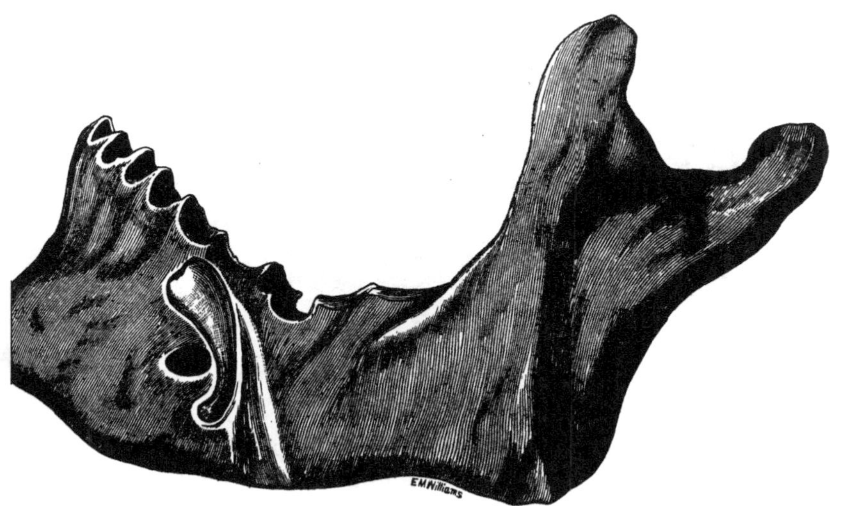

In the fifth volume of the "Guy's Hospital Reports" (1859), I published descriptions and illustrations of several examples of tooth-impaction; from the paper in question the following account has been copied:—

The first of these figures (fig. 95) illustrates a specimen in which the first bicuspid tooth of the lower jaw, on the left side, is impacted in the substance of the bone immediately behind and above the mental foramen: it has an oblique direction, the crown pointing upwards and forwards. The tooth is somewhat curved in form, and at its extremity there is a nodule of exostosis; it is of about natural length and size, and its upper extremity is about two lines below the edge of the alveolus.

On the right side of the same jaw, precisely the same condition existed. On this side, however, the bone has not been sufficiently chipped away to see the condition of the extremity of the fang. I have not thought it necessary to publish this second figure.

The second illustration (fig. 96) is that of an inferior maxilla of an adult, in which all the permanent teeth are present in their natural position, except the right canine; in its place, between

Fig. 96.

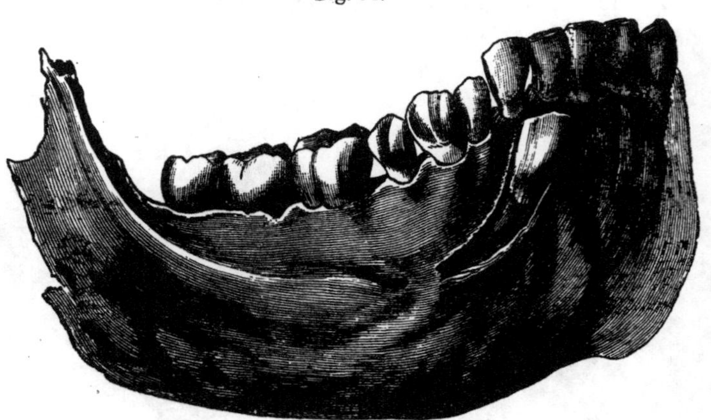

the lateral incisor and the first bicuspid, the temporary tooth is firmly retained. By removing the front of the bone the permanent tooth is displayed, passing obliquely upwards and forwards from just in front of the mental foramen to a position opposite the upper part of the fangs of the right lateral and central incisors; the point of the cusp, corresponding to the interval between these teeth, is about a line from the upper surface of the bone.

The third example (fig. 97) is of the lower jaw of a child, in which all the temporary teeth are present. Near the base of the jaw, scarcely two lines from its lower edge, at a position a little in front of the point intermediate between the chin and angle of the bone, is seen (by the removal of the outer table of bone) a molar tooth, in a horizontal position, the crown looking for-

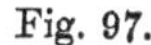

Fig. 97.

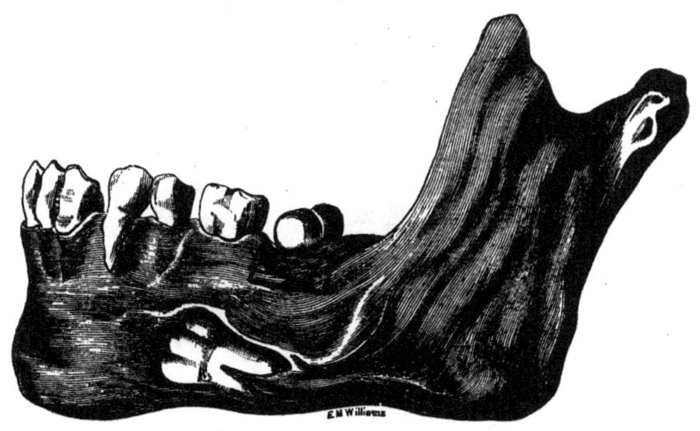

wards. The fangs seem perfectly formed, and the tooth matured. Apparently it is the second permanent molar. The distance of this tooth from the alveolar edge, and its direction, are very remarkable.

In the fourth specimen (fig. 98) the canine of the left side of the upper jaw is placed obliquely and almost hori-

Fig. 98.

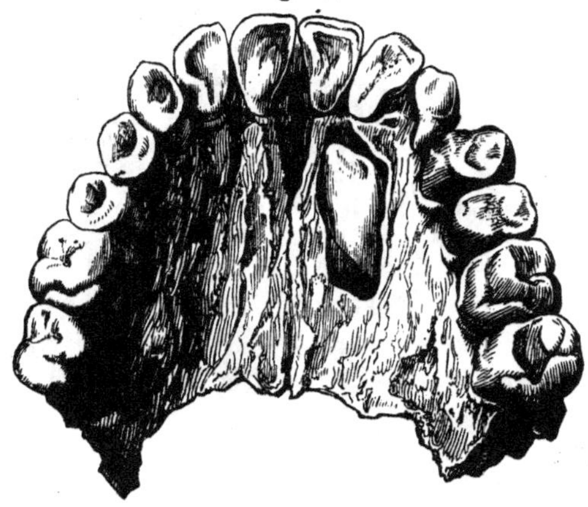

zontally in the substance of the maxilla. The tooth was originally covered by bone, which has been removed. The point of the cusp is immediately to the left of the incisive foramen, the crown of the tooth behind the fangs of the central and lateral incisors, the neck above and behind the fang of the temporary canine, in front of and above the first bicuspid. The point of the fang is situated just in front, and exterior to the antrum. The temporary canine remains. The tooth on the right side was normally situated.

Fig. 99.

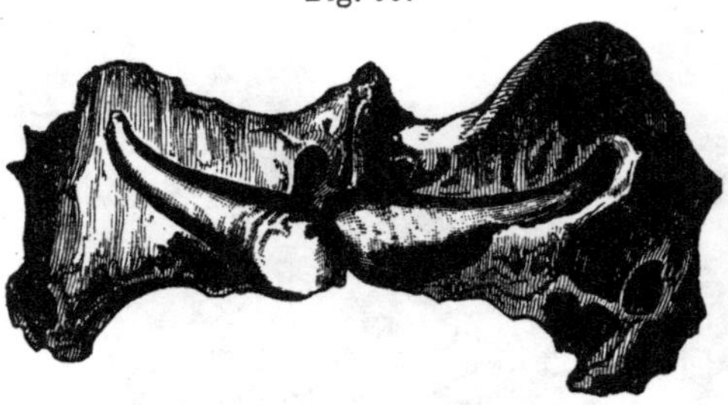

The fifth example (fig. 99) is essentially the same as the previous one, but affecting both sides. In this instance the points of the canines are in contact, immediately behind the incisive foramen. The jaw is that of an aged person, from which many of the permanent teeth were shed; and whether the temporary canines were retained during any period of adult life does not appear.

Fig. 100.

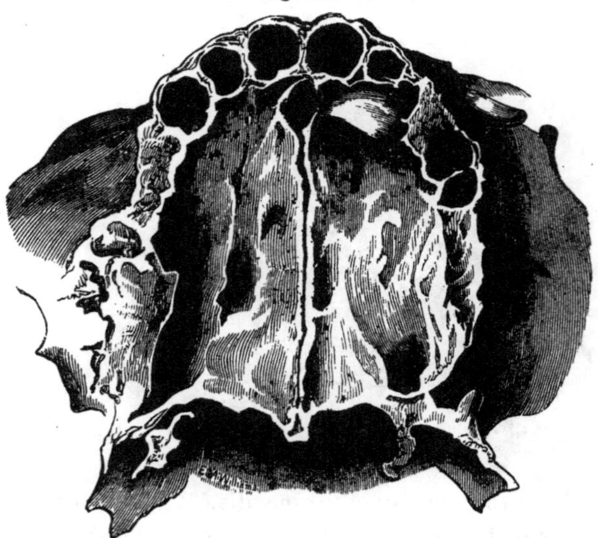

The sixth illustration (fig. 100) shows the left permanent upper canine embedded in the palatal process of the maxilla, immediately behind the alveoli of the central and lateral incisors; the fang of the tooth points backwards and slightly outwards.

In the previous cases the suppressed or embedded teeth have been displayed by opening up the surface of the jaw by artificial means; but it occasionally happens that the progressive absorption of the alveolar surfaces, frequently even after all the originally apparent teeth have been shed, exhibits these embedded teeth, at very advanced periods of life; and where, in unobservant persons, these members of the permanent dental series have not been missed from the set, the circumstance has given rise to the idea of a partial third set of teeth. Many examples of this condition (the appearance of suppressed teeth in the mouths of aged—otherwise edentulous people) have come under my notice.

In one of these, several years after the mouth had been edentulous, and when the patient had reached the seventieth* year of her age, an elongated elevation on the alveolar border of the upper jaw, on the left side towards the front of the mouth, was observed. In time the surface of the gum gave way, and displayed the left permanent canine tooth lying in a strictly horizontal position, and in the axis of the arch of the jaw. At the present time the tooth is attached to the surface of the jaw, for

Fig. 101.

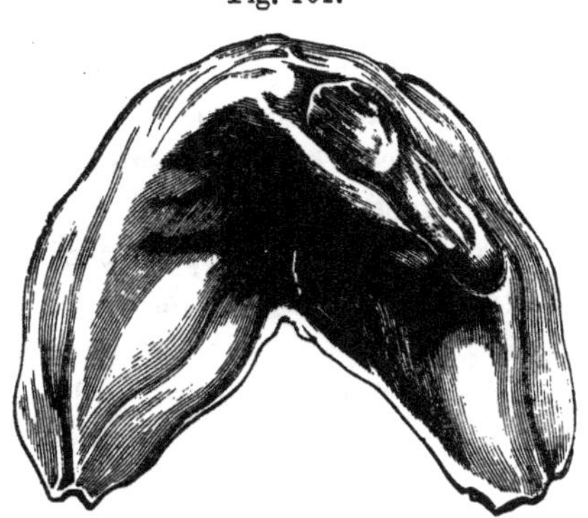

its whole length, by that which should be its anterior surface, while its posterior surface and sides, from the apex of the root

* M. Toirac mentions having seen the skull of a woman, who died at the age of 103; all the alveolar cavities were obliterated, but on one side of the lower jaw there was a wise tooth on the point of appearing.

to the summit of the crown, are exposed. The tooth is tolerably firm, and the patient still retains it. The case is in all respects analogous to the specimens figured in the fourth, fifth, and sixth illustrations of this series: its history however is defective. It is not known whether the temporary canine was retained for any unnatural time, but it is quite clear that the permanent tooth was never in its place. The accompanying figure (fig. 101) is from a plaster cast of the mouth, showing the position, *in sitû,* of this tooth on the otherwise edentulous gum.

The impaction of teeth in the jaws seldom causes inconvenience, and in the very great majority of cases the individual in whose mouth it exists is unconscious of the circumstance. Occasionally, however, the capsule around such a misplaced tooth becomes expanded into a fluid-containing sac, forming a dentigerous cyst, a subject to be considered presently.

But while an impacted tooth may not be associated in the minds either of the patient himself or by his medical attendant with any particular malady, it does not follow that such misplacement is always innocuous. The following cases, rare as they are, will I think sufficiently justify these observations:—

Impacted Canine Tooth producing violent Neuralgic Headache.—Miss B—— was under the care of Mr. Cartright, senior, in her childhood, and the shedding and succession of her teeth were carefully watched by him. All the permanent teeth appeared in due course, and in regular position, excepting the left upper canine, and the space which it should have occupied was obliterated by the contact of the lateral incisor and first bicuspid. At the time when the right upper canine appeared, a hard swelling was noticed in the palate on the left side, and towards the front of the mouth, and this slowly developed into a prominent rounded ridge, extending obliquely behind the left incisors, and left first bicuspid. Mr. Cartwright pronounced this to be the region occupied by the missing canine, and that the swelling was caused by its presence. No inconvenience was at first occasioned by this condition, and the patient was in good health up to the age of eighteen, when she was attacked with severe headache of a peculiar kind: it usually came on immediately after breakfast, and was attended with extreme prostration of strength: it continued the greater part of the day, and recurred sometimes three or four times a-week: the pain was always confined to one spot—the vertex of the head towards the left side, and over a circumscribed region, about the size of a crown-piece; it was attended with local heat, and was relieved for the time by pressure with the hand. This condition lasted for many years, from the time that the patient was eighteen years of age till she was twenty-six, and during this period she was under constant medical and surgical treatment for her painful affliction, but received no appreciable relief from any of the means adopted.

Every kind of tonic was employed, and *arsenic* was pushed to extremity without benefit.

The late Dr. James Johnson was consulted, and he prescribed the application of *Unguentum antimonii potassio-tartratis* to the region of the head where the pain existed. This was adopted, and carried to a painful extent, without, however, producing any mitigation of the patient's sufferings. Sir Astley Cooper recommended a repeated and even continued employment of the *Ceratum cantharidis* over the vertex, so as to establish, and maintain, for a considerable period, a continuous pus-discharging sore. This advice was followed, but the headaches were in no degree lessened. The patient still continued a permanent invalid. After many years of suffering, and ineffectual treatment, she conceived an idea, or rather, under the influence of certain not very accurately defined feelings, she had a strong impression, that the impacted tooth in the palate was in some way connected with her sufferings, and she desired to have it removed. The swelling in the palate had gradually become more distinct and prominent, though there was no attempt at tooth-eruption; indeed, the tooth was still covered in by compact bone. It was not the seat of actual pain; but upon the supervention of the headaches, the region about it became tender and hot, and, to use the patient's own expression, "I had an indescribable feeling that the tooth and the headache were connected together: when the hot throbbing came into my head, I always felt conscious of the existence of my shut-up tooth; at other times I did not think about it." At the urgent request of the patient, Mr. Cartwright removed the tooth; but to accomplish this a good deal of bone had to be chipped up so as to open the deep cavity in which it was embedded. The operation was a painful and a tedious one, and has left a marked depression in the palate. *The extraction of the tooth was followed by immediate, complete, and permanent relief: the headache vanished from that day, and never recurred.* It is now over thirty years since this case terminated thus favourably.

The lady herself from whom I received the foregoing history tells me that she is remarkably sensitive about the teeth, and that when she is affected with odontalgia it causes positive bodily illness; and upon the extraction of a tooth she suffers complete physical collapse, not fainting or becoming unconscious, but lying helpless, unable to stand, move, or speak, sometimes for hours. She tells me that this condition reminds her of the prostration which was associated with her former headaches.

A circumstance which adds great interest to the foregoing history is the fact that this lady's sister also had an impacted canine tooth in the upper jaw, though it gave rise to a totally different set of symptoms. This latter case was under my own care, and was as follows:—

Impacted Canine Tooth producing Maxillary Abscess.—Miss B——, senior, was nearly seventy years of age when the point of a canine tooth (right upper) first appeared through the gum. Her history was this: In early childhood she fell down stairs, and in the fall knocked out the right upper temporary canine tooth, inflicting at the same time a heavy crushing blow upon the corresponding region of the jaw. This circumstance was mentioned to me as a probable explanation of the impacted misplacement of the permanent successional canine. This lady was never aware, until the appearance of the canine late in life, that any of her permanent teeth had been previously deficient. She lost her teeth early, partly from decay, and partly from spontaneous loosening, and dropping out sound; and before fifty years of age was reduced to the wearing of a complete set of artificial teeth in the upper jaw, and many in the lower. The upper gum had a natural appearance, though, perhaps, it was rather full on the right side towards the front; this, however, was not sufficiently conspicuous to attract marked attention. After the patient had worn a complete upper set of teeth for nearly twenty years, a fissure was observed in the gum, on the prominence before indicated, and this disclosed a whitish body of bony hardness, which the patient considered at the time to be the remains of a tooth that had been imperfectly extracted at some previous operation. Matters continued *in statu quo* for some three years, during which period the artificial teeth were worn as before. At the end of this time, that is, in April, 1863, there was an attack of intense pain, and much swelling on the right side of the upper jaw, near and surrounding what proved to be an impacted canine tooth. The swelling was very large in the palate, bulging it out into a great convex mass: the local symptoms were attended with considerable constitutional disturbance, and the patient became quite ill. After the swelling had existed some ten days or a fortnight, a discharge of pus occurred; and the sufferings were, for the time, much mitigated. But the collection of matter recurred, and early in June became so considerable, and was attended with so much fever, and general illness, that the patient consulted me for her relief. The swelling in the palate was immense, blocking up the whole concavity on both sides; it was very hard, having a malignant aspect, and was scarcely to be recognised as an abscess. On the margin of the gum, but imbedded in the general swelling, was, what appeared to me, and ultimately proved to be, the apex of an impacted canine tooth. In the palatal tumour I traced deep indistinct fluctuation. Under these circumstances I determined to incise deeply the swelling, and attempt the extraction of the canine tooth: the former operation led to the discharge of much deep-seated matter, and the latter, which was accomplished very easily, was followed by an abundant outpouring of grumous fœtid pus. From that day the local and general symptoms rapidly disappeared. There can be no doubt that the impacted canine tooth had led to all the mischief in this case, and determined the maxillary abscess; the latter formed and discharged, but still continued as long as the tooth remained: when the tooth was extracted it vanished, and did not return.

The precise pathological relation of this tooth I am not prepared to declare. As regards the original displacement, it was probably a congenital, or rather an inherited, malformation, seeing that this patient's sister was similarly affected: the accident in childhood before mentioned may, or may not, have had some share in causing it. The relation which the tooth bore to the collection of matter I cannot exactly define; no part of the fang exhibited naked yellow crusta-petrosa which had been bathed in pus, such as we see in ordinary alveolar abscess; on the contrary, it was completely clothed with adherent periosteum. There is, however, nothing in this circumstance which militates against the idea that it was the tooth which caused the abscess, for the same fact is observed as regards impacted wisdom teeth in those cases in which maxillary abscesses are produced by them, in instances of their difficult eruption.

The antagonistic growth of crowded teeth is very apt to produce pain—heavy, aching, and diffused. One sees this when a *dens sapientiæ* is struggling into place against the resistance of a second molar. I have often seen similar suffering in children (who, unfortunately for them, can ill explain and ill define their pains), when a permanent tooth has been pressing forwards against an incompletely-absorbed and firmly-embedded temporary predecessor: I have noticed this especially as regards the advent of the second bicuspid tooth, whose predecessor, the second temporary molar, is apt to get firmly wedged between the first premolar and the first true molar.

But this suffering may arise from mere crowding of the teeth where they become jammed together in a jaw incapable of affording them proper accommodation.

Impacted Lower Bicuspid Tooth causing repeated Abscesses under the Tongue with Thickening of the lower Jaw.—Miss T——, 30 years of age, applied to me, March 1868, on account of a deep-set impacted tooth in the lower jaw. Many years ago she lost all her lower molar teeth from caries, and she had worn artificial teeth supplying their place for a considerable period. She was not aware that any of the permanent set had failed to appear; but she had been conscious of a swelling low down near the base of the jaw, and under the tongue on the right side behind the first bicuspid, where the impacted tooth had now declared itself. This swelling became so considerable and so painful, some three years previously, that she was obliged to desist from wearing her artificial teeth. The swelling towards the tongue then became tumid and painful; an abscess formed which burst under the tongue, and this was repeated again and again. The jaw-bone in this region became thickened, and there was a marked and very hard and pointed projection at the bottom of the cheek, close to the edge of the jaw. In 1866 Miss T—— consulted a dentist, who, by removing some mucous membrane over the swelling beneath the tongue, discovered the crown of a tooth, which he endeavoured but unsuccessfully to extract. The patient then remained as she was: no more collections of matter, however, formed—the crown of the tooth being free. The swelling outside the jaw slightly increased. When I saw Miss T—— in 1868, I found a considerable and hard swelling of the lower jaw at its base behind the first bicuspid tooth. The crown of the second bicuspid could be just felt projecting very low down into the floor of the mouth against the ducts of the sublingual gland. It appeared to me that for the extraction of this tooth, which caused much annoyance and disfigured the face, it would be necessary to remove a portion of bone, and for this purpose I was prepared with bone-nippers, gouge, saw, &c. But, upon removing the mucous membrane, the crown of the tooth was so exposed that I attempted its removal by forceps only, and I easily succeeded with a pair the blades of which were nearly at right angles to the handle. I drove home the blades to the neck as far as possible, and then with some torsion and pulling towards the tongue the tooth readily slipped out of its socket. The tooth lay directly across the axis of the jaw, the fang pointing outwards. The end of the fang was bent at right angles, as though it had had insufficient room to grow straight, which was doubtless the case.

Impacted Tooth producing Tumour mistaken for Cancer.—Dr. Forget* mentions the case of a woman 48 years of age, who had a large tumour in the right upper jaw and cheek: it had fungoid ulcerations, and was attended with lancinating pains. It was believed to be malignant; and it was determined to extirpate it. Soon after commencing the operation, a tooth was discovered in the axis of the tumour, which on removal proved to be the first molar; afterwards the second molar was found similarly situated. The patient then explained that several of the teeth in the upper jaw had never been cut. It was concluded therefore that the impaction of these teeth had alone constituted

* *Des Anomalies dentaires et de leur Influence sur la Production des Maladies des Os maxillaires*, par A. M. Forget, p. 36. Paris, 1859.

the disease. The teeth were directed obliquely inwards, had penetrated the inner portion of the alveolar arch, and had there lodged beneath the mucous membrane. The ulcerations on the jaw and cheek were repeatedly touched with nitric oxide of mercury, and the patient left the Hospital, in two months, cured.

CHAPTER XVI.

DENTIGEROUS CYSTS.

Collections of serum or sero-pus in the dental capsule, forming those fluid-containing tumours known as dentigerous cysts, are among the ill consequences which impacted teeth occasion; but they are very rare cases, particularly considering that this embedding of the teeth is by no means uncommon. These serous cysts may result from the presence of a supernumerary tooth, or teeth; but in the instances which have come under my knowledge, either by record or personal observation, with the exception of three, the tooth or teeth have been permanent and normal in their presence and serial character, though misplaced as regards position. I have heard but of one instance in which a temporary tooth has been the dental element in one of these cysts, and two in which it was occasioned by supernumerary teeth. These tooth-bearing serous tumours are therefore to be looked upon as the occasional complications of dentition, in which there is an accidental deviation in the anatomical position of some tooth or teeth. The cysts only arise when the tooth or teeth associated with them are embedded in the substance of the jawbone; they do not occur after the tooth has pierced the gum. The embedding of the tooth does not necessarily give rise to these serous collections, and why they should in any particular instance I cannot even suggest; though perhaps in some cases (as where a wisdom-tooth is impacted and held back behind a second molar) the irritation consequent upon a restrained position may account for it. But this explanation would not apply to the majority of cases.

When a tooth is impacted in the jaw its fang is enclosed in a bony socket lined by periosteum, as in ordinary circumstances, while the crown of the tooth is free in a little bony loculus lined with that which was the so-called "enamel-pulp." This structure is clothed with a sort of epithelium, which is apt to assume the function of secreting fluid. After the enamel is completely formed, the soft membrane which rests upon the surface of the crown of the tooth frequently separates from it, the interval being occupied by a sort of serum. This is probably the result of some irritation or difficulty in tooth-cutting; and where the irritation runs on to acute inflammation, as in some cases of tedious eruption of wisdom-teeth, the secretion may become purulent. In the cases of deep-seated impaction of teeth, the action is, I believe, always slow, and the secretion almost always serous. The recorded instances of this condition are so few, that it is scarcely possible to generalise upon them: it may, however, be said that they have usually happened in young persons; at least have commenced in adolescence, and shortly after, though sometimes before the maturation of the impacted tooth. In the cases narrated the upper grinders have perhaps been more frequently involved than other teeth, the serous cysts dilating into the maxillary sinus: but incisors, canines, bicuspids, and molars, have all been associated with this condition. In many of the cases where a description is given of the teeth involved, the crowns have been normal, but the fangs more or less abortive and defective.

M. Jourdain, in his very valuable "Treatise on the Diseases of the Mouth,"* describes three cases of dentigerous cysts, of which the following is a summary:—The first case he records is that of a girl about seventeen years old: it occurred in 1771. For some months the right cheek of this patient had been prodigiously swollen and hard to the touch, but without pain or change of colour in the skin; she was not able to blow her nose on that side; the palate was in a natural state; the maxillary bone extremely distended along the alveolar edge where the first and second molar were missing; the wisdom-tooth had not appeared. The bicuspids, canine, and incisors were altogether normal. The nose was thrown a little to the opposite side. There was no evidence of dental caries, nor the history of mechanical violence to the part. The tumour, which was the size of a hen's egg, was elastic on manipulation, yielding

* *Traité des Maladies de la Bouche,* par M. Jourdain; Paris, 1778.

and then returning to its previous shape, producing at the same time a kind of crackling, characteristic of fluid distending bony parietes. M. Jourdain opened the tumour by a simple incision; much serum escaped, and some passed through the nose. The swelling now flattened down under pressure. Injections of tepid water, which were used, passed partly through the nose. On exploring the cavity with a probe two foreign bodies were felt slightly moveable; when extracted they proved to be the crowns and bodies of the missing first and second molar teeth—the fangs not being formed. The treatment which was followed consisted in plugging open the orifice at the lowest part of the sac with a tent of lint; injecting with stimulating astringents, and applying firm compress on the cheek. The case was thus completely cured in three months.

In a second case described by Jourdain, the patient was sixty years of age, and the tooth causing the cyst was the superior second bicuspid. The tumour was the size of a pigeon's egg, rather in the front of the jaw on the left side; it pressed upon and completely closed the left nostril. There was a deep ulcer on the gum over the tumour, at the bottom of which a cusp of the tooth could be seen and felt; it moved under the pressure of a probe; and was easily seized and withdrawn by a pair of watchmaker's pincers. It was the second pre-molar tooth, the crown, with about a third of the fang, formed. "After the patient had rinsed his mouth, he tried to blow his nose, and this forced action produced immediately, through the aperture where the tooth had been removed, the discharge of about a dessert-spoonful of serum, a little turbid, though but very little fetid." Some pressure was applied over the tumour which caused it to collapse. In three months every vestige of the malady had disappeared.

A third case occurred in a girl thirteen years of age, in whom a large tumour had developed itself in the front of the upper jaw and occupying the bone over the region of the canines and incisor teeth. These teeth were all permanent, having normally replaced the corresponding temporaries, with the exception of one of the lateral incisors, which was wanting. On manipulation the tumour was found to contain fluid. One of the central incisors was loose. M. Jourdain removed this tooth, when from its alveolar canal issued two good sized dessert-spoonfuls of slimy yellow serum. The opening was then enlarged by a bistoury along the alveolar edges and the cavity stuffed with lint. "The cavity of the tumour was so considerable that I put into it five pads of dry lint the size and length of the little finger of an adult." When this treatment had been continued some days a body was discovered attached to the posterior wall inside the sac: pushing it with a probe was seen to make the palate bulge inwards. Under the continuance of the treatment the body became detached and free in the sac. It was removed with difficulty, and proved to be the missing lateral incisor tooth. The front of the crown of this tooth was normal, but behind it was bulbous, and at the inferior part of the bulb there were four cusp-like eminences: the root, in itself not otherwise than natural, was attached obliquely to the crown. The pads of lint were now diminished, and external pressure applied. In three months the case was cured.

Dupuytren, in his "Leçons Orales,"* mentions a case which was shown to him by M. Loir in which an osseous cyst had developed in the palatine process of the left upper jaw-bone, the parietes being formed by the two compact layers of this process: the immediate cause of the existence of this cyst was clearly the reversed position of a tooth. In fact, the left canine tooth, instead of piercing the alveolar edge of the corresponding superior maxillary bone, had opened for itself a passage through the inner wall of this bone, and had, by its presence, given rise to the formation of a cavity of at least thrice its own volume, in the diplöe of the above apophysis, where it had attained its full development; the rest of the tooth pressed against the outer plate of the alveolar system.

My late colleague, Mr. Bransby Cooper, informed me of a case of this malady in which great swelling occurred in the substance of the superior maxilla of a young man in whose mouth the first and second permanent molar teeth had never made their appearance. A free opening was cut into the expansion, when the wanting teeth were found inverted in the axis of a serous cyst, expanding into the antrum. No account of this case appears in Mr. B. Cooper's "Lectures on Surgery," but I took memoranda of its particulars when the history of the case was communicated to me by Mr. Cooper.

* *Leçons Orales de Clinique Chirur.*, Dupuytren; tom. iii. p. 8. Paris 1834.

Mr. Wormald operated on a boy about fourteen years of age, some time since, at St. Bartholomew's Hospital, in whom a serous cyst had expanded about the second bicuspid tooth in the lower jaw. The cyst was the size of a large chestnut, and was in the axis of the bone; the fang of the tooth was not fully developed, but the crown was complete. The interior of the cyst was lined with a thick vascular membrane, rather rough on its inner surface: it contained a glairy fluid. I am indebted to Mr. Wormald for these particulars.

One of the most remarkable examples of this malady which has ever been recognised was recorded in 1844, in an essay * published by F. E. Glaswald, at the University of Greifswald in Pomerania, where the case occurred.

The patient was a healthy girl about eight years of age when the malady first showed itself. About this time she was attacked every few weeks with violent pulsating pain of the right upper jaw, extending along the alveoli and teeth. These symptoms were relieved by fomentation and general treatment. But the same symptoms recurred after a year with swelling and redness of the right side of the face during the attacks, accompanied by fever. After the pain and redness had subsided no definite tumour remained, only a general fulness of the right cheek. During the following two years the patient had repeated similar attacks, with progressively increasing swelling, great hardness of the cheek, and tenderness during the existence of the inflammatory symptoms; and by the time she was ten years old the right cheek displayed large tumour-like prominence. At this time after exposure to cold the patient had an unusually violent attack of inflammation in the antrum, with fever; and after five days the sinus burst in the zygomatic region, discharging much pus. She was then taken by Dr. Warnekros into a hospital; the aperture was dilated, and this was followed by a fresh discharge of matter; the molar teeth were extracted, and as no matter escaped by their sockets, a fresh aperture was made in the canine fossa, when still more fetid pus came away. The swelling of the right cheek gradually diminished, and the apertures of discharge healed. After a lapse of five years the

* De Tumore quodam utriusque Antri Highmori, perversa dentium formatione exorta; Dissertatio inauguralis, &c. Auctor, Franciscus Edwardus Glaswald, Saxo, Gryphiæ. 1844.

girl was attacked with precisely the same symptoms on the left side, which continued till she was nineteen years of age, and at the same time the right cheek again became slowly enlarged. The left antrum was now tapped by Dr. Kneip, and much fœtid pus was evacuated. An offensive discharge was also found coming from the back of the mouth on the right side, but no dead bone could be discovered by a probe.

Fig. 102.

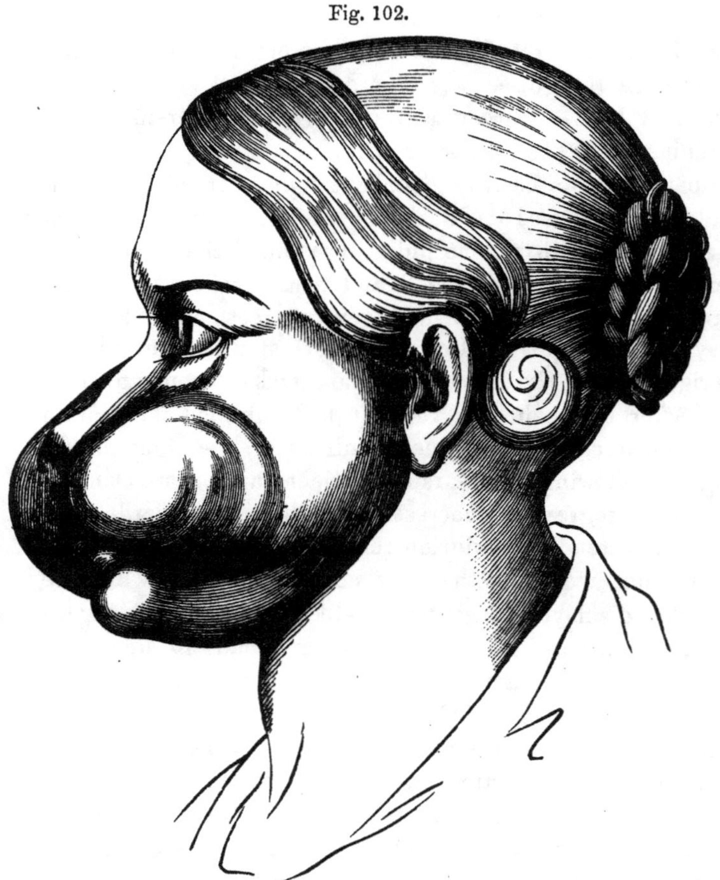

The patient was now excessively disfigured, and the antra remained permanently dilated and very prominent. The treatment she had undergone produced no satisfactory relief, and she ultimately came under the care of Prof. Baum, who opened each antrum and removed a portion of the wall. On the left side, the angle of the mouth being drawn aside, a crucial incision was made just below the canine fossa; this was followed by the discharge of about an ounce of fetid, yellow, clear serum. The covering of the sac at this part consisted of the mucous-membrane, some fibrous membrane, and a very thin layer of bone. On exploring the antrum with the finger a hard foreign body was discovered, which proved to be the crown of a molar tooth. The tooth was very firmly attached to the bone, and was extracted with great difficulty. On the right side the parietes were membranous also, and a little circle of the wall was cut out. In this sinus a canine tooth was discovered loosely attached to the wall, and easily removed. The right antrum contained fœtid pus.

The case was treated by injections into the antrum and external pressure. The ultimate issue of the case is not given, but it is stated that after many months little change had occurred: the swelling of the left side had diminished most.

Two very remarkable figures are given by Glaswald of this unfortunate woman, showing the deformity the disease had occasioned, and I have thought the interest of the case would warrant the copying of one of them (fig. 102). The drawing was made six months after the operation was performed.

In my own practice I have had some examples of dentigerous cyst; the following is an abstract of three of these cases:—

A young woman, æt. 18, applied to Mr. Cock, at Guy's Hospital, some years since, on account of a swelling of the upper jaw, immediately above the left central incisor tooth, and extending up to the base of the nose. The tumour evidently consisted of an expansion of the incisive bone in the situation indicated, and contained fluid. Mr. Cock requested my opinion of the case; and upon examining the mouth I found that the left central incisor was a temporary tooth, which had not been previously recognised. I at once suspected that the permanent tooth was imbedded in the jaw, and that its capsule was the seat of the cyst; and this turned out to be true. The temporary tooth was first extracted, and its root was found entire and unabsorbed; and upon removing the permanent tooth it was found to consist of little more than a crown, the fang having grown but about one-fifth of its natural length, and thus it was that it never reached the level of the contiguous teeth, and never extruded its predecessor. The accompanying figure, 103, is from a drawing of this tooth. Remaining embedded in the incisive bone, it either set up by its presence such irritation as caused the serous secretion in the sac that it occupied, or, irritation being set up from some other cause, its presence determined the development of the serous cyst.

Fig. 103.

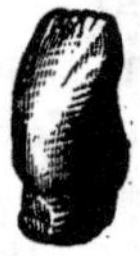

In another instance the tooth was an impacted *dens sapientiæ* of the lower jaw; and the particulars of this case are briefly these:—

The patient was a young man about twenty-two years of age. He had been admitted into Guy's Hospital on account of a large swelling of the left angle of the lower jaw. The swelling was tense and elastic, clearly contained fluid, and it occupied the centre of the bone which was distended by it. The cyst was first opened within the mouth and a large quantity of serum escaped; the swelling quickly subsided, and the patient experienced considerable relief. In a few days, however, the orifice closed, and the fluid rapidly re-collected. An incision was then made at the extreme angle of the jaw externally, so as to open the cyst at the most dependent part, but with exactly the same result. I was then requested to see the patient, and on inspecting his mouth I found that, while the right inferior wisdom-tooth was thoroughly through and in its right position, the left was wanting, and there was no indication of its approach whatever. I noticed that the second molar in front of the swelling was loose, and the surrounding gum much inflamed. From the first inspection of the mouth, I suspected that the serous cyst was the dilated sac of a misplaced tooth, and that the looseness of the second molar arose from the pressure of the sac of the *dens sapientiæ* itself. I determined, as the previous treatment had been of no avail, to remove the second molar, both to relieve the pressure which its condition indicated, and as a probable assistance in investigating further the nature of the case. When the second molar was extracted, it was found that a considerable portion of the posterior fang had been removed by absorption, presenting an even concave excavation, as seen in the accompanying figures, 104, 105, which display the tooth in two aspects, a posterior and an oblique side view. On passing a probe into the socket of the posterior fang, it immediately came in contact with the crown of the *dens sapientiæ*, which was thus exposed to the surface. The impaction of the tooth

Fig. 104.

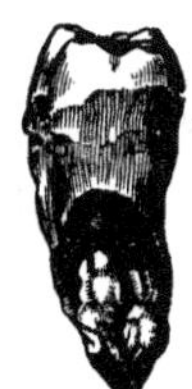

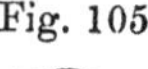

Fig. 105.

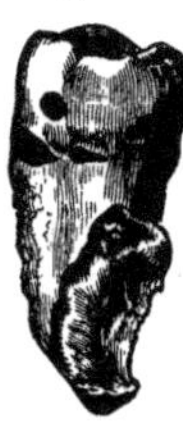

had now virtually ceased, and with that cessation the serous secretion vanished—the cyst no longer existed, and the patient left the hospital well.

In October, 1862, a gentleman about forty years of age consulted me respecting a tumour in the upper jaw on the left side, about the size of a pigeon's egg. It had been gradually coming for about a year, without any obvious cause. It had never pained him. Upon examining the mouth, I found the teeth in the locality of the tumour quite sound; but the second bicuspid was wanting, and he declared it had never been extracted. The first bicuspid and the first molar approached each other, but were not quite in contact. The tumour could, in the mouth, be easily demonstrated to be fluid-containing, and within bone. I evacuated the fluid by a small trocar; it was a thick serum, not exactly glairy, but syrupy and very dark yellow coloured; and it contained hosts of cholesterine plates,—small brilliant flat crystals. A probe passed into the cyst came upon a hard body, which, upon laying open the cyst with a scalpel, proved to be the crown of the missing second bicuspid tooth. It was hoped and expected that by this proceeding the tooth might come down and be more in reach, and might then be extracted. Nothing more was done on this occasion, and the patient promised to return in a short time; but he never came back.

A very singular case, in which the formation of supernumerary teeth was associated with the growth of a cyst, occurred in Stockholm in 1862 under the care of Mr. Tellander.

"In March, 1862,* a female, aged twenty-seven, applied to Mr. Tellander for professional assistance. He gained from her

* "On a Case of Supernumerary Teeth, treated by Mr. Tellander." In *Transactions of Odontological Society of London*, vol. iii.: London, 1863.

the following particulars respecting the history of her case. The temporary teeth attracted no attention, and it may be assumed that they presented no unusual characters. They were shed and replaced about the time common for the change of the temporary for the permanent teeth; and the process appears to have been completed, except on the right side of the upper jaw, where the first molar, the two bicuspids, and canine failed to make their appearance. A blank space marked the spot these teeth should have occupied, and at the age of twelve became the seat of a hard painless enlargement of the maxilla, causing disfigurement of that side of the face, but no further inconvenience. The patient applied to Mr. Tellander in consequence of an attack of inflammation in the enlarged part of the jaw, resulting, as she supposed, from the presence of the roots of a temporary molar, which in December last, for the first time, became painful, and from that time she dates the commencement of the present mischief. Mr. Tellander found considerable enlargement of the bone, with swelling of the contiguous soft parts, and a free discharge of pus from the gum about the roots of the temporary molar. These offenders were at once removed, and carious bone detected in the vicinity of their sockets. Three days subsequent to the first visit the diseased parts were again examined, and Mr. Tellander proceeded to remove the loose and carious bone which it was supposed formed the substance of the enlarged maxilla. It appeared, under the probe, to consist of large, hard particles of bone, amongst which the instrument might be moved, inclosed within a case of dead bone. After removing a few of these hard particles, Mr. Tellander found that he had come upon a cluster of minute teeth." The cavity was emptied, and twenty-eight *teeth*, or *cusps*, were found: probably some had escaped, and been lost before the nature of the case was detected. "There are nine single teeth, each one perfect in itself, having a conical root with a conical crown, tipped with enamel. Again we have six masses built up of adherent single teeth. Thus one is composed of three united cusps; two others are formed of two cusps each a fourth is but an irregular mass of dental tissues; a fifth consists of three similar masses united by membranes. In the sixth mass no less than nine cusps may be traced."

It may be doubted whether the aggregate bulk of the supernumerary teeth in Mr. Tellander's case would equal that of the teeth of which they held the place.

Mr. Tellander subsequently sent casts of his patient's mouth to the Odontological Society. "They show a supernumerary and a bicuspid tooth emerging from the gum in the situation previously occupied by the growth of supernumerary teeth."

In one instance only am I aware of a dentigerous cyst being associated with a *temporary* tooth. It occurred in the practice of my friend Mr. Alexander Edwards, of Edinburgh. The patient was a young man, in whose upper jaw, just below the orbit, a tumour had developed: the tumour consisted of exostosis from the maxilla, combined with a bony cyst: this contained a tooth which Mr. Edwards showed to the late Professor Goodsir, who pronounced it to be a temporary molar. A portion of this tooth was sent to me: it appeared to be the crown of the *second* temporary molar.

Fig. 106.

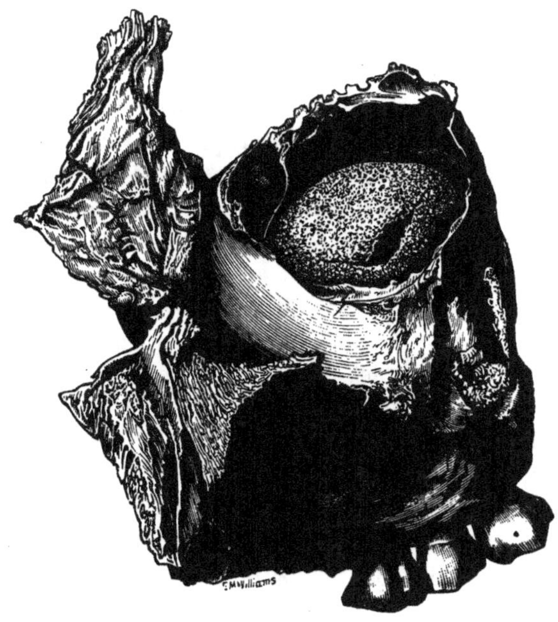

Pathological specimens of uncommon diseases, and those too not killing or shortening life, must necessarily be very rare. This applies to specimens illustrative of the disease we are now considering. One such specimen is in the possession of my friend Mr. Samuel Cartwright, and is valuable and instructive in many points. Through Mr. Cartwright's kindness I am allowed to figure it (fig. 106). The preparation consists of a right superior maxilla—an adult bone; the teeth that remain, and the alveoli from which others have been extracted, show that the normal number of permanent teeth had developed in their natural position. The turbinated bones are gone, and the antrum maxillæ is open. In the antrum, starting from its base, but not attached to its lateral walls anywhere, is an exceedingly thin delicate capsule of bone, about the size of a chestnut, white, with a granulated surface. The bony capsule contains nothing but a small *supernumerary* tooth, which is *loose* and *free* in the cavity. There are three important points in this specimen bearing on the anatomy and history of these cases: The tooth is a supernumerary one: it is free and wholly detached in the cavity of the cyst: and further, the expansion is not that of the antral wall itself with the tooth's crown uncovered within it, but a distension of that which was the bony loculus of the contained tooth, which, by its further dilatation, would have expanded the antral wall and probably have been confounded with it.

This latter circumstance appears to me to be of much anatomical interest in reference to those serous expansions of the antrum which are associated with inverted teeth. These have hitherto been described as expansions of the antrum itself: but I cannot conceive that a tooth being "cut" through the mucous-membrane of the antrum should produce such a result. The appearance of the crown of an inverted tooth in the nostril neither causes irritation nor increased secretion,—at least no such consequence followed in the three examples I have seen; and it seems to me to be far more probable that these cases have commenced as cysts within the bone of the base of the maxillary sinus, expanding into it, filling its whole cavity, and ultimately dilating its walls.

Two specimens in the Museum of St. Bartholomew's Hospital throw some further light on the pathology of this condition. One preparation (numbered I. 119) exhibits a thin bony cyst the size of a small Tangerine orange, with a thick membranous lining: it contained an inferior permanent canine tooth, *loosely attached* to its walls. It was removed from the lower jaw in the region of the contained tooth. The other preparation (I.

119*a*) is the superior maxilla of a young sheep, in which the central incisor is attached to the side of a large cyst; the *fang* of the tooth being *almost wholly destitute of bony covering.* This denudation of the fang does not appear to exist in the early stages of these cases, but seems to be brought about by great expansion of the cyst, and the progressive absorption of bone which accompanies it.

An unusually serious* case of dentigerous cyst was brought under the notice of the Midland Branch of the Provincial Medical Association, in June, 1864, by Mr. Fearn. A girl thirteen years of age was admitted into the Derby Infirmary, February 29, 1864. There was a large hard tumour occupying the whole of the horizontal ramus of the lower jaw on the left side, and there was much swelling on the right side. The tumour had been growing for six months. There was a fetid discharge from the surface, but a probe could detect no opening.

Fig. 107. Fig. 108.

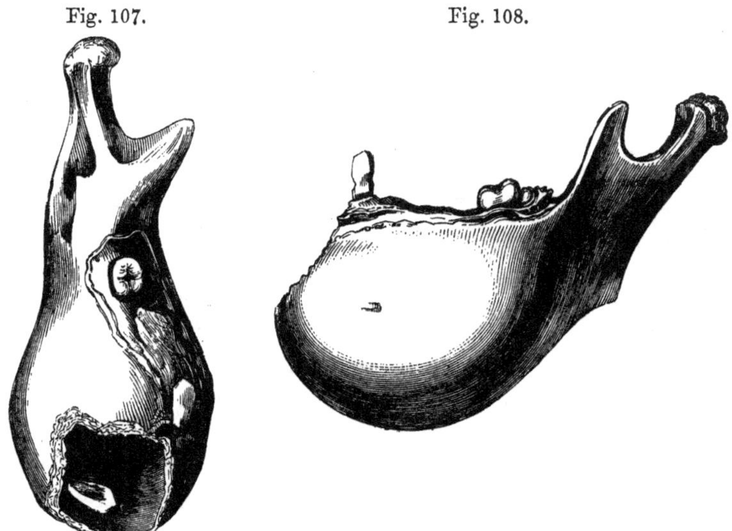

"The diseased mass was found to be essentially a large osseous cyst, of considerable thickness and density, separating the outer and inner plates of the jaw. The cavity was lined with a thickened pulpy, very vascular membrane; and the canine tooth was seen growing from its floor (fig. 107). The cyst extended

* "Case of Bony Dentigerous Cyst of the Lower Jaw," by S. W. Fearn. in *British Medical Journal,* No. 191, p. 241; Aug. 27, 1864.

from the ascending ramus of the left side beyond the symphysis for an inch and a half into the body of the jaw on the right side."

The cyst contained a considerable quantity of fetid pus. The accompanying figures, 107, 108, of this jaw are taken from the work on "Diseases of the Jaws," by Mr. Heath, to whom I am indebted for them.

An interesting and well-illustrated case of dentigerous cyst is recorded in the 5th volume of the "British Journal of Dental Science." It occurred in the practice of a French surgeon, Dr. Maisonneuve, and the particulars were narrated by Mr. Bennett at a meeting of the Odontological Society, December 1, 1862.

The patient, when twelve years old, received a violent blow on his chin. At thirty years of age a tooth, without a fang, came out whilst eating, leaving a hole at that part of the jaw struck in falling. For several years serum was discharged from this orifice, which then closed. A new swelling now made its appearance, and an opening formed behind one of the front teeth, from which a "saline fluid" escaped. Dr. Maisonneuve recommended an operation, which was consented to. A portion of the jaw was removed, and this illustration displays the parts. There was a cyst at the bottom of which was a canine tooth (fig. 109). The recovery was complete, and the lost parts were restored by an artificial substitute.

Fig. 109.

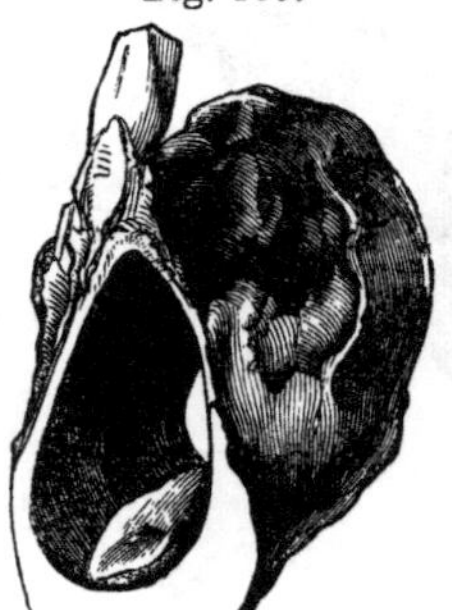

I have met with three cases of what might be called *incipient* dentigerous cyst in children who were cutting, with difficulty their bicuspid teeth. In each instance a second lower temporary molar was retained beyond its proper time for shedding: the capsule surrounding the imprisoned successor (the second bicuspid) expanded, with some bony enlargement, and contained a serous fluid. Upon the removal of the temporary tooth, the crown of the bicuspid was in view. In one of the cases, that of a girl thirteen years old, the swelling was very considerable, with external disfigurement of face, and considerable bony increase of the jaw. The temporary tooth was removed, and deep in the jaw the cusps of the premolar could be just discovered; slowly the swelling diminished, and the permanent tooth rose up, and six months after the mouth appeared as though nothing unusual had occurred.

A curious form of serous cyst-expansion over retàrded (not impacted) teeth has recently come under my care. Master T—, aged eleven, came to me, merely for inspection, about three years since. I had long before removed all four of the first permanent molars for caries and aching. The second upper molars had both pierced the gum, and the crowns were fairly through. The lower second molars seemed also about to protrude, and I told my patient that in a few weeks they would be cut also. Two years after this young gentleman came to me in much discomfort. He could hardly shut his jaws. The lower molars were still not through, but were each surmounted by a hemispherical cyst, the size of a large marble, the gum being thus distended over the teeth by fluid. The membrane covering in the fluid was nearly transparent, and very thin. I not only divided the membrane, but removed much of it. The discharged fluid was thin pale serum. The teeth were well up.*

* Other examples of dentigerous cysts have been recorded, to some of which I beg to refer the reader:—"Tumor of the upper Jaw depending on Cysts connected with the Presence of Teeth in a preternatural situation," by James Syme, Esq. In *Edinb. Med. and Surg. Journal*, vol. v. p. 381. Edinb. 1838. "Tumor formed by the Capsule of an uncut permanent Tooth," by Thomas Wormald, Esq. *Lancet*, vol. i. p. 756. 1850. "Dentigerous Cyst," in Stanley's *Diseases of the Bones*. Plate xviii. p. 20 of Illustrations. London, 1849. "Three Cases of Dentigerous Cysts," in Forget's *Des Anomalies dentaires*, &c. Obs. x., xi., xii., pp. 41–47. Paris, 1859.

The dentigerous cysts, which have been above described, are totally different in their origin and physiological meaning from those other tooth-bearing tumours, which are found, some in the ovaries of females, and others variously distributed in the bodies of either sex.

The dentigerous cysts occurring in the jaw are merely the result of misplacement of a tooth-germ or germs belonging to the jaw that contains them. The other two forms cannot be considered as strictly belonging to the individual in whom they are found, nor are they adventitious growths of disease, properly so called. Those dentigerous and many-tissued cysts found in the human ovary are evidently a modified form of reproduction, and apparently the physiological representative of parthenogenesis; whereas those other tooth-bearing growths which occur in either sex, and apart from the reproductive organs, seem to be associated with some entanglement of a secondary ovum within a primary one, or to some duplication of the latter. For the grounds upon which the author has arrived at these conclusions the reader is referred to a paper by him on *Dentigerous Ovarium Tumour*, in Guy's Hospital Reports, 3rd series, vol. vi.; also article "Surgical Diseases connected with the Teeth," in Holmes's *System of Surgery*, 1st edit. vol. iv. p. 32.

From the foregoing narratives one may thus far generalise that the *symptoms* of a dentigerous cyst are almost wholly local, consisting of an expansion of the jaw-bone at some particular spot, accompanied by a corresponding disfigurement of the neighbouring features, and a sense of weight and tension of the affected part. Where the impacted tooth has produced pressure upon a neighbour, the symptoms of pain and local distress have been more considerable, and have given rise to some constitutional irritation.

Upon manipulation, the fingers readily perceive that the tumour is a central expansion of bone, and that it contains fluid. The bony walls yield to pressure, and then return to shape with that peculiar kind of crepitation which Jourdain characteristically calls *craquement*, like the doubling of stiff parchment; and the bone is usually sufficiently thin at some parts to allow the production of fluctuation under the pressure of alternate fingers.

One of the most usual symptoms, which is also an important *diagnostic sign*, is the absence from the mouth of some tooth or teeth which should have appeared, and which have never been extracted. The presence of a fluid-containing tumour within the substance of a maxillary bone at the region of a tooth which is missing, and known always to have been wanting, would be well-nigh conclusive as to its being a dentigerous cyst, though the presence (or the past-known presence) of every mature tooth would not necessarily prove the reverse, for the dental element in the case may be a temporary or a supernumerary tooth. However, an impacted temporary tooth is a very great rarity, and one producing a serous cyst would be still more uncommon. The same may be said of a supernumerary tooth. The diagnosis may be further advanced by exploring the cyst either by means of a grooved needle or trocar, when a serous discharge will still further support the idea of a tooth-cyst. If the cavity be laid open, a probe will scarcely fail to discover the hard unyielding substance of the crown of the tooth—should one be there.

The *treatment* of these cases is obvious, and usually quite efficacious. It consists in evacuating the contents of the cyst, extracting the tooth or teeth embedded in it, and, where the expansion is large, in removing some of the dilated bone. The operations should be performed as early as possible, so as to prevent the necessity of cutting away much bone, and the prolonged and tedious absorption which would follow before the face could assume its natural form. All cutting should, if possible, be done within the mouth. Generally a portion of the wall of the cyst may be removed readily enough with a scalpel; but where the involved tooth is reversed, the expansion is likely to be away from the alveolar border. In that case, bone-nippers, the extraction of contiguous teeth, or even the employment of the saw, may be necessary. This has been especially the case where inverted teeth have caused cysts in the antrum. The tooth is likely to be found at the base of the cyst; furthest, that is, from the thinnest expansion. Some difficulty may be found in getting hold of and removing the embedded tooth; but various long-bladed extracting forceps may be readily devised to suit any case, if a difficulty should occur.

In some instances, from a persistence of the serous secretion after the tooth has been removed, it has been found necessary to inject the cyst with astringent and stimulating fluids.

Where the maxilla expands beneath the fangs of a temporary tooth too long retained in the jaw, it should be immediately removed: its permanent successor will be pretty surely discovered beneath it, and will advance into its place, the abnormal swelling at the same time subsiding. I have met with three or four such cases.

In some instances considerable portions of the jaw-bone, even as much as half the inferior maxilla, have been removed for dentigerous cysts. In all these cases, I believe, the operation was undertaken from an incorrect diagnosis. A knowledge of the real nature of the disease and an early interference would have rendered such proceedings quite unnecessary.

When properly treated the issue of these cases is, I believe, always satisfactory. They are very rarely associated with other bone disease. Forget mentions an example where, in an old and neglected case, a large osseous tumour mixed with much myelo-plastic material formed around the cyst.

In one instance which I saw, a fibrous tumour grew from the cicatrix of the wound some months after the first operation: it was removed, and did not recur.

CHAPTER XVII.

PAINFUL AND DIFFICULT ERUPTION OF THE WISDOM TEETH.

The eruption of the wisdom teeth is occasionally attended by very painful and distressing symptoms, and these may be protracted through many months, and even years, unless relieved by surgical interference. The frequent disproportion that exists between the size of the teeth and the jaws which hold them not only produces an irregularity of the teeth in the front of the mouth, but very often leaves so small a space for the last molar, the *dens sapientiæ,* that its advent is postponed, or may be prevented for a long period, and the repeated efforts at evolution become the cause of much suffering and even serious illness. In these cases the wisdom teeth, especially those of the lower jaw, have so little room that the front cusps of the teeth are frequently the only parts which are visible, the remaining portion of the tooth being covered by the mucous membrane where it passes up the ascending ramus and is reflected to the jaw and cheek; the imperfect room for the wisdom teeth, thus holding them back in their bony bed, also perverts their direction of growth and dislocates them. The painful symptoms which attend the cutting of the upper wisdom teeth where there is insufficient room are trivial to those which occur in similar conditions in the lower. In the upper jaw the wisdom teeth when misplaced are usually either directed backwards or outwards, or in both directions combined. When the tooth points backwards, every time the mouth is closed its crown comes in contact with the mucous membrane about the base of the coronoid process. When the direction is outward, which is more common, the tooth projects into the cheek, and, when the jaws are brought together, a portion of the mucous membrane in this region is nipped and pinched. This causes much pain, the surface ulcerates and is extremely tender. The submucous areolar tissue becomes infiltrated and stiff and hard, as well as painful. Beyond this the symptoms occasioned by the wisdom tooth in the upper jaw very seldom extend, and the removal of the tooth is always followed by complete and immediate relief. The position of the upper wisdom tooth thus impacted is sometimes such as to render it difficult of removal, and it frequently can only be accomplished by a pair of forceps with especially long and curved blades.

The difficulty which most commonly occurs with the inferior *dentes sapientiæ* is attributable to the comparative shortness of the horizontal ramus of the jaw. The tooth usually grows in the right direction and position as regards its neighbour in front, but from the imperfect lengthening of the jaw backwards the birth of the crown is only partial and incomplete. The tooth is upright, but only the front portion is able to emerge. This produces a terrible pinching of the mucous membrane over the tooth every time the jaws are brought together. Before, however, the enamel eminences of the crown make their appearance, the soft structure behind the second molar become much inflamed, and even suppurate, the pus secretion appearing to be within the enamel sac of the tooth between the tooth crown and the membrane covering it. This produces considerable inflammation in all the surrounding parts, the cheek and fauces suffer, the movements of the jaw are stiff and painful, swallowing is difficult, and attended with suffering like that of sore throat. Occasionally the resistance which is offered to the vertical growth of the wisdom tooth produces a dislocation in its direction, and it grows horizontally forward, more or less. This is often attended with serious consequences. The direction is sometimes combined with the inward leaning of the crown as well. This is uncommon, but I have seen it in the worst case of impaction that has occurred in my practice.

There is one peculiar symptom which is frequently associated with difficult eruption of the lower wisdom teeth, but which may also arise from the inflammation produced by periostitis in caries or other teeth diseases affecting the posterior molars, second and third. The symptom in question consists of a spasmodic contraction of the muscles of the jaw, especially the masseter muscle. The contraction is continuous and persistent, and appears to be the result of contiguous irritation. It is not a spasm which varies in intensity, but is of a truly *tonic* character, the muscles being permanently set so as to keep the jaws nearly closed, and susceptible only of very slight separation. The jaw can usually be opened to a small extent, and then is definitely fixed so as to give the impression that some hard substance prevents further movement. Such, however, is not the case, for directly the cause of the irritation is removed the spasm rapidly ceases, and then the mouth can be fully opened.

The pain which accompanies and precedes the cutting of a wisdom tooth, when this is retarded, is of a dull, aching character, not unlike rheumatism, and it often extends over a considerable area, over the side of the head and down the shoulder. The parts on the side affected in the immediate neighbourhood of the tooth frequently swell to a considerable extent, and the lymphatic glands behind the jaw are sometimes enlarged and tender.

But far more serious consequences may arise from impaction of the lower wisdom teeth in the development of abscess, which is sometimes considerable, and extends along the cheek and jaw. It is not unfrequent even where there is sufficient room for the eruption of the tooth for pus to be formed, and it has appeared to me that it occurs in the capsule of the tooth, the pus being secreted by that which was the enamel pulp. I may mention that when I cut my lower wisdom teeth at the age of sixteen, a little sac of pus formed over each tooth before its appearance, and though, from the early age at which the teeth were cut, there was some crowding, still it was not of a nature to render the evolution of the teeth a matter of much difficulty. In severer cases the pus burrows among the areolar tissue along the periosteum of the jaw; the neighbouring soft structures become infiltrated with lymph, and the integument is glued irregularly to the bone. Pus may burrow in these cases to a considerable extent, and sinuses open here and there along the track which the fluid takes, leaving afterwards a series of red shining cicatrices. I have seen the side of the face from the tragus of the ear and the angle of the jaw behind to the angle of the mouth and mental foramen in front, a web of pus-discharging sinuses, and which, after their cure by the removal of an impacted wisdom tooth, left an integument, thin and bound down to the bone with the glossy, tense, cicatrix-like aspect of a recently healed burn—a great and permanent disfigurement.

The accompanying illustration (fig. 110) is the portrait of a patient whom I attended for this malady, and the appearance is very characteristic. He was twenty-two years of age, and had long suffered from pain and swelling of the face on the left side with nearly complete closure of the lower jaw. He had been attended in the country by a general practitioner who had not apprehended the real nature of the case, and mistook it for one of diseased bone. When he applied to me he exhibited on the left side of the jaw, and for a considerable distance down the neck, a large glossy scar exactly resembling the cicatrix of a burn, which might have occurred a few months previously. Near the centre of this scar was a mass of pouting granulations about the size of half-a-crown, on the centre of which pus was discharged from two or three orifices. Upon exploring these orifices with a probe, I was able to pass backwards through a canal, so as to strike a hard body at the extremity of the jaw, which proved to be the crown of the wisdom tooth. After some difficulty I succeeded in getting the jaw sufficiently open to observe the state of the tooth. I found that the wisdom tooth was deeply impacted at the base of the coronoid process, and there was much perversion of direction. The tooth pointed forwards and outwards. I had considerable difficulty in getting the mouth sufficiently open to reach the wisdom tooth, and only accomplished it by the continued process of wedging open for a period of three weeks. I then succeeded in laying hold of the wisdom tooth with a pair of long-bladed forceps, and ultimately removed it. The operation, however, was accomplished with very great difficulty indeed. The tooth was sound. A probe passed backwards from the external orifice into the mouth about the region of the extricated tooth and appeared within the mouth, but whether it entered the socket or not I could not positively say.

Fig. 110.

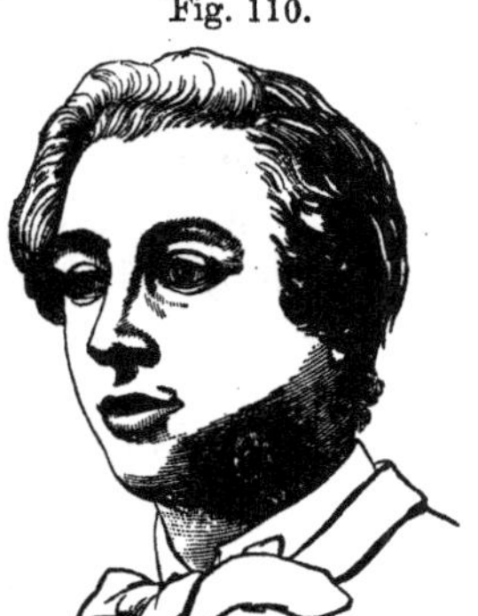

There was nothing about the fang of the tooth to indicate that matter had formed within the alveolus; indeed, after examining a large number of cases, I have come to the conclusion that the pus does not form, as in alveolar abscess, in the socket of the tooth, and immediately connected with the fang, but that it begins either in the areolar tissue of the gum, or, as I have already suggested, within the enamel sac, and that the farther progress of the abscess is due to the subsequent burrowing of the matter, and its *pocketing* in a downward and onward course. As long as any part of the crown of the tooth is covered by the gum, pus may be secreted by the under surface of the overlying portion. I have seen an impacted wisdom tooth give rise to that form of serous cyst known as dentigerous cyst, a case of which will be found described in the chapter on that subject. Where the wisdom tooth is impacted in such a position that its crown points forwards, the second molar often suffers. The posterior fang is apt to be eroded by absorption, and the fang may be so much absorbed as to open the pulp-cavity of the tooth, and even to pass through it and erode the posterior surface of the front fang. I have met with several instances of this, and in one case the second molar was completely necrosed. The periosteum was completely stripped from both fangs, and the tooth remained in its socket bathed in pus. When this condition arises, it usually produces extreme pain, but I have had an example in which I found it necessary to extract the second molar from the mere looseness of the tooth in which no pain had arisen. Upon extricating it I found the posterior fang entirely removed by absorption, and its socket occupied by the crown of the wisdom tooth, which was lying horizontally in the bone, and had never made any appearance whatever in the mouth. These affections of the second molar should be taken into consideration in balancing the merits of the plans of treatment which may be contemplated in any particular case, and will, I think, favour the course of proceeding which I believe ought in many cases to be followed, but which is not now usually adopted, namely, the removal of the second molar instead of the wisdom tooth itself.

The French surgeons have been particularly alive to the interest and importance of these cases, and have published valuable contributions to their illustration.

Velpean delivered an interesting lecture on this subject at the Hospital of La Charité, a translation of which appeared in the *Journal of the Provincial Medical Association* for 1841 (vol. ii. p. 104), in which he fairly remarks that the subject has been "too much neglected by medical men." I beg to refer the reader to this interesting memoir. Another and more recent lecture on the same subject has been published by M. Nélaton in the *Journal de Médecine et de Chirurgie Pratique*, tome xxxiii. p. 61, Février, 1862, entitled "Accidents produits par l'éruption des dents de sagesse."

In this lecture he refers to a memoir of Toirac, who appears to have been the first person to have written on this subject. Nélaton remarks that the symptoms produced in this painful cutting of wisdom teeth have been mistaken for scrofulous caries of the jaw, for syphilis, and for cancer.*

Besides the local symptoms which the impaction of the wisdom tooth may produce, others of secondary nature occasionally arise. I have seen an instance in which the arm of the affected side was partially paralysed. These symptoms vanished upon the removal of the wisdom tooth. Instances have occurred also in which the impaction of the tooth has occasioned epilepsy and delirium; and Velpean records, on the authority of M. Esquirol, a case in which a lady was brought to La Charité Hospital labouring under mental derangement. She was quite restored by the liberation of an impacted wisdom tooth by means of simple lancing of the gum.

Treatment.—When the wisdom tooth of the upper jaw is misplaced or impacted so as to produce inconvenience or painful symptoms, the treatment is very obvious and very simple. The tooth is useless, and worse than useless, and it may be removed without hesitation. I do not remember ever to have met with an instance in which a misplaced upper wisdom tooth was associated with locked-jaw complication, which is so common when the lower wisdom tooth is the subject of this condition. The teeth may be generally got at without much difficulty, provided suitable forceps are employed. In one instance, I was unable to reach the upper wisdom tooth, which had grown forward in a horizontal direction, producing absorption of the second

* See also the Paper by M. Robert in the 4th chap. of the *Conférences de Clinique chirurgicale faites à l'Hôtel Dieu*, 1858-59.

molar fangs. In this case I was obliged to remove the tooth in front; the wisdom tooth was afterwards extracted with ease. In the treatment of the inferior wisdom teeth much will depend upon the degree of the impaction of the tooth and the age of the patient. If the tooth is simply covered over by dense gum, the free lancing of the latter is all that may be needed. Where painful symptoms arise in young subjects whose wisdom teeth push forward at a precocious period, and before the jaw is large enough for their reception, it should be remembered that time will do much to accommodate them by the increased size and posterior elongation of the horizontal ramus of the jaw; and a good deal of inconvenience ought to be borne in such cases rather than sacrifice a sound tooth. At the same time, if such a patient have a carous first or second molar, considerable relief will be obtained by its extrication. And, indeed, this remark would apply to patients of any age, though with less effect in those who are older. As regards lancing the gum, it is well not only to lay bare the crown of the tooth, but to remove the flaps of gum which have overlaid it.

M. Nélaton, in the clinical lecture already referred to, recommends that the gum should be divided by a crucial incision with a bistoury, and the four flaps afterwards removed with curved scissors, and he states that the same suggestion had previously been made by Toirac and Robert. Where lancing the gum and time do not liberate the tooth, it will be necessary either for the wisdom tooth itself or the second molar to be extracted, so as to relieve the crushing tension which exists. The question now arises, which of the two should be taken out? *Cœteris paribus*, it is better to sacrifice the third than the second molar. The wisdom tooth is less useful for mastication, and more liable to decay. But the circumstances of the two teeth may not be equal: the second molar may be carous, or it may be loose or necrose by the pressure of the tooth behind it. In either of such cases it would be better to extract the second molar. Again, the wisdom tooth may be so situated that its extraction is a physical impossibility, or nearly so, as is frequently the case where it grows horizontally forwards deep down in the jaw. Another reason—the locking of the jaws by reason of the masseter spasm—may render it impossible to reach the tooth; then the second molar should certainly be extracted. The painful symptoms which occur when the lower wisdom tooth is thus placed, obviously depend upon the antagonism between the third and second molars, the former pushing forward, the latter resisting its progress. The extraction of either tooth destroys this condition, and the patient feels an equal amount of relief whether the second or third is taken out. The extraction of the second molar, moreover, permits the wisdom tooth to come into a more forward position, and it has a wonderful faculty, when thus liberated, of altering its direction of growth, and an oblique or nearly horizontal tooth will so change its attitude as to become nearly or quite vertical, and a fair opponent to the upper second molar. In this condition, moreover, it is not only useful for mastication, but is less liable to caries. When an abscess has been formed, and suppuration has been fairly established, especially if any burrowing of matter has occurred, it is of the greatest importance to take out the wisdom tooth, as extraction of the second molar under these circumstances frequently fails to arrest the discharge of pus. I have in more than one case recently found this to be the case, and have been disappointed at the result of extracting the second molar. The removal, however, of the front tooth may become necessary in such cases, the wisdom tooth being too deeply imbedded to be otherwise reached by instruments. The closure of the jaws is often so complete that it is impossible to get at either of the molar teeth until that condition has been combated. The jaws can be opened without much difficulty by means of a wedge gradually pushed between the teeth. It is sometimes necessary to continue this operation for many days, but I prefer, if possible, to do it in one day by the diligent perseverance of the patient, as the jaws are apt to close again somewhat in the night, so that the patient has to do much of the work over again. Steel instruments have been devised on the principle of the ear speculum, composed of two shafts or blades which separate slowly but forcibly by the action of a screw. I prefer a wedge of hard wood, such as beech or box wood, which is pushed further and further into the mouth as the contracted masseter yields before it. If this is followed up from early morning until the afternoon the mouth will generally be sufficiently opened to allow the operator to reach the tooth which he intends to extract. Another arrangement, however, invented by Mr. Maunder, seems to possess especial advantages. It is a conical wedge, upon which is cut a spiral screw-worm, gradually increasing in diameter and thickness of the worm. It is shown in the accompanying illustration (fig. 111). It resembles the shell of a univalve mollusc, such as a whelk shell, but the spiral is more elongated and drawn out. Where the contraction of the mouth is the result of an impacted wisdom tooth, occurring as it does in early life, the teeth in front of the mouth are almost always firm, and will bear the use of this instrument. Upon introducing the point of Mr. Maunder's gags between the incisors or canines or præmolars, and slowly turning the instrument, it evenly and regularly progresses, separates the jaw, and, as I have thought, with quicker results than any other method. In removing a deeply impacted lower wisdom tooth, one rather serious accident has been known to occur on several occasions, namely, crushing of the inferior maxillary nerve, leading to sentient paralysis of the nerve and lip of that side. Cases of this casualty will be found recorded in the chapter on accidents occurring in tooth extraction.

Fig. 111.

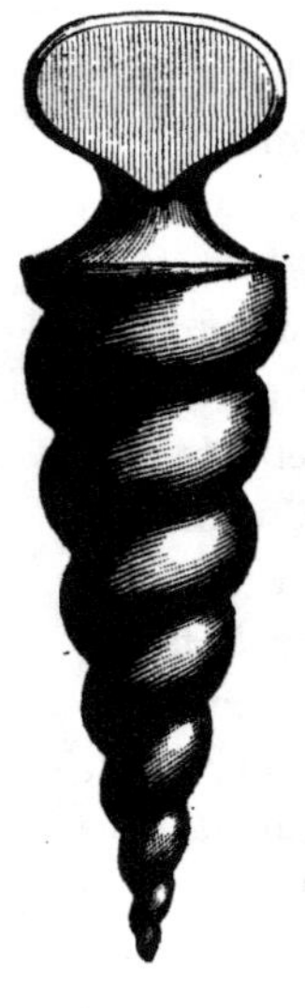

CHAPTER XVIII.

ALVEOLAR ABSCESS. GUMBOIL.

The periosteum immediately surrounding the fangs of the teeth is very prone to inflammatory action, dependent on diseases of the teeth themselves. These may be divided into suppurative and plastic inflammation. Suppurative inflammation of the periosteum around the fangs of the teeth produces that disease known by the name of alveolar abscess, and more popularly, but less correctly, gumboil. Plastic alveolar periostitis is mostly the result of the same causes as suppurative, and is an approximation to that disease, but stopping short of its results. Alveolar abscess is a very common affection; its pathology, however, is often ill-understood. The very name which is popularly given to it—"gumboil"—is a proof of the mistaken notion entertained of its nature, and is a means of perpetuating the error.

The gum is, in fact, only secondarily affected, the cause being situated within the alveolus, and where the disease has reached its consummation, "alveolar abscess" is the best term that can be applied to it.

The *causes* of alveolar abscess are various. Now and then, though very rarely, it is the result of inflammation in the periosteum of a sound tooth, from cold or some local irritation; or it may arise from mechanical injury to a tooth, as its being loosened or partially dislocated by a blow. Fracture of a tooth exposing the pulp, generally ends in alveolar abscess. But the presence of dentinal caries is its most common cause by far, and it may or may not be preceded, or accompanied by tooth-ache.

From whatever source, however, the irritation may arise which produces alveolar abscess, the progress of the disease is, in all essential points, similar, and the indications of the treatment the same.

The first effect produced by the irritation of a diseased tooth, or a dead root which is leading to alveolar abscess, is a thickening of the periosteum of the alveolar cavity, which raises the tooth in the socket, and renders it a little loose, and susceptible of pain on pressure; an effusion of lymph then takes place around the extremity of the fang, which becomes condensed into a sac, within which pus is formed. The sac will be found closely embracing the root, just above the extremity, which is bathed in pus—the pus not being in the substance of the lymph, but between it and the exterior of the fang, the latter itself having frequently undergone change; in some instances consisting of an increased deposition of crusta petrosa, in others of erosive absorption, by which the extremities of the fangs are diminished in length, and rendered ragged on their surface.

Fig. 112.

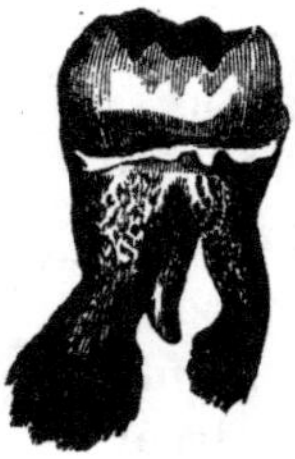

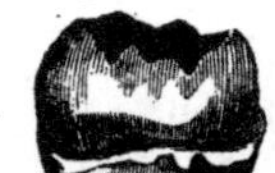

These sacs assume different appearances, depending mainly on the nature of the teeth upon which they have been formed. Thus at the extremity of a cylindrical root, as in the foregoing figure, 112, the sac is simple and of an oval or pyriform shape: but in the case of its being formed on a bicuspid tooth, the root of which is longitudinally contracted, so as to separate the internal cavity into two, having each a distinct foramen at the point, the sac is often double, and has the appearance of two small globular sacs united together. Occasionally the sacs are marvellously elongated, approaching an inch in length; and it will be very frequently observed in teeth with more than one fang, that the sac is attached to that fang on the side towards which the tooth is most decayed. The same holds good in reference to the erosion of the ends of the fangs.

As the morbid phenomena attendant on the development of the alveolar abscess progress, the irritation increases and extends to the neighbouring parts, which become affected with severe throbbing pain, redness and thickening of the gum; and frequently a greater or less degree of tumefaction of the face occurs. These symptoms, both as to the physical suffering of the patient with consequent constitutional sympathy, and amount of swelling and pus-secretion, are often very disproportionate to one another. Occasionally a very small abscess is accompanied with the most agonizing pain, and with great constitutional disturbance and fever. At other times the whole side of the face becomes suddenly and prodigiously swelled, and, when in the upper jaw, causing ecchymosis and œdema of the lids; and yet there may be scarcely any pain or symptomatic fever. These symptoms are but the more palpable demonstrations of what is going on within the jaw. The first deposition of plastic lymph about the extremity of the fang is associated with a concurrent absorption of the cancellated bone around; it is held in a little excavated bony cavity, but when suppuration takes place the cavity rapidly dilates, both by expansion and bony absorption; the investing parts thin and expand, the whole of the bone in one part or other becomes absorbed and the abscess points; it forms for itself an outlet, in some cases externally, either in the cheek or opposite the base of the lower jaw, but more frequently within the mouth through the gum; at other times, in less severe cases, and especially where denudation of the necks of the teeth exists, the matter may burrow along the tooth, stripping off the periosteum from the fang for a small part of its circumference, and pour itself out at the edge of the gum between it and the tooth. This, when it does occur, most frequently happens with the inferior incisor teeth.

The direction in which the matter points in these respective cases, though involving no distinction of pathological principle, bears with it the most important practical considerations. The matter usually finds its way to the surface by the shortest and most direct route. It very readily burrows along the course of a tooth's fang, and, especially where denudation has occurred, escapes at the edge of the gum. The common lateral gum-boil is the most simple and obvious issue of the dilating alveolar pus capsule. If, however, on account of a preternaturally long fang, or from the abscess sac burrowing unnaturally deep into the substance of the jaw, or from the reflection of the mucus-membrane from the gum to the cheek being more than usually superficial; if, from either of these causes, the abscess, instead of pointing within the mouth, burrows deep, and, piercing the cheek, approaches or reaches the surface of the face, the malady then becomes a much more serious matter, entailing, as it does, marked and permanent disfigurement.

In all instances where pus passes from an abscess towards the surface, whatever tissues may be involved, the course of its progress is limited and directed by a surrounding deposition of lymph. When lymph has once been deposited, the inevitable consequence is the contraction of the structures infiltrated by it. Now, when an alveolar abscess points, and opens itself, or is opened, on the surface of the face, directly the first inflammatory swelling subsides, contraction between the skin and the suppurating part commences, the integument is drawn down into a more or less funnel-shaped cavity, at the deepest part of which is usually situated a little mammilla of red granulations, pouring forth pus from its patulous point, which is so characteristic of superficial fistulous opening. It is an unsightly appearance, only to be exchanged, when the causing tooth or stump is removed, for a deeper depression starred in its centre by a cicatrix. There is no condition connected with the diseases of the teeth which has been so commonly misunderstood as this form of alveolar abscess, and there is none which can be more surely prevented when the case is seen early.

I have already said that one of the earliest circumstances connected with the formation of alveolar abscess is the production of a cavity around the apex of the fang. The enlargement of this bony sac, by the pressure of the pus, is sometimes very great; and the absorption (according to the direction in which the abscess points) of the external or internal alveolar plate — by far more commonly the external — is frequently very considerable. Of this, a remarkable specimen is preserved in the museum of Guy's Hospital, of which the accompanying is an illustration (fig. 113).

Fig. 113.

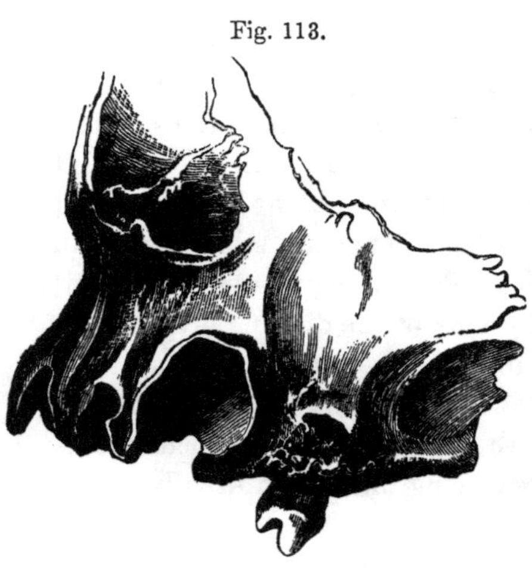

A still greater dilatation of the abscess occasionally occurs, and such a case is recorded in the chapter on the casualties that may arise in tooth-extraction, p. 361.

The course which the matter takes in coming to the external surface is usually short and direct, the canal single and the surrounding indentations circumscribed. Occasionally the orifices of discharge are multiplied and the canal burrowing: one orifice may close and another appear more remote from the cause. I have seen a remarkable example of this latter condition: in this case the abscess first discharged immediately below the lower jaw on the right side; this orifice closed, and was succeeded by another lower down; this also closed, and was followed by another in the neck. The burrowing continued, and when I saw the patient, many months after the first discharge of pus, there were two sinuses opening about an inch below the right clavicle. A carious first molar had caused the suppuration, and its removal was followed by the immediate healing of the sinuses.

Alveolar abscess is usually a trifling matter as regards its ultimate consequences, but occasionally it becomes a very serious malady. An unusually severe instance is recorded by M. Robert.* His patient was 22 years of age, and had long suffered from tooth-ache in the left lower *dens sapientiæ*. When he applied to M. Robert he had stiffness of the neck, with considerable swelling extending from the jaw down to the shoulder and the upper part of the breast. The jaws were closed. There was obscure fluctuation in the front and upper part of the neck. This became more evident, but it was diffused over the whole of the swollen parts. Two incisions were made into the neck, and from them issued a quantity of fetid sero-pus mixed with gas. Suppuration went on increasing, and the patient died a week after admission into the hospital. The post-mortem examination showed that the whole of the muscles from the left side of the neck and shoulder had been dissected by purulent inflammation. There was matter in the subclavicular triangle, and under the trapezoid muscle, and it had passed behind the clavicle even to the armpit. It was shown that the suppuration had originated at the angle of the jaw immediately in contact with the decayed wisdom tooth.

* *Conférences de Clinique chirurgicale.* Par M. A. C. Robert. Paris, 1860, p. 145.

Occasionally the matter, in alveolar abscesses, points at the posterior extremity of the hard palate, though the abscess has been occasioned by one of the front teeth, usually the upper lateral incisor. Why this should arise I cannot say: the pathological anatomy of the affection is essentially the same as in ordinary cases, only the canal of the abscess is lengthened out in the narrow cancellated bone between the two compact plates of the palatal process of the superior maxilla. This condition may readily lead to mistake, and suggest the presence of necrosed bone. A critical scrutiny of the front teeth will, however, scarcely fail to clear up the difficulty.

The characteristics and history of those alveolar abscesses which open externally deserve the closest attention.

Any tooth, except, I believe, the upper *dens sapientiæ*, may give rise to an outward opening alveolar abscess. It is rare with the upper canines and incisors. I have, however, seen an instance in which an abscess connected with a central incisor burst just within the nose; and another, in which the lateral was at fault, where the opening occurred by the side of the nose an inch below the inner canthus. In the upper jaw the external opening of an alveolar abscess, when connected with molars or bicuspids, is usually on the cheek under the edge of the malar bone. In the lower jaw the orifice is somewhere along the lower edge of the buccinator muscle, where a molar or premolar tooth is the cause; but when occasioned by the inferior incisors (canines also?) the matter points frequently beneath, or sometimes in front of the chin.

Before the bursting externally of an alveolar abscess the surface becomes red, distended, and glistening; the skin is thin and papery, and the epidermis scales off. If the surface be kept dry, the breaking of the abscess is often tardy and delayed; but it ultimately bursts through a jagged opening, which soon changes into a small fistulous orifice, surrounded by a pouting circular lip of granulations, that sink into a depression, surrounded by the adhesions which limit the pus-discharging canal. Sometimes the lip of granulations becomes elongated into a papilla, and is covered with cuticle. I have seen one more than half an inch in length. The apex of this papilla has an orifice, which is the outlet of the fistulous canal communicating with the abscess; it frequently closes for a time, but bursts repeatedly as the matter accumulates. When once this papilla forms, it returns again and again, after excision by the knife, till the cause of the whole malady (the diseased tooth) is removed. Another curious modification of the external orifice of the alveolar abscess is occasionally seen when it pierces the under surface of the chin; in such cases a *pad* of granulations sometimes forms, as large as the area of one's thumb-nail, from the centre of which the discharge flows.

In children, with the milk-teeth, alveolar abscess very seldom opens on the surface of the face. I have, however, seen a few such cases. On account of the extreme thinness of the alveoli in them, the end of the affected fang frequently appears through the orifice of the discharge within the mouth, and often projects so far as to wound and ulcerate the mucous membrane of the cheek or lip.

It sometimes happens, that after the first evacuation of the pus of an alveolar abscess the secretion becomes serous. I have known some instances in which the sac of the abscess has remained as a serous cyst even after the extraction of the tooth upon which it originally depended, the secretion recurring again and again after the cyst had been lanced. In one case, where it had happened in a child in connection with an upper incisor tooth, I found it necessary to remove a portion of the wall of the cyst, when it granulated from the interior, and was obliterated.

The *diagnosis* of alveolar abscess is really very simple, though, as I have said, it is often mistaken for diseased bone in those examples where the orifice occurs on the surface of the face. The tooth is the equivalent in these cases of a bone-sequestrum; and it is, as far as the pulp-vitality goes, a dead organ. The fistulous canal leads to the dead tooth, as a sinus to the dead bone; thus far the two conditions are the same, and their appearances are much alike; but there are obvious differences. In alveolar abscess there is less general swelling, except at first in acute cases, and there is an absence of the diffuse indurated lymph-infiltration of the cellular tissue, which is present in bone-necrosis; the canal leading to the abscess is single, usually short and direct, and not burrowing and complicated as is commonly the case in bone-disease; moreover, there is an absence of that fœtor in the discharge, which is so characteristic of necrosed bone. The locality in a doubtful case, being the neighbourhood of the jaw, is in favour of the idea of a tooth being the cause; and an appeal to the state of the teeth seldom fails to settle the question definitively. Sometimes, however, a difficulty may arise from the fact that the cause of the abscess is a mere stump, overlapped by prominent gum; or, what occasions still more obscurity, the abscess may consist of a large excavated cavity in the substance of the jaw, into which the stump has fallen and become loose and free. A probe and the elevator will in either case complete the investigation.

While alveolar abscess, when connected with the integument of the face, is very apt to be mistaken by surgeons for diseased bone, the reverse has happened where a dentist has attributed to carious teeth morbid conditions which have been coincident with them, though not produced by them. I have known this occur in an instance where the patient was suffering from scrofulous caries of the malar bone near its suture with the superior maxilla—a mistake which led to the extraction of two slightly damaged teeth in no way connected with the disease. Again, I have seen one of the submaxillary lymphatic glands, rather adherent to the bone and in an early state of suppuration, mistaken for an outward-pointing alveolar abscess. Such errors as these, leading at most to the extraction of carious, though innocent, teeth are trivial in comparison with those more frequent mistakes, in which alveolar abscess is confounded with bone-disease, and an easily cured malady is allowed to run its course unrestrained, and permanently disfigure the face.

The *treatment* of alveolar abscess depends upon the stage at which the case is seen. In the earliest period, when suppuration is rather impending than established, the malady may be cut short by the extraction of the affected tooth, or by the removal of the stopping in a stopped tooth. Often it is undesirable to extract a particular tooth that may be threatening or causing the abscess; and in that case recourse should be had to leeching the gum freely, the administration of brisk purgatives, and abundant hot fomentation of the face at the swelling part. This mode of treatment, when it does not arrest the malady, much mitigates the attendant suffering. When matter has formed, and the wall of the abscess has sufficiently thinned, the pus should be evacuated by a puncture made through the gum with a narrow thin scalpel. This is followed by immediate and complete relief, and the general swelling associated with the advent of the attack rapidly subsides; but the disease, in the very great majority of cases, remains in the form of a continuously pus-discharging fistula. It is very rare indeed for the pus-secretion to cease: it may be so diminished that the external orifice may close for a time, but it is pretty sure to burst out again and again; though I am confident (contrary to the general published opinion) that in a few exceptional instances the disease ceases altogether, the offending tooth still remaining in the mouth.*

When an alveolar abscess shows symptoms indicative of external pointing, immediate and active treatment is necessary. The offending tooth should be taken out: and in case it breaks in extracting, every vestige should be sought and removed. If matter has formed, and there has been decided thinning of the integument, showing its near approach to the surface, not only should the tooth be extracted, but a vertical incision should be made between the cheek and the jaw, so as to cut across the pus-containing canal; else the matter is apt to *pocket*, and cause progressive absorption to the surface; and though the tooth be removed, the abscess may thus still open externally. This vertical incision between the cheek and the jaw is also useful after the removal of a tooth, even when the external opening has occurred; it cuts across the bands of lymph which glue the integument down to the bone. In this case a piece of oiled lint should be introduced and kept in the wound, to prevent the adhesion and reunion of the cut surfaces. In all cases of alveolar abscess, extraction of the diseased or dead tooth is *the* cure; and I know but of two circumstances which peremptorily interdict this mode of treatment. First, where a strongly pronounced hæmorrhagic diathesis forbids the extraction of teeth altogether; and secondly, in those cases where the abscess is associated with the upper incisor teeth of young people in whom the jaws have not yet assumed their adult form, and where the permanent dentition is as yet incomplete. In this latter case it is of much importance to retain the teeth, even if reduced by

* I have never seen this spontaneous form of cure when the abscess has opened externally on the face.

ecay to mere fangs, till the adult form of the jaws is established, hough at the cost of much suffering and discomfort. The earlier removal of the teeth would be followed by such contraction of the maxillary arch as would be incompatible with a proper replacement by artificial teeth of the natural ones missing.

There are some varieties of alveolar abscess and the circumstances attendant on them which deserve notice here.

Large palatal abscess in children of a very distinct character sometimes occurs. I have generally seen it in children about two or three years of age, whose temporary teeth have decayed early. When the abscesses caused by temporary teeth point on the labial or buccal surface, there is seldom, I believe, anything remarkable about them, excepting that they are apt to denude and free the extremity of the tooth's fang. When, however, the matter is formed towards the palate, the swelling is often much more considerable than in an adult, and from its great size and formidable appearance, might convey an erroneous impression as to its nature. I have seen one of these swellings completely fill the hollow of the palate, passing across the median line and leaving but a narrow space between its convexity and the concavity of the palate on the opposite side. The amount of suppuration, as far as I have seen, is disproportionately small in relation to the size of the tumour; which indeed appears to be mainly produced by a sero-plastic effusion beneath the mucus-membrane and fibrous tissue covering the palate.

Removal of the offending tooth, with or without a scission of the tumour, speedily relieves it.

Suppuration in the eyelid and cheek.—The extreme irritation of a forming alveolar abscess, especially in the upper jaw, occasionally leads to such intense inflammation of the integument of the face as to put on an appearance of erysipelas, and often produces considerable ecchymosis. These results usually subside upon the bursting of the abscess. But occasionally the inflammation is so intense as to lead to suppuration in the subcutaneous areolar tissue.

I have the notes of several such cases which occurred in my own practice.

In one, an abscess appeared in the lower lid of a child four years old, following diffuse erythematous inflammation of the cheek, associated with alveolar abscess. This was not connected with dead bone, and had no direct communication whatever with the teeth which had caused the inflammation: it was an independent and outlying result.

In an adult I have seen suppuration arise in the cheek under similar circumstances: in this case the inflammation was of a phlegmonous character, and resulted in a sort of boil.

A young lady, nine years of age, was brought to me with acute abscess of the cheek, following intense inflammatory toothache, occasioned by a first permanent molar. And in another instance I saw a middle-aged lady in whom the inflammation ended in carbuncle of the cheek. In all these instances the suppuration was independent of any direct connection with the alveolus.

Gumboil, not connected with the alveolus.—There is a particular kind of gum-boil (not, as I believe, described in books) in which suppuration occurs within the substance of the gum, and altogether superficial to the alveolar process. The first example of this that I saw, or at least that I recognised, occurred in my own person, and I had consequently an opportunity of observing it closely. In this instance the tooth, a second lower molar, was loose, but free from decay; it was causing extreme irritation, and the gum was much swollen; the alveolar process was absorbed in some degree. A collection of matter formed again and again quite superficially. On one of these occasions I had the tooth extracted, and there was no evidence on its fangs of matter in contact with them.

I have since occasionally seen this form of superficial gumboil, and I have noticed that it has always been associated with loose teeth, absorbed sockets, and tumid gums.

CHAPTER XIX.

ABSCESS OF THE ANTRUM.

THE antrum maxillare is one of those anatomical regions immediately contiguous with the teeth, which is prone to be affected in a secondary manner by their maladies. But of these only one, that which is called abscess of the antrum, fairly comes under the consideration and treatment of the dental surgeon. The large mucous sinus, known as the antrum Highmorianum, occupies the body of the superior maxilla immediately over the bicuspids and molar teeth; but it varies considerably in its size, form, and relation to the teeth in question. In some instances it extends from the canine to the *dens sapientiæ*, and in others it may correspond only to the first molar. This extreme variation in the size of the antrum is not mentioned in ordinary text-books of anatomy, but it has been pointed out by Otto.* Moreover, the cavity is liable to be divided by bony septa, as shown by Mr. Catlin,† a circumstance which modifies the management of certain contingencies that may arise in extracting the stumps of upper molar teeth. The floor of the antrum is very thin, and in some cases the fangs of the molar teeth pierce it, simply being covered by periosteum, and the mucous lining of the sinus. More often, however, the palatine and external roots diverge, so as to leave an interval between which the more depending sulcus of the antrum is excavated. The antrum opens by a small orifice into the middle meatus of the nose, and through this the secretion of the mucous lining of the sinus is normally discharged. This orifice varies considerably

* *Lehrbuch der pathologischen Anatomie des Menschen und der Thiere,* von Dr. A. W. Otto, p. 180. Berlin, 1830.

† *Des Maladies du Sinus maxillaire,* par M. Giraldès. Paris, 1851.

in size. In some instances it would admit the point of the little finger, and in others it is barely sufficient to allow the passage of a probe. It is always much smaller in the living state when the mucous membrane lines and fills up the opening, and it is the pouting of the tumid mucous membrane which closes the orifice in inflammation.

The term abscess of the antrum conveys a wrong impression as to the real nature of the disease. It is not the suppuration of inflamed parenchyma, but the shutting up of a purulent secretion within the mucous cavity. The lining membrane of the antrum is liable, like all mucous membranes, to inflammation and altered secretion; mucus being impregnated with or replaced by pus, and accumulating in quantity. This may occur in different degrees both as to amount and rapidity of development. The lining membrane of the antrum may secrete and discharge pus through the nose without any of the severe symptoms which occur in the so-called abscess of that cavity. But if the orifice communicating with the middle meatus of the nose becomes occluded by the swelling and turgescence of the mucous membrane around it, then, that which was merely a catarrhal inflammation, spending itself in the discharge of pus, becomes a shut sac full of pus or muco-pus, and in many respects equivalent to a deep-seated abscess, but the pathological history and absolute anatomy of the condition are by no means the same.

The *causes* of abscess of the antrum are, in the majority of cases, some affections of the teeth, the commonest being alveolar abscess dependent on caries. In some few cases, especially those of a mild character, the affection appears to arise from catarrhal inflammation. An instance has been recorded which occurred in a new-born child, and apparently originated from pressure on the cheek during a hard labour.

The symptoms of pus secretion within the antrum vary almost indefinitely. There may be a discharge of matter into the nose producing scarcely any discomfort or consciousness, and, on the other hand, an acute case of so-called antral abscess may occasion the severest local and constitutional suffering. Such cases as the latter are comparatively rare at the present time, and many practitioners of dental surgery seldom see the malady in its severest forms. But half a century since, when diseases of the teeth were less attended to, these severe cases of abscess of the antrum were comparatively common; and Mr. Bell informs me that at that period, and for long after, he was seldom without a case under treatment at Guy's Hospital. Where symptoms are marked they usually commence with an aching pain in the cheek, which is hot and flushed and somewhat swollen. When the orifice into the middle meatus is closed, there is little or no purulent discharge from the corresponding nostril. As the case advances, and the matter accumulates within the antrum, the pain increases in extent, and becomes throbbing in character, and frequently the patient has symptoms like those of acute abscess, with rigors and fever. The physical condition of the jaw gradually undergoes change. There is a general expansion of the whole bone; the malar bone becomes lifted up, and the depression beneath it full and prominent; the molar teeth on the affected side are depressed, so as to seem too long, and interfere with the closure of the mouth. The secretion still increasing, the cavity of the palate, instead of being concave, becomes flat or even convex, the nostril of the affected side is encroached upon, and in severe and protracted cases the floor of the orbit may be so pushed up as to protrude the eye, the vision of which is affected by stretching the optic nerve. Some rare instances have occurred, in which the inflammation resulting from antral abscess has extended backwards and upwards, so as to involve the motor as well as the optic nerves entering the orbit, producing blindness and fixedness of pupil on the affected side.

Such cases are very rare; but one has occurred in my own practice at Guy's Hospital; * a second was under the care of Mr. Pollock; and a third is mentioned by Dr. Brück, in Casper's *Wochenschrift.*† Necrosis of part of the jaw is one of the rarer accompaniments of this malady; but when any portion of the

* "Case of Amaurosis from Abscess of the Antrum, caused by a Carious Tooth," by S. J. A. Salter. *Med. Chir. Trans.*, vol. xlv.

† Wiederholte Entzündungen des Antrum Highmori und Amaurose, &c., mitgetheilt vom Dr. T. H. Brück, in Casper's *Wochenschrift*, März, 1851, Berlin. A case of a similar character was described by Professor Galenzowski, in *Archives Générales de Médecine*, tome xxiii. p. 261. Paris, 1830. These cases are referred to in detail in the chapter on Affections of the Nervous System dependent on diseases of the teeth.

bone is affected, it is usually either the alveolar processes, or the nasal plate of the maxilla.

When the disease has advanced so as to produce thinning of the bony walls of the sinus, manipulation assists the diagnosis by giving evidence of fluid fluctuation, and this may be completed by exploring the cavity with a minute trocar or a curved needle: the fluid then discharged through the slender canal will establish the nature of the malady.

If the case is left to itself the pus will ultimately find a vent somewhere. According to Hunter, the most frequent course of the matter is to burst through the cheek, but it may find its way into the nose, or it may burrow along the side of the fang of the tooth in the alveolar cavity, and the fluid be discharged into the mouth. Occasionally the floor of the orbit gives way, and the pus is discharged somewhere along the lower eyelid. I have known more than one instance in which there has been a temporary yielding of the orifice into the nose, the discharge taking place for a time, and then ceasing.

As regards the treatment of this malady, one cannot do better than follow the often quoted injunctions of Hunter.

"The first part of the cure, as well as that of all other abscesses, is to make an opening, but not in the part where it threatens to point; for that would generally be through the skin of the cheek.

"If the disease is known early, before it has caused the destruction of the fore part of the bone, there are two ways of opening the abscess: one by perforating the partition between the antrum and the nose, which may be done; and the other by drawing the first or second grinder of that side, and perforating the partition between the roots of the alveolar process and the antrum, so that the matter may be discharged for the future that way.

"But if the fore part of the bone has been destroyed, an opening may be made on the inside of the lip, where the abscess most probably will be felt; but this will be more apt than the other perforation to heal, and thereby may occasion a new accumulation, which is to be avoided, if possible, by putting in practice all the common methods of preventing openings from healing or closing up; but this practice will rather prove troublesome; therefore, the drawing of the tooth is to be preferred, because it is not so liable to this objection." *

But the surgeon may have an opportunity of seeing the patient when the antral abscess is imminent, and before it has become established. There are sufficient premonitory conditions to indicate this condition, and then it is possible to avert the malady by early and active treatment. Any carious tooth in the neighbourhood of the antrum should be removed. Further, bleeding may be accomplished by leeches, and hot fomentation should be used, and purgatives administered. When, however, pus is actually formed and is shut up in the cavity, as Hunter has remarked, it is necessary to make an opening for its evacuation, and for many reasons the extraction of the tooth is the best method of commencing that process. It enables the operator to enter the antrum at its most dependent part, and to remove what is the probable cause of the disease. In the great majority of cases it will be found that the first permanent molar is the offender. It is more apt to decay than any other tooth in the jaw, and it occupies a position which usually leads to the sinus most readily. But if any other tooth appears to be the cause of the disease it should be removed, even a canine, for in such case not only is the cause removed, but the absorption of bone which has occurred around the fang of the carious tooth renders the perforation of the antrum more easy than if a sound tooth immediately at its base were taken out. However, it is a safe rule to extract all the carious teeth from the side of the upper jaw affected.

The mere removal of the tooth will in many instances be followed by the discharge of matter, but it is desirable to increase the size of the cavity so as to complete the evacuation of the purulent fluid, and allow the further operation of washing out the antrum by means of a syringe. Perforating the antrum sometimes requires very considerable force, and this force should be applied with great caution and reticence. While the operator pushes the trocar upwards with rotating motion, the forefinger of the right hand should be placed far forward on the shaft of the instrument, so as to be prepared for any sudden giving way of the floor of the antrum, as in that case the trocar

* *Practical Treatise on the Diseases of the Teeth,* by John Hunter, pp. 45, 46. 4to. London, 1771.

may traverse its cavity, and strike hard upon the floor of the orbit, and even pierce it. I have once witnessed this accident in the hands of a young operator, but fortunately it was not followed by any injurious results.

Occasionally the antral abscess is associated with necrosis of a portion of the upper jaw. When this is the case, the alveolar process is most often affected, and the amount of dead bone inconsiderable. In such cases the presence of the necrosed bone is attended with purulent discharge having the characteristic odour so familiar to every surgeon. The pus, which is simply pent up in an antral abscess, has merely the putridity of staleness, which is quite distinct from the fetor indicative of the presence of dead bone. Though the amount of necrosis is usually inconsiderable, it sometimes involves a large portion of the jaw. In the case under my own care, already referred to, besides several smaller sequestra, one mass was brought away, consisting of a considerable portion of the floor of the orbit and the cheek surface of the maxilla involving the infra orbital foramen, and also a long thin plate of bone from the outer wall of the nose. In this case it was necessary, for the removal of the sequestrum, to make a crescentric cut from below the outer canthus of the lid to a similar point below the inner canthus. The loss of this bone so completely opened the antrum that all further occlusion of matter ceased, and the case, so far as it was an antral abscess, quickly came to an end. But the loss of substance which occurred in the front of the cheek was so considerable that it was necessary, after some months, to close a large remaining opening into the antrum by means of a plastic operation, at the expense of some of the integument of the cheek. It is not always easy to remove dead bone at once, but where there is necrosis it is advantageous to make a perforation in the neighbourhood of the dead bone, which will allow the discharge of the matter, and afterwards assist in the shedding of the sequestrum. If antral abscess occurs in a case where the teeth have long been removed, the *osteal cicatrix*, which forms the floor of the antrum, will be extremely dense and compact, and it may be difficult to enter the cavity through its hard substance. In such case it may be desirable to open the antrum on the side below the malar bone. To do this the mucous membrane should be divided down to the bone, and the latter pierced either with a trocar, or, as Sir B. Brodie suggests, with a strong pair of scissors closed and held firmly in the hand, and these should be bored into the part chosen for perforation, the same care being used, as before suggested, to prevent the instrument from passing across the cavity and injuring the parts on the other side.

It has been suggested by more than one surgeon to open the antrum by means of a bent *sound*, by forcing it through the natural orifice. This plan was originally advised by M. Jourdain, who in 1795 read a memoir on the diseases of the maxillary sinus before the Academy of Surgery of France. He proposed first to introduce a sound, and having re-established the orifice, to pass a catheter into it, and by this means to syringe it and remove the discharge. A Committee of the Academy was appointed to investigate the feasibility of this plan, but their verdict was rather adverse. Some experiments in the same direction were made many years since by Mr. Bell on the dead subject at Guy's Hospital, but I believe his trials led to no definite result. Still the idea does not seem otherwise than reasonable and practical.

When the antrum has been opened, by whatever means, it should be thoroughly washed out by injections. Warm water abundantly employed will at first remove the matter and any inspissated secretion that the sinus may contain. This process is usually followed by immediate relief; the swelling and inflammation subside. If the secretion of pus continues, some astringent solution should be employed. The injection of sulphate of zinc, or a weak solution of nitrate of silver in distilled water, will be found efficacious.

I am in the habit of using a glass syringe with an ivory nozzle, to the extremity of which a bent silver tube is fitted. In employing this apparatus, the silver tube is introduced into the opening in the antrum, and kept there while the syringe is filled and used, and withdrawn, refilled, and used again many times. When the washing out of the antrum is completed, both the syringe and the silver tube are withdrawn; and now, unless some means are taken to prevent it, accidents of two kinds may occur; first, food may pass through the orifice into the maxillary sinus; and, secondly, the aperture thus artificially made may close and cicatrise over. To frustrate these results, the plan usually adopted has been to plug the orifice with a piece of wood, which effectually prevents both ill consequences. This is, however, a clumsy method: the same and further advantages may be gained by adopting a plan which I have followed in some recent cases. After the perforation through the alveolar cavity has been made, I have taken a model, and a plate has been prepared to pass over the space occupied by the extracted tooth, and fastened to the contiguous teeth by the customary metal bands. Through this plate a hole has been bored, which corresponds to the orifice into the antrum; and to the applied surface of the plate a very short tube has been soldered, sufficiently long just to enter the antrum, to occupy the perforation, and prevent its closure. This plate has been permanently fixed during the active treatment of the case, and the orifice in the tube has been kept closed by a plug of cork in the intervals between using the injection. By the removal of the cork, the nozzle of the syringe, which fitted the tube, could be applied, and the injection used any number of times, the tube being sufficiently short to allow the complete washing out of the cavity and the escape of the fluid. This plan of treatment has the additional advantage that, when there is no further need of keeping open the artificial orifice, the plate over the gum facilitates its closure. By removing the tube, and closing the hole by a little sheet of metal soldered on, the passage of air and fluid from the mouth to the antrum is suspended, and the healing of the wound is thereby facilitated, as will be hereafter explained. (See Chapter on the Application of Obturators, &c.)

It has sometimes happened that the fang of a tooth associated with an antral, or an alveolar abscess, has passed into the antrum at the time of its attempted removal. This has occurred to myself on two occasions, and in both of these the fang again appeared at the orifice on the floor of the antrum and was easily removed. Such, however, is not always the course of events when this casualty has arisen. As has been before mentioned, the sinus is sometimes divided by partial septa of bone projecting from its walls. In such a condition the fang may be pocketed in one division of the cavity, and so remain a source of permanent irritation not to be removed by mere syringing with fluid. An instance of this kind occurred in the practice of Mr. Catlin, and the particulars are described in the second volume of the "Transactions" of the Odontological Society. In this instance it was necessary to remove the foreign body by means of a curved scooping instrument which was introduced into the antrum. In any doubtful case of obstinate and prolonged inflammation this possible condition should be remembered.

CHAPTER XX.

AFFECTIONS OF THE NERVOUS SYSTEM DEPENDENT ON DISEASES OF THE TEETH.

SCATTERED through Medical and Surgical literature, and occasionally recorded in works specially devoted to Diseases of the Teeth, are to be found cases in which some portions of the nervous system have been affected by dental irritation, or have been implicated by the inflammatory results of tooth disease. I do not here allude to the centric and reflex nervous diseases incident to the first dentition of early infancy, which have already been abundantly recognised, and have formed a conspicuous part of all treatises on the diseases of childhood; but to those less regular and generally much more obscure affections, which have in many instances been proved to depend on certain faults of second dentition, or have been traced to morbid changes in the tissues of the teeth themselves. Such cases are far less common than those in early childhood, or, perhaps it may be more properly said, have been less often recognised; for I suspect that many such instances of disease occur without their being attributed to their real cause.

In the following pages I have principally narrated examples of nervous disease, dependent upon the teeth, which have occurred in my own practice; but in some instances I have selected from the writings of others such cases as I have thought would best illustrate the subject.

The affections of the nervous system dependent on the teeth naturally divide themselves into those which are reflex—secondary and remote; and those which are direct—immediate and from contiguity. In the former category would rank epilepsy, neuralgia, paralysis; in the latter local pain, facial palsy, some forms of amaurosis, &c. In other instances, such as the exalted sensibility of the tegumentary nerves of the face, erratic pains through the maxillary nerves, associated with tooth-ache, it might be difficult to say whether the phenomena are mostly reflex or direct: they probably comprise both conditions.

The situation of the teeth, their abundant supply of nerves, and the great and diffuse swelling which their diseases produce in contiguous structures, inevitably involve much nervous disturbance and complication. The inferior lower molars are but little removed from the tonsils and Eustachian tube, from the parotid region, and the external auditory passage. The fangs of the upper back teeth are close to the orbit, and its all-important contents; and more posteriorly they approach the spheno-maxillary fossa and fissure. Thus it is easy to account for the nervous complications which are directly entailed by the spread of inflammation from the periosteum of diseased teeth.

The reflex nervous disturbances dependent upon tooth irritation are not a little remarkable, and their variety and importance are in keeping with the large bulk of nerve supplied to these organs, and the conditions for extreme irritation to which they are exposed in them.

By far the commonest reflex nervous disturbances, to which dental irritation gives rise, are neuralgic pains of the head; and this is especially the case where the upper teeth are implicated: the supra- and infra-orbital nerves, the globe of the eye, the temple, and particularly a spot near the vertex a little on one side—the side of the affected tooth—in all these regions "dental neuralgia" is really very common: and I have observed not unfrequently that, where the pain has continued long, the integument, at the painful spot, has become hot and tender and red. I have noticed this in my own person when suffering from a carious upper molar tooth: the induced tenderness of the brow was such as to render the disturbance of the hairs of the eyebrow intensely painful.

The several branches of the trigeminus appear to be the most susceptible of reflex affection, caused by the dental irritation of one of them: but next to the different elements of the fifth nerve, the branches of the cervical and brachial plexuses are most commonly involved—pains of the neck, shoulder, acromian process, insertion of the deltoid, bend of the elbow, are by no means uncommon, and with them occasionally a loss of motor power, a weary sense of fatigue in the flexor muscles, and an inability to grasp firmly with the hand. It would really seem that there is occasionally and in some individuals a special and exceptional communication between the fifth nerve and those of the arm. Dr. Anstie * has seen two instances in which wounds of branches of the ulnar nerve have caused reflex neuralgia of the fifth nerve. And he remarks upon this circumstance:—"That the mental perception of the patient should in each of these cases refer the pain, not to any point in the course of the injured nerve, but to branches of the trigeminal, affords, in my opinion, a strong suggestion that that portion of the central nervous system with which the trigeminus is directly connected, presents some congenital or acquired peculiarity of organisation." This idea is fully borne out by what one occasionally, but only occasionally and exceptionally, sees in the occurrence of brachial neuralgia and paralysis caused by dental irritation of the branches of the fifth nerve.

Reflex nervous irritation dependent upon dental disease is most uncertain and capricious in its manifestation. One person will suffer much from a comparatively slight cause, while in others the same condition more severely developed will produce no such result. There is unquestionably in some persons a neuralgic diathesis; and it is not improbable also that in some individuals there may be a congenital, or induced, peculiarity in the centric, or perhaps collateral, relations of certain nerves, by which the exalted polarity of one may be passed on and so reflected upon another with exceptional facility. In persons obnoxious to these forms of neuralgia from dental irritation, nothing is so liable to induce an attack as exhaustion or depressed nutrition: and patients will often say that the attacks only come on when they are very tired, or have gone long without food.

Pain is only one of the phenomena of reflex dental nerve irritation. It may induce *muscular spasm, muscular paralysis, paralysis of some of the nerves of special sense, perverted nutrition.*

As regards the teeth themselves which excite this exalted

* Lettsomian Lectures on Painful Affections of the Fifth Nerve. By Dr. Anstie. *Lancet*, 1866, vol. ii. pp. 31, 32.

nervous irritability, nearly all their diseases appear capable of causing this condition :—

Caries, with or without exposure of the pulp. Exostosis—hypertrophy of the crusta petrosa. Nodular developments of dentine in the pulp cavity. Periostitis, plastic or suppurative. Impaction of permanent teeth in the maxillary bones. Crowding of teeth from insufficient room.

Each and all of the above enumerated abnormalities of teeth have caused manifestations of reflexed nervous irritation, though, as I have remarked, they may exist in the severest forms without producing any such result.

I will now proceed to illustrate the foregoing observations by narrative cases, selected from very many, some of them of more than ordinary interest.

Reflex Affections.

Facial Neuralgia from Dentine-excrescence in Pulp Cavity.—During the year 1854, a woman applied to me at Guy's Hospital on account of severe neuralgic pains obviously connected with one of the central incisors of the upper jaw. The pain was described as of a gnawing character, abiding, but not constantly severe; frequently amounting to a mere consciousness of the presence of the tooth, and at other times sharp and darting. In the former condition it was confined to the region of the tooth; in the latter, it flashed up the side of the face, and through all the branches of the superior maxillary division of the fifth nerve of that side. Sudden pressure, or a tap upon the tooth, or a marked change of temperature, produced a considerable augmentation of pain. The tooth itself was sound, to all external appearance; it was somewhat elongated beyond its fellow, and was very slightly loose. The patient was not aware that the tooth had ever received a blow. When I extracted it, no exostosis (which I had expected) was found upon the root, and, with the exception of some patches of half-organised lymph, it appeared quite healthy. Upon making a section of the tooth (vertical, from side to side), I found an oval pearl-like excrescence of dentine growing from the side of the pulp cavity, so as to encroach much upon it, and occupying, for a short space, more than half its diameter.

The removal of the tooth, though accompanied with a violent

paroxysm of neuralgic agony, was followed by a total cessation of pain. Pain never recurred.

Cranial Neuralgia from an Impacted Canine Tooth.—The particulars of a curious and severe case will be found at page 202, in the chapter on Impacted Permanent Teeth.

Intense and General Neuralgia from Exostosis on Fangs of Teeth.—Miss B. P—— was from her early childhood a patient of Mr. Bell's. Nothing occurred during her first dentition to attract attention. On the advent of the permanent teeth there was some crowding, and four bicuspids (one on either side above and below) were extracted to make room. During adolescence, Miss P—— being in delicate health, was attacked with pains of a neuralgic character, affecting the maxillary nerves and their terminal branches. These attacks appeared associated with certain teeth from which the pain seemed to emanate, and this association became more and more manifest. At first the neuralgia was confined to the branches of the trigeminus, but, as it increased in intensity, it spread to the arms, legs, and, indeed, nearly the whole body. The teeth themselves appeared quite sound; they had, however, a tendency to elongate and spread, as though by filling-up of the sockets, and this was especially the case with the front upper teeth, with which, indeed, the pain was principally associated at first. The offending teeth always gave pain on being slightly struck. The neuralgic suffering became so severe, and its connection with the teeth so distinct, that Mr. Bell removed those most obviously involved. The loss of the teeth was followed by complete cessation of pain, though this was only of temporary duration. The teeth themselves were quite free from caries, but the fangs were in each case encrusted with small nodules of exostosis.

A brief period of immunity from pain having passed, the same neuralgic symptoms recurred, and the same association with some particular tooth or teeth; and as the suffering became greater, and at last unbearable, Mr. Bell extracted more teeth, followed by the same temporary relief. And this succession of suffering, of tooth-drawing and of short-lived ease, was repeated again and again. In every instance the teeth exhibited the same nodular exostosis. At length, when some twenty teeth had been lost, the young lady's friends had misgivings respecting the treatment that had been adopted, and determined to take the opinion of an eminent surgeon as to its propriety. Miss B. P—— was taken to Sir Benjamin Brodie, and the teeth that had been removed were also submitted to his inspection. Sir Benjamin deprecated the treatment which had been followed, expressing a positive opinion that the teeth had had nothing to do with the neuralgic suffering, and that their removal had been altogether unnecessary. The patient herself was, however, so satisfied that Sir Benjamin was mistaken, that, at her urgent request, a further opinion was sought, and she was taken to the late Mr. Samuel Cartwright: the history of the case was narrated to him, and the teeth, which had been extracted, were placed in his hands for inspection. After examining the teeth with great care and minuteness, he separated them into two lots: four bicuspids he placed on one side, declaring his belief that they were sound in every respect, and could not have been associated with the painful affection which had been described to him: as regards the remainder, he considered that each and all of them might have occasioned the neuralgia, and he pointed out to his patient and her friends the nodules of exostosis on the fangs of the teeth as the reason for his coming to that conclusion. Miss P—— then explained to Mr. Cartwright that the four bicuspids he had pronounced sound were removed in early childhood in the regulation of her second dentition, and that the others were all of them extracted by Mr. Bell for her relief during her long and painful illness.

When I saw Miss P—— (in 1851), only two teeth remained in her mouth, the two lower left bicuspids. They were causing the same distressing pain that the others had done. I extracted them, and on the fangs of both were the expected nodules of exostosis. The neuralgia again entirely ceased after the teeth were gone.

At this time Miss P—— was in a condition of extraordinary anœmia: her gums were like wax stained of the palest pink; and on extracting the bicuspid teeth, the empty alveoli remained white and bloodless; it seemed some seconds after the teeth were out before blood oozed from the broken vessels, and then there was not enough to fill the hollow sockets. I never saw anything exactly like it before or since.

Neuralgia of the Arm from Carious Teeth and from undue

pressure of Artificial Teeth.—Mrs. E——, the wife of a medical practitioner, has been under the care of Mr. Bell and myself for many years, and has now (January 1867) lost all her teeth, and wears a complete artificial set. One curious fact was constantly observed during the progress of her case—when any of the teeth in the lower jaw on the left side became irritable or tender from caries, she was immediately attacked with severe neuralgic pain at a spot, small and circumscribed, on the front of the left forearm, about two inches below the line of flexion of the elbow joint. And what is more remarkable is, that when her artificial teeth hurt the lower jaw on that side, the same symptom manifests itself. The right side has never been similarly affected.

Chronic Trismus from Impaction of Lower Dens Sapientiæ.—A. B——, aged 23, with large teeth and comparatively small maxillary bones, had been suffering for the last three years from recurrent attacks of pain and swelling within the mouth, and in the angles of the lower jaw, where the wisdom teeth were deeply embedded, and unable from want of room to come into place. For four months there had been persistent "lock-jaw," which at first alarmed the patient and his friends exceedingly. It supervened suddenly, and appeared to be occasioned by contraction of the left masseter muscle. At present the patient could barely force a tobacco-pipe between his incisor teeth. I directed him to use Maunder's screw gag * to force open the jaws, and after its employment for a week I was able to extract the second molar tooth of the left side, the wisdom tooth being altogether out of reach. The posterior fang of this tooth was much eroded by absorption. The trismus did not recur, and the jaw had lost all its stiffness in four and twenty hours.

It may be a question whether the muscular spasm, in this and similar cases, is caused by contiguous irritation, or is the result of reflex nervous action.

Wry-neck from Carious Teeth of Lower Jaw.—Mr. Hancock has published † the following interesting case:—

"A young woman was brought to me at the Charing Cross Hospital with *wry-neck*, the head being drawn down nearly to

* For further particulars on this subject, and an illustration of this instrument, see Chapter on Difficult Eruption of the Wisdom Teeth.

† *Lancet*, 1859, vol. i. p. 80.

the left shoulder, accompanied with considerable pain. She had suffered in this way for above six months, and had been treated with blisters in the spine, leeches, various liniments, and internally with quinine, calomel, various preparations of iron, valerian, &c., but without benefit. I was informed that with this exception she was in good health, and I therefore concluded the mischief must depend on some local cause. An examination of the spine in the cervical region showed that there was no disease in that situation, but upon looking into her mouth a stump and a partially decayed tooth were seen in the lower jaw on the left side. When I decided to have these extracted, she assured me they caused her no inconvenience. Nevertheless she was induced to have the operation performed, and she got well in a few days."

Epilepsy from Carious Tooth.—Dr. Ramskill gives a very interesting case of epilepsy from a carious tooth—conclusive as to its cause—in a clinical lecture published in the "Medical Times and Gazette" for 1862.*

"A boy, aged thirteen years, has had frequent attacks of epilepsy for the last eighteen months. Latterly his mother has noticed that some days he rubs his left cheek, complaining of faceache, after which the fit follows. On examining the mouth, there is to be seen a molar tooth considerably decayed, with a swollen gum around it, and partly growing over into the cavity; it is not very tender to touch, and the examination does not give rise to toothache. On questioning, I find the sensation, which the boy experiences before a fit, does not seem to be one of pain, but rather of an indefinite uneasiness. He always has a fit the night this comes on. Has never felt it during the day: it is always about seven or eight o'clock. I desired the mother to have the tooth extracted, and ordered a simple saline with a quarter of a grain of belladonna, to be taken twice daily. This was in June. The tooth was extracted next day. I saw this boy once a fortnight from that time for four months, but he has had no recurrence of the fit.

"In this case I believe an unfelt aura commenced about the gum surrounding the tooth, and was not recognised till some degree of inflammation arose, and thus a modification of pain became associated with the aura and directed attention to it."

* *Medical Times and Gazette*, 1862, vol. ii. p. 216.

Tetanus from Mechanical Irritation of the Pulp.—The fracture of a tooth leaving bare a healthy and uncalcified pulp, exposes one of the most intensely sensitive, and (anatomically speaking) one of the most nervous structures in the body.

The mechanical irritation of the tooth-pulp under such circumstances causes the most acute pain; but it may excite also exalted nervous polarity, extended to the cerebro-spinal nerves, eventuating in fatal tetanus. Mr. Tomes, in his "Lectures on Dental Surgery," gives the following brief but graphic account of a terrible example of fatal lock-jaw, induced by pivoting with a gold peg an artificial tooth upon a tooth-fang with a newly-exposed, raw pulp.*

"The following statement was placed in my hands by a medical man, who had some knowledge of the case which is related. —— —— Esq., aged twenty-five years, tall and thin, but apparently in very good health. On his marriage trip he visited Paris, and there had the misfortune to break off a front tooth. Wishing to conceal the accident from his wife, he went immediately to a dentist. The tooth was pivoted (and I have no doubt carefully, for the dentist was one with a great and just reputation), and the necessary concealment seemed insured. From the time of the operation, however, he had severe pain in the stump, which pain increased for four or five days, when he left Paris for Rouen. Upon arriving there the pain had become excessively severe: he consulted a medical man, but it was too late. Trismus came on within twenty-four hours, and was soon followed by tetanus and death."

I am indebted to my late brother, Dr. Hyde Salter, for the following account of his own sufferings from neuralgia caused by a decayed tooth:—

Neuralgia of Neck and Arm from Carious Molar.—"Many years ago, when about seventeen years of age, I suffered a great deal for many months from symptoms caused by a carious tooth. The affected tooth was the lower anterior molar on the left side. It must have become carious when I was about ten or twelve years of age, I think, and at the time that I speak of was little more than a large crater of enamel. The upper surface was gone, but the four lateral walls were perfect, except on the inner side, which was partly broken away. The tooth was quite firm.

* *Lectures on Dental Surgery.* By John Tomes. London, 1848, p. 321.

"For some years previously I had had occasional acute attacks of inflammation in it, accompanied with swollen face, but these for two or three years had ceased, and there was nothing beyond an occasional grumbling uneasiness in it. But, about the time that I speak of, neuralgic pains of a dull aching character began to extend from the tooth down into the neck on the left side, and thence over the collar-bone down the left arm. These aching pains were not constant; for some days I would be perfectly free of them, and then for several days together they were so constant and so wearing as to be almost insupportable. There was no actual pain in the tooth itself, nor any tenderness in it, nor in the adjacent gum, nor any appearance of inflammation; but I had a feeling (not a mental conviction, but a bodily sensation) that all these pains down the side of the neck and left arm were connected with this tooth. The situation of the pain in the neck and clavicular and supra-mammary region was exactly that of the descending cutaneous branches of the cervical plexus, and the part in the arm where the aching was the most intense and intolerable was the insertion of the deltoid. There were certain times of the day, I forget which, when for a period the pain came on with punctual regularity. There was one curious circumstance that I well remember, and that is, that the pain was always brought on by playing on the piano. The longer I persisted, the more intense the aching became, till after an hour or so I was obliged to give it up. This tendency of playing on the piano to induce the pain increased so much at last that I could not play for a quarter of an hour without the aching becoming almost unbearable. It was this circumstance that chiefly compelled me at last to have the tooth out. From the moment of its extraction all these symptoms ceased, and I have never had the slightest return of them since."

Paralysis of the Arm from an Impacted and Carious Wisdom Tooth.—Miss B——, aged twenty-four, consulted one on the 15th of October, 1864, respecting the left lower wisdom-tooth and the symptoms to which it had apparently given rise. The tooth had pierced the gum, but it was low down and placed horizontally, the crown pressing forwards against the second molar. The tooth was carious. From the first attempt at the eruption of this tooth there had been much pain of the ordinary kind about the angle of the jaw; latterly it had been intense, and for a fortnight there had been paralysis of the left arm: the patient complained of total inability to use the arm, to raise it or to grasp with the hand: she could not employ the limb in dressing herself, and could not hold her fork at dinner. There was also a continuous pain of the whole arm resembling rheumatism. I extracted the tooth, but with extreme difficulty. As soon as the patient recovered from the pain of the operation, she declared that the arm-symptoms had vanished completely. A casualty arose in extracting this tooth, which sometimes will occur in removing the inferior *dens sapientiæ*. The inferior maxillary nerve was crushed, or at least bruised, so that the teeth on the left side of the lower jaw, and the integument of the lip around the region of the mental foramen, were numb. This, however, passed away in a few days.

Neuralgia of Face, Neck, and Arm, with partial Paralysis of the latter from Carious Wisdom Tooth.—Miss W——, residing at Southampton, applied to Dr. Wilks, January 16, 1865. She was suffering from constant aching pain on the left side of the face and neck and of the left arm. The pain sometimes became intensely severe. The arm had nearly lost all muscular power; the patient could not raise it to her head, or squeeze any object in her left hand. This state of things had existed two years, and the patient had been under medical treatment all the time.

Upon examining her mouth, Dr. Wilks observed that the left inferior *dens sapientiæ* was carious. He sent the patient to me, and I extracted the tooth. She immediately felt great relief, and in a few hours all the symptoms had completely disappeared.

Amaurosis caused by crowding of Teeth.—The following interesting case is from Mr. Hancock's paper in the "Lancet" of 1859, already referred to. "J. K——, aged eleven, admitted into Charing Cross Hospital, November 11, 1854. About a month previously, upon waking one morning, he found he was entirely blind. Previously, he had nothing the matter with his eyes, and when he went to bed on the preceding night he could see distinctly. He consulted a surgeon in the country, who prescribed medicines, blisters, and subsequently cupping, but as he did not derive benefit therefrom, he was, at the expiration of a month, sent up to me at the hospital. His pupils were dilated, fixed, and uninfluenced by light, which he could not distinguish from darkness. The suddenness of the attack, and the absence of the usual premonitory symptoms, led me to conclude that the mischief was functional rather than structural, and I consequently examined his teeth. I found these much crowded and wedged together; the jaws, in fact, not being sufficiently large for them; and I therefore suspected that the amaurosis depended upon this cause. I accordingly ordered him to be shown to Mr. Roberts, the dentist to the hospital, who, on November 17, extracted two permanent and four milk molar teeth.

"On the same evening the boy could distinguish light from darkness, and on the following morning could make out objects. From this time his sight rapidly improved, and he was dismissed cured on the 28th, the only treatment beyond the removal of the teeth being two doses of aperient medicine."

Dr. Watson * mentions a very similiar case. But the blindness was confined to one eye: it recurred two or three times, and was on each occasion cured by tooth-extraction.

Deafness from Carious Tooth.—Mr. Cattlin describes † a case of deafness, in which the loss of hearing was evidently reflex paralysis, caused by a carious tooth.

"In the month of September 1843, a lady in the second stage of consumption consulted me concerning a diseased right lower molar. She had for about three months suffered acute pains in the tooth, ear, and side of the neck. When I saw her she had become deaf for four days. The inflamed tooth was extracted, and hearing returned within an hour after the operation."

Perverted Nutrition from Nervous Dental Irritation.—If the nervous irritation caused by diseased teeth can be reflected upon nerves of sensation, motor nerves, and nerves of special sense, exalting, or depressing, or perverting their functions, the same would also be expected as regards those nerves which are distributed to the blood-vessels, and which (as is well known) largely influence the vascular circulation, and, as a consequence, the nutrition of contiguous tissues. And such is unquestionably the case.

* *Lectures on Physic.* 4th edit. vol. ii. p. 351. London, 1857.

† *Transactions of the Odontological Society*, vol. iii. p. 308. London, 1863.

Mr. Hilton * enumerates some interesting examples of perverted nutrition dependent on dental nervous irritation, the irritation being propagated to remote parts by some collateral branch of the fifth nerve.

He narrates three cases in which the tongue has been decidedly furred on one side, and only one side, and that corresponding with carious or painful teeth.

Another instance, in which the hair of the left temple had turned grey, the change occurring coincident with, and apparently dependent upon, severe neuralgic pain of the side of the head; the painful affection having been caused by a carious molar tooth. The hair of the right temple remained black.

Another example, in which ulceration of the auditory canal was the complication, is so interesting that I shall quote Mr. Hilton's account of it. "In a previous lecture I mentioned that a professional friend of mine had long suffered from a condition bearing on the subject of the influence of nerves upon the structures supplied by them. That friend, unfortunately, is no more. It was Dr. Addison to whom this happened. The case is of some interest, and I will repeat it in a few words. Some years ago Dr. Addison had a very offensive discharge from the auditory canal of one of his ears, which annoyed him very much, and below the external ear was a small gland, enlarged in the upper part of the neck. He had tried various remedies for this discharge, and had gone, I believe, to some surgeons who attended especially to the ear; but, as far as I could learn, no good resulted from any of their applications. Upon examining the ear from which the offensive discharge proceeded, I found a slight ulceration upon the floor of the auditory canal. On arguing the question out between us, we came to the conclusion that the ulceration probably depended upon a diseased molar tooth in the lower jaw on the same side. We had that tooth extracted, and in a very short time the ulcer healed: the discharge and morbid secretion disappeared from the auditory canal; and as soon as that ulceration was cured the enlarged gland subsided."

Intense Neuralgia of the Eye-ball and Face: Alteration of

* *On the Influence of Mechanical and Physiological Rest, &c.* By John Hilton, F.R.S. London, 1863, pp. 194–8, 9.

the Colour of the Iris: Carious Teeth.—Mrs. C——, a lady aged about thirty years, was sent to me by Dr. Oldham on the 21st of June 1867. She was suffering from neuralgia of extraordinary severity, affecting the left eye-ball and the left side of the head and face. She had suffered almost continuously for ten years, the attack commencing on her recovery from a bad confinement; and no medicines had given her distinct relief. The most singular and interesting part of the case is, that the iris of the affected eye has completely changed colour under the influence of the continued pain. Both her eyes were originally of a deep and bright 'hazel' colour: the iris of the right eye remains as it was, but the left has changed to a dull grey, without any trace of the original hue. This change has occurred progressively, till the eyes are now as if belonging to two people of totally different complexion. No artificial painting could exhibit a more strange and striking contrast.

When this lady came to me she was in a pitiable condition, suffering such agony as I have seldom witnessed, and worn out and exhausted by the continued sleeplessness which the pain had occasioned. Upon examining her mouth I found that the left lower *dens sapientiæ* and the first upper bicuspid were badly carious. I removed these teeth, and the operation was attended by a terrible paroxysm of neuralgia; but upon recovery from this the patient expressed her conviction that the extraction of the teeth had cured her; and so it proved. From that day till the 8th of October, over three months, she was free from pain:—she had scarcely known such immunity even for three days, since her neuralgic sufferings commenced ten years before. As she expressed it—it was like "a new life" to her.

On the 8th of October the old pain came back again, and my patient came to me on the 10th, just in the condition she had been at first. I now found that the second upper bicuspid was carious and intensely tender. Upon its removal a considerable exostosis was seen on the root. The pain vanished with the tooth, and the patient wrote to me, a week after, saying she was quite well. The iris of the left eye has, however, never gone back to its original colour, but remains a leaden grey. The eye does not appear to have undergone any other nutritional change: its vision has not been affected.

Superficial Sloughing of the Cheek caused by a Carious Tooth-stump.—Many years ago a young woman applied to my relative, Mr. Bell (to whom I am indebted for these particulars) on account of a remarkable slough of the skin and cellular tissue about the size of a shilling, but of an oval form, just beneath the orbit. It was nearly black and detached from the edges when he first saw it. Mr. Bell removed the slough, but the sore only partially healed, and soon afterwards the same appearances recurred.

Upon examining the mouth, a diseased stump was found on the same side of the upper jaw, which appeared to be causing irritation. This Mr. Bell removed. The slough separated, the sore healed, and it never recurred.

Ulceration of the Neck, resulting from a Carious Dens Sapientiæ.—M. S——, aged twenty-two, a servant girl, residing at the watering-place, Bournemouth, in Hampshire, applied in 1846 to my late father, Mr. Salter, of Poole, on account of an ulcer in the neck behind and below the angle of the lower jaw on the right side. The account she gave of the affection under which she was suffering was, that, more than a year previous she was attacked by a painful red spot at the place now ulcerated, that it occurred quite spontaneously and without any apparent cause, that it speedily became ulcerated to about the size of a shilling, and that this has continued without change ever since. She had been under medical and surgical treatment almost continuously, but without benefit.

Her state, on applying to Mr. Salter (and I speak from personal observation), was this :—She was a remarkably fine young woman, rosy and robust; general health perfect. Some fourteen lines behind and below the angle of the jaw on the right side of the neck, there existed an ulcer about the size of a shilling; it looked thoroughly unhealthy, with sharp cut but irregular edges : it discharged pus. Applications of every kind, soothing, stimulating, &c., had been had recourse to, but without result. Medicines of various kinds, tonics, alteratives, &c., had been taken without the slightest modification of the patient's condition. Mr. Salter then examined the mouth, and found that the lower wisdom tooth on the right side was carious, in a very bad condition, with much neighbouring irritation. He extracted this tooth : in eight-and-forty hours the aspect of the sore had changed, in a week or ten days it had healed, and remained a firm cicatrix ever after. Various opinions had been expressed as to the nature of the sore: it had generally been considered scrofulous. The ulcer was quite superficial, and had no fistulous connection with the tooth.*

DIRECT AFFECTIONS.

Direct affections of the nervous system caused by tooth disease are far less common and less varied than those which are reflex, and their mode of production is more obvious and intelligible. As far as I am aware, the portio dura of the seventh nerve and the nerves which enter the orbit are those only which suffer in this way; are entangled, that is, in their course by those inflammatory influences and products which tooth diseases engender. It might have been expected, *à priori*, that alveolar abscess would, in some instances at least, so involve the maxillary nerves in their course through the jaw bones as to paralyse their more distal parts, and produce numbness at the region of their tegumentary distribution. But I am not aware that any such case has ever been observed, though similar consequences, the result of accidental mechanical injury in extracting teeth, do sometimes occur, as will be found mentioned elsewhere.

The consequences of the direct implication of nervous trunks by the inflammatory results of tooth disease are so very grave, especially when affecting the nerves of the eye in their course to the orbit, and the ultimate results so permanently serious, when relief is not speedily given, that it is impossible to exaggerate the importance of these cases. And I would lay the more stress upon this subject because I fear that such cases are very likely to be misunderstood, and injuries may thus become permanent and irremediable which, if correctly interpreted and properly treated at first, might be easily removed.

The following cases have appeared to me worthy of record and of quotation.

Facial Paralysis &c. from Carious Dens Sapientiæ.—Mrs.

* For other interesting examples of serious reflex affections of the nervous system, brought about by dental irritation, the reader is referred to records published by Sir A. Cooper, *Lect. on Prin. and Pr.* of Surgery, 1824, vol. i., p. 6; Dr. Castle of New York; *Lancet*, 1846, vol. ii. pp. 266–7. Dr. Parsons; *American Journal of Med. Sc.*, Oct., 1854, p. 423.

Barnard, a healthy married woman, frequently suffered from toothache in the right superior *dens sapientiæ* during the years 1863 and 1864. There was no swelling, and pain was the only symptom. The tooth was carious.

On the 27th of December 1864, she had violent toothache in this tooth: it was extremely severe, and at first strictly local. Rather more than a week afterwards, namely, on the 5th of January 1865, the pain, still very distressing, became diffused and erratic, wandering along to the front of the jaw and up to the eye: there was also pain in the throat on the right side. The right arm was seriously affected: it became nearly powerless, and was constantly in a state of aching pain: the patient could hardly grasp or hold anything in the right hand.

On the 7th of January symptoms of facial palsy displayed themselves: the patient noticed that the mouth was drawn and the features generally towards the left side: this increased, and became complete in two days. At the same time the vision of the right eye became very dim, and there was a dull aching behind the globe.

The woman at this time applied to my late brother, Dr. Hyde Salter, at Charing Cross Hospital, and he, after some unsuccessful treatment, suspected the cause of her malady to be dental, and requested her to see me.

She came to me on the 14th of January, and I then found her suffering from complete facial paralysis of the right side: the features were drawn to the left: she was unable to bring the lids of the right eye together, and she could not corrugate the right brow—could not frown on that side. The right superior *dens sapientiæ* had a carious cavity opening the central pulp chamber. The patient complained of all the before-mentioned symptoms—severe toothache, pain wandering along the jaw and down the throat, with an aching painfulness and powerlessness of the right arm. There was some deafness of the right ear. But little distinct swelling was visible within the mouth, nor much outside; still in the parotid region there was some fulness, extending back to the ear and up to the temple: it was hard and continuous, a dense infiltration, though inconsiderable in amount. I now removed the *dens sapientiæ*: with it came away a piece of alveolus. The fang of the tooth was covered with patches of red lymph, but there was nothing unusual or excessive in the appearances.

The removal of the tooth was followed immediately by marked relief, and before the patient left the house she said that the pain of the right arm and its feeble powerlessness had quite vanished. The patient spoke of a grateful sense of easement.

On the 18th of January the dimness of vision had much diminished, and she could see nearly as well with the right eye as the left. All pain had ceased. The drawing of the mouth towards the left side was not half so much as four days before, when the tooth was removed. The report in my note book continues:—Jan. 23. The patient presented a marked change to-day. I could not detect any obliquity of the mouth; but the angle of the lips was perhaps a little sharper on the left side than on the right. The sight of the right eye was completely restored. Every feeling of pain had vanished.

February 8.—The patient called on me to-day. Facial paralysis quite gone. She complains of wandering pains about the right side of the face and eye: right globe somewhat congested; the right pupil certainly, though slightly, less active than the left: the vision of the right eye not quite so clear as when I last saw her, and the deafness, which had much diminished, is now rather more marked. She complains of pain in the lower jaw on the right side: the right second lower molar is badly carious, tender, and somewhat loose. I extracted the tooth, and directed the patient to call again on the 13th, on which occasion the injection of the eye had quite disappeared, and the vision was perfect: the only remaining symptom was slight deafness. The patient did not call on me again, but I subsequently learnt that she was quite well.

It should be mentioned that Dr. Salter had given this woman iodide of potassium, and had applied a blister behind the ear, four times repeated, dressing with unguentum sabinæ, but not the least relief was afforded till the tooth was extracted.

I never saw a more distinct or more severe case of facial palsy: the cure by the removal of the tooth was equally marked. The symptoms appear to have resulted both from immediate implication of nerves and from their reflex action. The facial palsy was no doubt produced by entanglement of the portio dura in plastic inflammatory products about the parotid region: the blindness may have been caused by a similar implication of the optic nerve in its course. The painful paralysis of the arm wa sunquestionably reflex. The deafness perhaps arose from some tumefaction of the auditory passages.

Amaurosis consequent on acute Abscess of the Antrum, produced by a Carious Tooth.—Eliza Foley, aged twenty-four, a domestic servant, had been in perfectly good health up to the 25th of April 1860, when, without any new or special cause, she was attacked with violent pain about the remains of the first right upper molar tooth, the crown of which had been lost by caries. Enormous swelling of the side of the face came on rapidly; infiltration of the lower lid, which nearly closed the eye; protrusion of the malar bone, and a thrusting over of the nose to the opposite side. The patient described as fearful the pain of the whole of that side of the face and eyeball, which latter became protruded. A few hours after the occurrence of those symptoms, she observed that she was quite blind in the right eye, which had hitherto been perfect in all its functions. About twenty-four hours after the supervention of this great and extended swelling, matter pointed just below the inner canthus, and the general practitioner, who was attending the patient, evacuated it by means of a lancet-puncture. This orifice closed at once, and after the lapse of another twenty-four hours a fresh pointing of matter was observed below the outer canthus, which was evacuated in the same way. No further treatment was adopted, and the patient remained in great suffering for two or three weeks, the blindness of the right eye continuing, and the swelling and protrusion of the cheek being only mitigated by occasional discharges from the two orifices which had been punctured, and sometimes also by a flowing of purulent matter from the nose; but this latter did not occur till many days after the distension had been relieved by the bursting of the antrum at the corners of the eye.

At this juncture the girl was sent to Guy's Hospital, and was admitted on the 23rd of May under the care of Mr. Cock, at whose suggestion I was consulted.

The patient presented herself to me with her face covered up in a handkerchief, upon the removal of which she exhibited the most horrible disfigurement. The left side of the face was natural. The right was enormously swollen over the whole cheek, but especially about the region of the malar-bone, which was protruded and tilted forwards; the lids were œdematous and closed, while from the orifice just below the outer canthus and in the lower lid streamed a profuse discharge of grumour pus. The surface here was livid-red or purplish, and the surrounding skin polished and glistening. So remarkable was the patient's appearance, that I had a water-colour drawing made of her at the time, and before any surgical interference had taken place. Upon examining the mouth I found that the second right upper bicuspid had been recently removed, and that the fangs of the first molar, whose crown had been destroyed by caries, and a carious *dens sapientiæ*, remained. The hard palate on the right side was full and convex into the mouth.

I determined to remove the stumps and the carious wisdom tooth. Upon applying the elevator to the former they were very readily extracted. The pressure of the instrument caused pus to pour from the orifice near the corner of the eye, and more from the right nostril, while the withdrawal of the molar fangs opened the floor of the antrum and led to an abundant purulent discharge into the mouth. The performance of this operation conveyed to my touch a perception that the whole maxilla was implicated; there was a general bogginess and a soft yielding of the entire bone; and further, the hæmorrhage which followed the extraction of the stumps, and which was rather considerable, led to blood-discharge from the cheek-fistula and nose, as well as from the tooth-socket. Upon examining the extracted fangs of the molar tooth, the two outer ones were found naked of periosteum at their extremities, having been free and bathed in pus within the antrum.

The condition of the eye of this patient constituted the most important and the most distressing of the symptoms. The sight was utterly gone; the globe prominent, rather less so than at first, and slightly everted; there was extreme conjunctivitis both of the eye and eyelids; films of inspissated mucus covered the front of the eye; but the cornea, aqueous humour and chamber, and the iris, were nearly healthy. There was general deep inflammation of the fibrous textures of the eye. The pupil was large and rigidly fixed; it did not move in co-ordination with that of the other eye under any circumstances.

On the 7th of June, ten days after the previous report, some abatement of the inflammatory symptoms was said to have followed the extraction of the teeth; there was still very abundant discharge through the orifice on the cheek, from the nose, and into the mouth; the relative amount that escaped from the two former being determined by the position of the head; if laid on the right side, the chief flow was from the orifice in the cheek; if on the left, from the nose. The passing of a probe through the upper aperture distinctly indicated the presence of dead bone, which I had suspected to exist.

On the following day a considerable sequestrum was removed, consisting of part of the floor of the orbit and the cheek surface of the maxilla, involving the infra-orbital foramen, and also a long, thin plate of bone from the outer wall of the nose. The bone was removed by a crescentic cut from the orifice below the outer canthus to the scar of one that had existed below the inner canthus.

The removal of this dead bone was followed by an immediate and complete cessation of all inflammatory symptoms: the integument about the eye paled down to a normal colour, and the general inflammation of the eyeball rapidly disappeared, but the eye remained sightless, and the pupil still rigidly fixed.

It is unnecessary to detail the frequent reports which followed this date. The discharge continued, and was fetid, and nothing remarkable occurred till the 12th of July (five weeks after the removal of the dead bone and the cessation of the general inflammation), when, for the first time, I noticed that the pupil of the implicated eye moved in accordance with that of the seeing eye, though vision had not returned. A small flake of bone came away at this time through the orifice made in the removal of the large sequestrum, and this aperture had now assumed a definite shape: it was oval, about the size of a horse-bean, with clean edges deeply adherent to the subjacent bone, and continuous with the mucous lining of the antrum.

I had the patient's portrait taken at this time, as contrasted with her condition during the acute stage of the case, and the artist well succeeded in portraying the vacant, meaningless stare of the sightless eyeball. During the remaining five months of the year nothing of importance occurred in the patient's condition beyond the exfoliation of six small flakes of bone (three in September and three in November), and the gradual diminution and ultimate cessation of the discharge. The affected eye remained totally blind, but the left eye had never in any way sympathised with its damaged fellow.

On January 3, 1861, the patient was discharged, and was taken into the hospital as a night-nurse, and she continued under observation for a long time. The loss of vision in the affected eye remained permanent, and the necrosis of bone below the orbit produced a persistent opening into the antrum. Neither of the eyes has exhibited any inflammatory or textural change; the movements of the two pupils are coordinate; the axis of the blind eye has remained slightly everted.

On several occasions I have examined the blind eye with the ophthalmoscope; the humours are all perfectly transparent, and the retina healthy. The only abnormal appearance which this method of examination has displayed has been extreme *anæmia of the optic nerve* at its abutment on the retina. Instead of exhibiting the ordinary yellowish-pink disc, it has presented a white, circular area, characteristic of anæmia of the optic nerve, so constantly associated with suspension of the function of vision dependent upon causes external to the globe.

In making these examinations I have availed myself of the assistance of my accomplished colleague, Dr. Bader, whose long-continued and extended investigations with the ophthalmoscope give great weight to his observations.*

Amaurosis—Antral Abscess—Carious Molar Tooth—Splinter of Toothpick embedded in Alveolus.—In 1830, Professor Galenzowski published the particulars of a somewhat similar case † in the "Archives Générales de Médecine," of which the following is an abstract:—

F. P——, aged 30, possessed a good constitution and usually

* The particulars of this case were published in the forty-fifth volume of the *Transactions of the Medico-Chirurgical Society*, with a Chromolithographic illustration (Plate viii.) of the optic nerves and retinæ of the two eyes.

† Cas extraordinaire d'Amaurose produite par la carie d'une dent. *Observation communiquée par M. le docteur Galenzowski, Prof. adj. à l'Université de Wilna.* In *Archives Générales de Médecine Journal.*, tome xxiii. p. 261. Paris, 1830.

had good health. In the autumn of 1825 he suddenly experienced violent pain, extending from the left temple to the eye and that side of the face. It diminished and recurred with renewed force at intervals. About two months afterwards the pain suddenly became very intense, especially in the eye; the globe had a painful sense of protrusion. The patient now discovered that he was blind of the left eye. The pain then diminished; at the end of six months it again increased, the cheek swelled, and some spoonfuls of sanious pus were discharged through a spontaneous opening in the lower lid; then the swelling went down, and the pain nearly vanished. The blindness remained complete. The discharge was renewed from time to time: there was no great suffering. But in the autumn and winter (1826) the pain, especially in the eye, became so severe, that F. P—— came to Wilna in the commencement of 1827, determined to have the globe extirpated, if no other remedy could be discovered. Professor Galenzowski found the left eye totally insensible to light, and the pupil dilated; there was no other visible alteration. The pain, less severe, consisted in pricking and darting sensations in the left temple and around the eye: the discharge through the lower lid continued. The first upper molar tooth was carious; it had not caused much pain, and the tooth-ache, when there was any, was not coincident with the pains in the temple and eye. This carious tooth was now extracted, and at the end of the fang a foreign body was found, which upon examination proved to be a splinter of wood, probably the end of a toothpick; it was a quarter of an inch in length. The alveolar cavity communicated with the antrum, and some pus escaped from the sinus. The pain now ceased almost entirely, and on that same evening the eye became sensible of light. Vision gradually improved, so that, on the ninth day after the extraction of the tooth, F. P—— could see as well with the left eye as with the right, after a blindness of thirteen months: on the eleventh day he left Wilna to return to his family.

A case, in some important particulars analogous to the foregoing, occurred a few years since in the practice of Mr. George Pollock, of St. George's Hospital, to whom I am indebted for the following summary:—

Amaurosis caused by a Carious Molar Tooth.—A gentleman, aged about 35, was attacked with intense, deep-seated inflammation of the superior maxillary region and orbit, more specially the latter, involving the eye in universal congestion of its tissues. The globe was protruded, the sight completely gone, and the pupil dilated and fixed under all circumstances. Upon examination, Mr. Pollock found that there was much tenderness on pressure, extending downwards from the inner edge of the lower margin of the orbit towards the jaw on the affected side, and upon scrutinising the condition of the mouth, some carious teeth were found, which, for want of any other evident cause, he considered might be the origin of the existing mischief. He therefore directed that any of them which could possibly be implicated should be removed. This was done by Mr. Vasey, the Dental Surgeon of St. George's Hospital, who informs me that he extracted the fangs of the first premolar and the first true molar teeth, and that the latter exhibited indications of great irritation about its roots. The removal of the teeth was followed by the immediate and complete subsidence of all the inflammatory symptoms, and in about ten days all heat, redness, and apparent ophthalmic inflammation had vanished.

The eye was sightless. At first the pupil remained as it had been during the inflammatory action, fixed and dilated; but it subsequently resumed its contractile function in coordination with that of the seeing eye.

I learn from Mr. Pollock that there was no "abscess" of the antrum, but there was sufficient evidence that active inflammation pervaded the whole soft structure connected with the maxillary bone.

The eye has remained perfectly natural to external appearance, though entirely blind, and its suspended function has given rise to no textural change in itself, or, by sympathy, in its fellow. The latter has been tried severely, as the patient, not long after his recovery, was exposed to great bodily exertion and physical hardship in a naval expedition.

Another published case, resembling those here described, is recorded by Dr. Brück, in Casper's "Wochenschrift" * for 1851,

* "Wiederholte Entzündungen des Antrum Highmori und Amaurose" &c. Mitgetheilt vom Dr. A. Th. Brück. In Casper's *Wochenschrift für die gesammte Heilkunde.* Berlin, März, 1851.

and an abstract of it is given in the "Annales d'Oculistique" * for 1856.

Amaurosis—Antral Abscess—Carious Teeth.—The patient was a healthy man, aged 45. He had suffered for many years from chronic inflammation of the mucous membrane of the nose and maxillary sinus on the left side, with frequent acute attacks of great severity. On the occasion of the acute attacks, the inflammation involved the whole maxillary bone on the affected side, the teeth, the tongue and throat, and extended up the scalp, which became intensely sensitive. There was great injection of the eyelids, the globe protruded, and there was much and severe tooth-ache. After a few days, matter, previously pent up in the antrum, burst through the left nostril, and the patient recovered from the acute symptoms, which, however, again and again recurred.

The interesting point of this case is the relation of the affection of the eye to that of the antrum. The former appears to have followed and been dependent upon the latter. On the occasion of the acute attacks the globe was protruded, as Dr. Brück says, by the vaulting of the roof of the maxillary sinus from its distending contents, and all the structures within the orbit appear to have shared the inflammation. In an early stage of the case *vision was entirely lost, and the axis of the eye diverged.*

Under treatment, the symptoms of the antral affection gradually disappeared, and with their disappearance the sight of the affected eye returned.

The function of the right eye never suffered, either intrinsically or by sympathy with its fellow, and the sight was only imperfect in calculating the perspective. The general meaning of this case is sufficiently obvious, though some of its details are deficient. The fixedness or mobility of the pupil in relation to that of the other eye is not given, nor is the condition of the teeth distinctly defined, though dental caries is implied from the repeated allusions to tooth-ache on the affected side.

More recently (December 30, 1865) Mr. Charles Gaine, of Bath, published † the particulars of a very similar case.

* "Amaurose coincidant avec une Inflammation de l'Antre d'Highmore." In *Annales d'Oculistique*, p. 90, tome xxxvi. Bruxelles, 1856.

† *British Medical Journal.* Part cclxi. p. 683.

Amaurosis—Antral Abscess—Carious Tooth.—E. B——, aged twenty-two, was admitted into Bath Hospital, August 7, 1863, on account of defective vision of the right eye. There was *ptosis* of the right upper eyelid, also much swelling of the face, with an alveolar, and, as it proved, an antral abscess associated with the first right upper molar tooth, which had been broken off in an attempt to extract it. The patient could not be persuaded to have the fangs of the broken tooth removed. By September 16, the sight of the right eye was entirely lost. The stumps of the broken tooth were then extracted, the antrum pierced, and a large quantity of pus evacuted. The optic nerve, as seen by the ophthalmoscope, was very anæmic. When seen by Mr. Gaine on May 5, 1864, the third nerve had recovered; the ptosis had disappeared, and there was a fair action of the pupil. The optic nerve was still anæmic, and the right eye entirely blind.

When we consider the degree of inflammation which often attends alveolar abscess from carious teeth, it seems strange, rather than otherwise, that neighbouring parts do not suffer more often deeply and destructively.

The manner in which the consequences of tooth inflammation may wander to a remote region is shown in those instances where a tooth in the front of the mouth may give rise to an alveolar abscess, which will point far back in the palate. The pus in such an instance burrows among the cancelli which separate the two (nasal and palatal) layers of compact bone constituting the hard palate: the occasional, though rare, development of osseous septa which traverse the cavity of the antrum would, by connecting the floor with the roof of the maxillary sinus, form a course, which might possibly bring the inflammatory products of a suppurating periodontal membrane to the immediate region of the eye, instead of the soft palate. General and diffused inflammation of the whole maxilla, brought about by the same cause, would, however, render such an explanation unnecessary.

In none of these cases did the loss of vision appear to depend upon damage done to the structures of the eye itself: when the inflammation of the globe subsided, which it did rapidly upon the removal of its exciting cause, the humours at once exhibited a perfect transparency. In my case, moreover, as in Mr. Gaine's, when the eye was examined with the ophthalmoscope, the retina itself presented no textural change which would account for the loss of vision. Again, in neither case were there any *cerebral* symptoms during any stage of the disease, so that the blindness cannot have depended on disease of the brain. These negative reasons, and all the positive circumstances of the cases, tend to show that the mischief occurred to the nerves themselves, whose functions were damaged, in their course external to the cranium and before they reached the globe. The stretching of the nerves by the protrusion of the eye may have had some temporary share in the suspension of their function; but, were this the only influence bearing on them, the blindness would probably have been in each case partial, and perhaps transient, as the mechanical protrusion of the globe, by tumours not involving the optic nerve, does not necessarily entail blindness; and where that does occur, the restoration of the eyeball to a tolerably natural position is usually accompanied by a return of sight.

In the case of Eliza Foley, the loss of bone from the floor of the orbit does not explain the suspension of vision, as the sequestrum came from the front of the eye-socket, and could not in any way have entangled the nerves of the eye. In all the five cases which I have referred to, the pathological condition (as far as the ophthalmic complications are concerned) appears to have been *a plastic inflammation*, involving the fibrous tissues which surround the nerves passing from the cranial cavity to the eye. Whether the inflammatory products had simply enclosed the nerves, and affected only their fibrous coverings—thus, as it were, strangling by pressure the softer nervous elements—or whether the plastic exudation had been intrinsic in the nerves themselves, can only be matter of speculation in the absence of anatomical observation. It is an interesting fact, both in Mr. Pollock's case and my own, that the different nerves entering the orbit have been similarly affected; the optic nerve was hopelessly implicated from the first, blindness was complete and final; the third nerve was involved in the early stage of the disease, as evidenced by the temporary fixedness of the pupil, which afterwards recovered its contractile function; while the eversion of the axis of the globe showed that the sixth nerve (*abducens oculi*) had escaped injury or had suffered less than the third.

In Mr. Gaine's case, the third nerve recovered itself, while the optic nerve was hopelessly lost.

As regards the anæmia of the optic nerve, was its bloodlessness the result of mechanical obstruction to the circulation, or did it simply depend upon, and was it secondary to, suspended function? A circumferential plastic exudation encasing the nerve might possibly strangle by pressure the circulation within it, or an interstitial deposit of lymph between the fibrillæ might effect that consequence more readily and completely. Then, on the other hand, it is well known that a suspension of the function of sight by causes external to the globe itself, even so remote as disease of the brain, will entail complete anæmia of the optic nerve. The precise relation, therefore, of the sightlessness of the eye and the anatomical condition in question must remain matter of doubt.

CHAPTER XXI.

PHOSPHORUS DISEASE: MAXILLARY NECROSIS FROM PHOSPHORUS FUMES.

THE most remarkable of all the secondary consequences dependent upon tooth-disease, is probably that terrible malady, necrosis and exfoliation of more or less of the maxillæ, which attacks the makers of lucifer-matches.

The relation of the phosphorus poison to the disease in question, and its method of introduction, or rather application, are among the most distinctly proved of any of the circumstances connected with the history of disease. Probably there is nothing in pathological history where clear data, and simple induction from those data, have more lucidly illustrated the questions of cause and effect. To bring about the "phosphorus disease," phosphorus in some form must be applied to the periosteum, or, what is equivalent to the periosteum, to some raw vascular surface in immediate connection with the nutrition of bone; and the application must be prolonged, must be under particular circumstances of temperature, and probably of oxidisation. These conditions alone occur in those manufactories where phosphorus is employed in the making of lucifer-matches; and there alone (or with few exceptions) it is that this disease is manifested. But the circumstances which connect the outward cause with the disease that follows it, is a predisposition in the individual, consisting of some exposure of the periosteum, or what is tantamount to such exposure. The only manner in which this occurs, at least in which phosphorus appears to be effective in causing bone-necrosis, is where caries of a tooth exposes the pulp to the poison-influence, the bone necrosis being that of the jaw. It is the poisoning of the tooth-pulp that is the essence of the disease; the severe combinations of bone-affection, which give all the importance to the malady, are but contingent and secondary consequences.

This relation of tooth-disease to jaw-disease has been generally looked upon as unique and exceptional; but I believe it has really, as regards cause and effect, the same contingent sequence as occurs in those cases where portions of the maxillary bones die, and are shed, after exanthematous fevers. The tooth is poisoned first; the jaw-bone suffers afterwards.

It is this fact in the essential nature of the disease that links it (as I think) to that other form of maxillary necrosis which occurs in children after attacks of the eruptive fevers; only that, whereas in the phosphorus disease the poison is applied to the tooth from an extraneous source—from without, in the jaw-necrosis of eruptive fevers the poison is generated within, and alights upon the teeth and tooth-pulps, by virtue of their being dermal organs, members of the tegumentary system, upon which system generally the eruptive fever-poisons spend their chief destructive force.

The necrosis and exfoliation of portions of the jaw-bones, dependent on phosphorus fumes as its cause, is so entirely associated with the manufacture of lucifer-matches, that not only are all the particulars we know of the malady derived from the victims of that occupation, but the disease itself was not known to have an existence until some years after these light-producing agents had taken the place of the old tinder-box, and by the large demand for them had given rise to extensive laboratories for their production.

Though the manufacturers of phosphorus, and those who have employed it in medicine and the arts, have been more or less exposed to its fumes, since its discovery by Brandt in 1669, no case of jaw-disease occurred from it, or at least was attributed to it, till after the manufacture of lucifer-matches: a circumstance which is no doubt attributable to the fact, that under no other conditions than in the making of these matches are persons so much exposed to the deleterious influence of phosphorus.

The earliest published account of the disease which we have, is by Lorinser,* of the *Besisks Krankenhause Wieden*; and the

* I have had no opportunity of consulting Lorinser's original writings: they are referred to by Geist as—"in den medicinischen Jahrbüchern des K. K. Oesterreichischen Staates, Jahrgang 1845, Märzheft."

first case which fell under his notice occurred in 1839, about eleven years after the opening of lucifer-match manufactories in Vienna. In this country, as far as I am aware, the malady was first recorded by Dr. Wilks, in Surgical Reports of Guy's Hospital, from April 1846 to March 1847, where he remarks, "Of the other diseases of the lower jaw, one occurred in a lucifer-match-maker, with suppuration and exfoliation of bone."* It is, however, to the continental surgeons, and those principally of Germany, that we are indebted for the complete and early account of this malady, from which, indeed, all subsequent notices have been mainly derived. Besides the original memoir by Lorinser, before referred to, important contributions have been added by Strohl,† Heyfelder,‡ Roussel and Gendrin,§ Sédillot,|| and, above all, by Von Bibra and Geist,¶ whose exhaustive treatise, their joint production, has given the clearest elucidation of this new disease.

In this country an admirable digest of the subject has been published, in the shape of a review of Von Bibra and Geist's work, in the "British and Foreign Medico-Chirurgical Review" for April 1848.

In 1862 I wrote the article on Phosphorus-disease in "Holmes's System of Surgery;"** containing a general summary of the subject, and some original observations and suggestions of my own. And in 1863, the most important article on this disease that has appeared in our language was published by

* *Guy's Hospital Reports*, 2nd series, vol. xii. p. 163, Lond. 1847. This case occurred in the hospital practice of the late Mr. Aston Key, who, as Dr. Wilks informs the author, was already aware, from his own observation, of the essential nature of the disease and its relation to its peculiar cause.

† *Gazette Médicale de Strasbourg*, cinquième année, no. 11, 20 novembre 1845.

‡ *Vierteljahrsschrift von Roser und Wunderlich*, Jahrgang 1845, Heft 3; and *Medicinische Zeitung des Vereins für Heilkunde in Preussen*, Jahrgang 1845, no. 45.

§ *Recherches sur les Maladies des Ouvriers employés à la fabrication des Allumettes chimiques*, &c., Mémoire présenté à l'Académie des Sciences, le 16 février 1846.

|| *Comptes Rendus des Séances de l'Académie Royale des Sciences de Paris*, mars 1846.

¶ *Die Krankheiten der Arbeiter in den Phosphorzündholzfabriken*, &c., Erlangen, 1847; also *Die Regeneration des Unterkiefers nach totaler Necrose durch Phosphordämpfe*, von L. Geist, Erlangen, 1852.

** "Surgical Diseases connected with the Teeth:" in Holmes's *System of Surgery*, vol. iv. p. 40.

Dr. Bristowe in the form of a Report* to the Privy Council, on "The Relation of Phosphorus and its Manufactures to the Question of Public Health."

This terrible malady has been observed in all countries where phosphorus is employed in match manufactories: the association is nearly constant: it is seldom otherwise manifested. Cases are recorded with this association as having occurred in Vienna, Nürnberg, Prague, Berlin, Wurzburg, in Saxony and Wurtemburg, in Switzerland, France, England, and America.

That the actual *cause* of the jaw-disease which attacks the workers of phosphorus is that substance, or some of its compounds, is beyond all controversy. Other opinions have been advanced, but were easy of refutation.

Drs. Jüngken and Helfft considered that the association of the malady with the particular employment was merely an accidental coincidence; and the former especially suggested that it might be a rheumatic affection brought about by the atmospheric conditions (heat, cold, and moisture) to which the artisans were exposed.

A more serious objection was advanced by Professor Martius, of Erlangen, and Dupasquier, of Lyons, who asserted that arsenic, as an impurity in the phosphorus employed, was really the deleterious agent. But this supposition was not found to hold good under more critical and extended examination.

Dr. Bristowe very fairly summarises the evidence on the question as follows:—

The *primâ facie* evidence is that the disease is due to the inhalation of the fumes of phosphorus. "The proofs of this are manifold: 1st, phosphorus is the only article, universally employed in match-making, which gives off vapours, the effects of which have not hitherto been tested by experience; 2ndly, those persons who are most exposed to these vapours, are just those who are found to be most liable to the disease; and, 3rdly, it is in those manufactories in which the composition employed is

* "On the Manufactories in which Phosphorus is Produced or Employed," in the fifth *Report* of Medical Officers of the Privy Council, p. 162, Lond. 1863. I cite my paper as anterior to Dr. Bristowe's from the fact, that though the volume containing it was not published till 1864, it was finally committed to the press in 1862 (see note by Mr. Holmes in his *Surgery*, vol. iv. p. 7), and Dr. Bristowe was furnished with a copy of my paper (from which indeed he quotes), before compiling his *Report*.

richest in phosphorus, and those which are worst ventilated, that jaw-disease chiefly occurs."

And this has been further confirmed by Von Bibra's experiments on rabbits. He extracted teeth, and in some instances slightly fractured the jaw. The parts were then exposed to the fumes of phosphorus, and pathological changes occurred, identical with those observed in the jaws of lucifer-match-makers.

The actual agent in producing the phosphorus-disease is doubtless oxidised phosphorus, probably in the form of phosphorous or phosphoric acid, dissolved in the saliva. The precise nature of the fumes is not, however, exactly known: they consist principally of phosphorous acid (H_3PO_3), which by mixture with air becomes phosphoric acid (H_3PO_4); and probably minute quantities of phosphorus-vapour (P), phosphuretted hydrogen (H_3P), and hypophosphorous acid (H_3PO_2) are also present. Any vapour of phosphorus and hypophosphorous acid would be speedily converted by the air into phosphorous and phosphoric acids. Phosphuretted hydrogen would be more slowly oxidised into the same products. At any rate, nearly, if not quite the whole of the fumes when inhaled by the work-people would be in a state of some acid of phosphorus.

The chemical compound employed in making lucifer-matches, and from which the noxious fumes are evolved, consists essentially of a mixture of phosphorus and chlorate of potash:—the former originating, by friction, the fire, and the latter supplying immediate and abundant oxygen for its sustenance.

There is, however, a curious modification of phosphorus known as "amorphous" phosphorus, which does not emit the noxious fumes when heated sufficiently for its employment in match-making. This kind, however, is not mixed with the chlorate of potash for the tipping of the matches, but is employed to coat the rubber on the surface of the box, and it is by rubbing the chlorate of potash match against the amorphous phosophorus that the fire is produced and the match catches alight. Amorphous phosphorus is only employed by one firm of match-makers.*

* Messrs. Bryant and May, of London, hold a patent for the manufacture of matches in this way. These matches deserve universal adoption; for not only are they made without possible injury to the work-people, but they are perfectly safe, being incapable of accidental ignition.

The effects of phosphorus-vapours upon its victims are not immediate. It is only when the cause has been long in operation, and under circumstances of great intensity, that the disease is developed; it is confined almost entirely to those who are employed in the process of *dipping* the matches into the fused and reeking phosphorous compound, and those who dry them in the same apartment. Moreover, a long exposure to the influence is necessary for the production of the disease. Lucifer-manufactories had existed eleven years in Vienna, when in 1839 Lorinser observed the first case which attracted attention; and the shortest known period in which the malady has developed itself is a little under a year. A case is recorded by Gendrin, that occurred in Paris, in which the patient had been employed in the occupation two years before the first symptoms appeared.

A circumstance of curious import, though not invalidating the generally-received doctrine of local poisoning, is, that the sufferer may have been removed from the baneful influence for a considerable period, and nevertheless be subsequently attacked by the disease. Strohl gives an instance of a girl who had worked as a *dipper* at a lucifer-match manufactory for five years; she left that employment, and adopted a totally different and a healthy occupation, when, after three months, she was for the first time attacked with unmistakable symptoms of the phosphorus-disease, ending, after fifteen months, in exfoliation of portions of the superior maxilla.

It is very seldom that others than those employed in making lucifer-matches suffer from this malady; but that this may happen should not be lost sight of. Pluskal* mentions an example of a little girl seven years of age, who was in the constant habit of playing with matches, standing before a wall and discharging them in the dark for amusement, so that her face was bathed in their fumes; in time she was attacked with necrosis and exfoliation of small portions of the front of the lower jaw, with the ordinary attendant symptoms. Simon narrates a case in which the disease appears to have been brought on by a person chewing pieces of ginger, which he kept in his pocket with some lucifer-matches. And Sir James Paget † describes an in-

* *Oesterreichische Medicinische Wochenschrift*, no. 30, Wien, den 25 Juli 1846.

† *Medical Times and Gazette*, vol. i. p. 41, 1862.

stance in which a patient had necrosis of the palatine and alveolar portions of the upper jaw. He had never suffered from syphilis, nor taken mercury. nor had he been employed in match-making. He had, however, been exposed to phosphorus-vapour in preparing medicine for himself containing that drug.

The influence of the phosphorus fumes upon the jaw is undoubtedly local.

Lorinser, who has the merit of discovering this disease, held a modification of this view. He considered that the blood is first surcharged with phosphorus which has an affinity for the osseous tissues, and that the immediate action of the poison is localised in the jaws by their direct exposure to its application.

Dr. Ebel holds the same view, in a very interesting memoir published by him in Casper's "Wochenschrift." * However, Roussel, Geist, and indeed subsequent writers generally, have adopted the opinion, which all the evidence upon this point seems clearly to establish, that the disease is local in its causation.† I have not space here to enter upon the argument of the question; I may, however, mention one telling fact; it is, the necessity of dental caries in the individual before the disease can be produced. It has never been known to occur, excepting where the sufferer has had carious teeth; and many persons have worked in the manufactories for a long series of years with perfect impunity, who, upon the supervention of dental caries, have been attacked with the malady. Dental caries, by opening the central chamber of the tooth and exposing the pulp, seems to offer a direct channel for the poison to be communicated to the subjacent periosteum, and this, no doubt, is why tooth-destruction is a necessary pre-existing condition.

Dr. Bristowe, in his collection of evidence on phosphorus disease laid before the Privy Council, disputes the fact that the local application of oxidised phosphorus to the exposed tooth-pulp is the primary and essential cause of the malady; and he bases his opposition to the generally received opinion

* "Ueber den Einfluss der Phosphorzündholzfabrication auf die Geshundheit der Arbeiter," Mitgetheitt von Dr. Ebel, in Casper's *Wochenschrift.* 15 Mars. 1851.

† The arguments bearing upon this question, and the conclusive inference to which they lead, are stated with cogent force in an admirable clinical lecture on this subject by Mr. Simon, in the *Lancet* for 1850, p. 41.

upon the circumstance that some of those who have been afflicted with the disease, have told him that they had not previously been the subjects of dental caries. If, however, Dr. Bristowe were, as a dental surgeon, practically acquainted with the neglected condition of the mouths of the poorer classes, and their ignorance, and utter indifference as to the state of their teeth, he could not, I am sure, have adduced the mere assertions of these people as of the slightest value in discussing the question. A large majority of the poor, between the ages of fifteen and forty, have carious teeth, and very many of them remain entirely ignorant of the circumstance till the fact asserts itself by the occurrence of tooth-ache. I would go further:—I am confident that, in any given number of the poor artisan class, who, upon being asked, asserted that their teeth were sound, a considerable proportion would be found to have dentinal caries. No such assertion therefore by the patient, unless endorsed by the careful scrutiny of a surgeon, *skilled in tooth-disease,* would be of the slightest value as a matter of evidence. Indeed it requires a particular and special knowledge and habit of search to discover many of the points of dental caries, which would be overlooked by an ordinary practitioner of medicine or surgery.

What the precise nature of the action of phosphorus-oxide thus absorbed may be upon the bone, is a matter of speculation; but the particular nature of the poison, entering as it does so largely into the composition of the skeleton, is a suggestive circumstance: perhaps, if accumulated by the periosteum, it may generate on the bone's surface a condition of chemical *superphosphate,* inconsistent with osteal vitality.

The *symptoms* of phosphorus-necrosis do not differ essentially from other forms of necrosis in the same parts: they are, however, not infrequently accompanied by bronchial and pulmonary irritation from inhalation of the fumes: this has been especially pointed out by Sédillot, Gendrin, and Dupasquier.* And one of the patients whom I have seen, affected with this malady, has detailed to me symptoms of *spasmodic asthma* which occasionally supervened, when he was employed for many continuous hours "*dipping,*" while suffering from a common

* *Gaz. Méd. de Paris,* 1846, no. 49.

"cold" in winter weather. Barring this occasional manifestation of pulmonary irritation, the general health of these work-people seems to be remarkably good.

The symptoms of the jaw-disease usually commence with what is supposed to be tooth-ache, the pain being at first pretty much localised to some one tooth that is carious, and which is probably the channel by which the poison is introduced. The advance of the disease is generally slow at first, and, as it were, undecided—indeed, indefinitely chronic : the pain is inconstant, and not early attended with more serious symptoms; presently, however, it becomes more severe and erratic, extending vaguely about the side of the head and down towards the shoulder, and with this severer pain, swelling, and extreme tenderness occur; the integument near the affected region becomes red, tense, and distended, while the teeth feel elongated and extremely painful when brought in contact with their fellows of the opposite jaw, and they become loose. The gums are swollen and livid, and this condition extends to the mucous membrane of the cheeks. All these symptoms increase till suppuration is established, and with them, more or less symptomatic fever is developed in proportion to the severity and extent of the disease : the patient has rigours and pyrexia, and is often thoroughly ill. The point at which the pus finds its discharge varies a good deal : the soft parts become very boggy, especially the gums, and matter often escapes early around the necks of the loose dead teeth; when pointing externally, its approach is accompanied by intense glistening erysipelas-like redness of the integument. The discharge of the pus is attended with great mitigation of the patient's suffering. The pus itself is often sanious at first, and always very fetid; having the odour characteristic of the presence of necrosed bone. The orifice of discharge frequently leads to long burrowing sinuses, especially where the lower jaw is affected; and through these the dead bone may be detected by a probe. The swelling which attends the disease is often very great, particularly when the lower jaw is necrosed : it is diffuse and wide-spread, encasing the external and under surface of the bone in a prodigious, dense, plastic exudation. In very severe cases, previous to the discharge of pus, while the inflammatory symptoms are at their extreme height, the whole head, except the summit of the scalp, is involved—the eyes are closed, the nose, and even the forehead, swollen; the cheeks, lips, neck, and throat, are one continuous area of florid intumescence.

It is a curious circumstance, that in the lower jaw the necrosis is attended with a very large and complete development of ossifying callus, whereas none is formed when the upper jaw is affected. The large plastic exudation which surrounds the base of the lower jaw becomes converted into a mass of supplemental bone, supporting the sequestrum, which is, for the most part, naked and bare within and behind, and connecting sound portions of bone at its extremities when the whole of the maxillary arch is not involved. Geist assumes that the particular region occupied by the osteophytic incrustation about the lower jaw is the result of gravitation—an idea altogether too mechanical: it is rather to be looked upon as a physiological manifestation, and one element in that marvellous exhibition of the *vis medicatrix naturæ* which this lower jaw-repair displays: the supplemental bone thus placed forms the best support for the sequestrum and the least interferes with the functions of the mouth; while the absence of an ossifying callus at the upper and inner region of the maxillary arch offers the readiest escape of the dead bone through the thin mucous membrane which there alone covers it, and this without damaging the integument of the face.

As the bone becomes laid bare by alteration of the soft parts, it is observed bathed in ichorous pus, ragged and irregular on its surface, and of a dirty blackish grey colour. Heyfelder has pointed out this latter as a characteristic element of the disease: but it is certainly not so, though very general. I have seen specimens of phosphorus necrosis white and clean, and with the compact external layer of bone intact. And I have seen syphilitic necrosis of the lower jaw in which the sequestrum was much coated with this particular black-grey incrustation.

To return to the symptoms of the disease. When the extent of necrosis is very great, the constitutional disturbance is correspondingly severe; and in the early stages of the malady the patient may have intense fever, with delirium and agonising local sufferings, the more distressing from the region which the affection occupies—interfering with or altogether suspending the action of the mouth, and, by the secretion of foul and fetid pus, producing nausea, ructus, vomiting. The looseness and projection of the dead teeth is another source of annoyance and distress: as the sequestra containing them emerge from the surrounding parts, their elongation and angularity much irritate the gums and cheek in contact with them. In the severest cases, general sphacelus of the soft parts about the jaw, with œdema of the face and neck, may supervene, accompanied, or not, by erysipelas; and death may then close a scene of terrible suffering. In other instances with a fatal issue, life is drawn out through many months of tedious illness, varied by different degrees of local irritation; till at length the patient, with vital endurance inadequate to the requirements of the disease, sinks, tabid and exhausted, under continuous hectic, and not infrequently with tubercular complications.

But the pathological changes may be even more terrible than those already mentioned. Dr. Ebel describes a case, which occurred in the practice of Dr. Hervieux at the Hospital *Necker*, in which the patient, a lucifer-match-maker, had first necrosis of the lower jaw, then of the upper, afterwards of the palate bones, and the orbits, and lastly of the os frontis. He died with brain symptoms. Pus was found between the dura-mater and the brain.

When the malady progresses to a favourable issue, which it does in the majority of cases, the dead bone gradually loosens and becomes detached; and this is generally anticipated by the falling out of some of the necrosed teeth. In the upper jaw the sequestra are usually more broken up and smaller than in the lower, and they are shed easier, not being held in and detained by ossifying callus, which is always wanting in the upper jaw. In the lower jaw the sequestra are usually more extensive, often including large portions of the body of the bone, not infrequently the ascending rami, and sometimes the coronoid processes, and even the articular condyles. The shedding of these sequestra is often hindered by the large surrounding ossifying callus which always forms when the lower jaw is the subject of this disease.

I may here mention that some stress has been laid upon the circumstance that the lower jaw has been more frequently observed to be affected than the upper. The learned reviewer *

* *British and Foreign Med.-Chir. Review*, before cited.

of Geist and Von Bibra's work has given much detail bearing on this point; he enumerates twenty-five examples in which the lower jaw was affected, to twenty-one in which it was confined to the upper jaw. In five cases which I have seen, the lower jaw was diseased in four and the upper in one; whereas, four, which occurred in the practice of a surgical friend, were confined to the upper jaw. In seventeen instances of which I have obtained particulars or seen specimens, nine were connected with the superior, and eight with the inferior maxilla.

Dr. Bristowe, in his investigations, met with evidence of thirty-nine cases in the lower jaw,* twelve in the upper, and five in both.

The results of phosphorus-necrosis, in cases which get well, are very various. As regards general health, the patient usually recovers with an elastic convalescence after the dead bone has been removed; but the physical condition of his maxillary apparatus is often terribly mutilated. When the front part of the upper jaw is affected, it is an absolute and unrepaired loss, miserably disfiguring the patient, altering the physiognomy most painfully: when it affects more hidden parts of the jaw, the loss is not less complete, though less conspicuous.

If the affection is confined to the inferior maxilla, the removal of the sequestrum leaves a supplemental bony representative, which, for a time, more than makes up for the loss of dead bone, and for a long subsequent period efficiently performs the office of edentulous mastication, and supplies the wants of personal comeliness.

In some instances the whole of the lower jaw has been lost, excepting the articular condyles; and these, apparently connected with the new bone, have established the joint requirements of the supplemental jaw; but in other instances (cases in St. Bartholomew's Hospital, and those mentioned in Geist's later work †) even the articular ends have been shed with the rest of the sequestrum; still there has been joint movement, doubtless from a ligamentous attachment of the new bone.

* This circumstance tallies with the idea that the disease is produced locally by the action of the phosphorus-oxide dissolved in the saliva. The lower teeth and inferior maxilla are far more exposed to this influence than the upper:—in evidence, observe the accumulation of salivary calculus on the lower teeth.

† *Die Regeneration des Unterkiefers nach totaler Necrose*, v. L. Geist, 1852.

The supplemental jaw does not always remain as a complete compensation for the loss of the original. I once had an opportunity of examining a patient who had lost his lower jaw ten years before from phosphorus-disease. The new bone was diminished by absorption to a mere narrow arch: there was scarcely bone enough to keep out the lower lip, and the chin was entirely lost.

Dr. Bristowe, however, mentions two instances, one after six and one after ten years, in which the supplementary bone remained large and well formed: but he describes another in which, after eight years, the new jaw was scarcely bigger than the hyoid bone.

How far this loss, by absorption of the new bone, may be prevented by supplying it with a function, through the means of artificial teeth, is a question of theoretical interest and of practical importance.

The *prevention*, however, of phosphorus-disease is so easily accomplished that its occurrence is discreditable to the sanitary laws of any country where it occurs. If the employment of amorphous phosphorus were decreed, and the use of ordinary phosphorus prohibited, by statute, the disease, in all probability, would cease to exist. But if this could not be enforced, the employment of ordinary phosphorus might be rendered almost innocuous.

There should be scrupulous cleanliness; large rooms and abundant ventilation—the dipping stones and mixing apparatus being placed under hoods communicating with shafts. Those who are exposed to the fumes should work short hours, and but few days a week. The amount of phosphorus employed in the mixture should be a minimum.

I would suggest, moreover, that in all lucifer-match manufactories there should be a periodic and rigid scrutiny of the mouths of all the work-people employed. Those having faulty teeth should be excluded from the rooms (the *dipping* and *drying* rooms) where the obnoxious fumes are being developed. All carious teeth should be extracted or plugged. What is more important, a very simple and effectual respirator for the mouth might be worn by the employés: it would be unnecessary over the nostrils. It should be constructed on the ordinary plan of respirators, but its centre consisting of a porous diaphragm, such as sponge or some woven fabric, linen or cotton, which should be daily dipped in a solution of one of the fixed alkalis or their carbonates. This would arrest nearly, if not quite, all the acid fumes of the phosphorus. Or the respirator devised by Mr. Graham for persons exposed to carbonic acid vapour would probably be as efficacious. It consists of the mixture in equal bulk of fresh-slacked lime and sulphate of soda, through a cushion of which it is easy to breathe. The wearing of some such respirator should be compulsory with the dippers and dryers. Again, the acid vapour might be neutralised and rendered innocuous by keeping the atmosphere of the apartment ammonuretted. I believe, if these precautions were adopted, the disease would seldom, if ever, manifest itself.

The *treatment* of phosphorus-necrosis of the maxillæ divides itself into that which is common to all bone-necrosis, and that which specially applies to the particular local affection in question. Upon the latter head alone I would remark.

In the early stages of the disease, when as yet it is not established, but its supervention feared, it would be of the last importance to remove the patient from the cause of the malady: pure air should be sought, abundant cleanliness, with urinary and alvine excretants, resorted to, and all suspicious teeth extracted. When, however, the local symptoms—extreme pain, swelling, and indurated infiltration of the soft parts—develop themselves, and the disease has already passed its premonitory stage, it will be advisable to have recourse to more active measures. Upon this point I cannot do better than quote Mr. Simon's remarks in his admirable Clinical Lecture, already referred to, and in the justice and propriety of which I entirely concur: "So soon as the second or inflammatory stage of the disease has thoroughly set in, the bone seems in every case to be irrevocably doomed to necrosis; and I would therefore recommend you, in the event of your being called to a case at the transition period between the two stages, when hypertrophy is passing into inflammation, to adopt without hesitation the most active measures for relief of the periosteum and bone. Leeches and general antiphlogistic treatment *may* do good; but the consideration of the pathology of this disease, together with the analogy of other periosteal affections, leads me to believe that the only real chance of doing good would be still more energetic measures: and I would recommend you in any such instance to make, with your scalpel, free vertical incisions through the gum wherever tenderness and swelling exist; extending your line of cut upwards in the upper jaw, or downwards in the lower, as far as the structure of the parts will allow, bringing your incisions as near together as circumstances may require, and in every point carrying them clearly down to the bone, so as to afford the utmost relief and relaxation to the overloaded and tense periosteum. I believe that this method of procedure would be the nearest approach to an effective one for checking the inflammatory stage of the disease before it has reached an intensity which must inevitably destroy the jaw."

When the stage of threatening has past, the extent of the inflammatory mischief usually asserts itself at once—the whole of that portion of bone which is subsequently the sequestrum appears to be stricken from the first. But occasionally different parts of the jaws are attacked in succession. When, however, pus has formed, it should be early conducted to the surface; and by judicious interference external scars may often be prevented by means of well-directed punctures within the mouth. The whole of the teeth implanted in the dead bone become loose, and apparently elongated; their doom is already sealed, and they should be extracted without delay, as they cause much irritation to the tongue and cheeks.

When the discharge has established itself, and the fetid pus is pouring from the sinuses that communicate with the dead bone, abundant rinsing of the mouth should be had recourse to, not only in the form of washes of water to remove the filthy secretions, but astringent and deodorising lotions, such as decoction of cinchona and solution of alum, solution of chloride of lime, and, still better, solution of permanganate of potass. As has been pointed out by Mr. Simon, the unhappy patients are sometimes so disabled as to be incapable of gargling out their mouths, and then little pieces of sponge may be used by them to wipe away the stinking discharges.

As regards the sequestra, little can be done. Sharp projecting pieces of bone may be cut off by nippers; but the bulk of the dead bone must take its own time to be shed—often a very long time. It is a period of miserable suffering to the patient, and terrible constitutional exhaustion; but it cannot be shortened, or its results anticipated.

In March 1862, there was in the London Hospital, under the care of Mr. Adams, a patient whom I then examined, who had been suffering from the disease, affecting the entire inferior maxilla. It had been going on two years and a half; the latter four-fifths of the time with the lower jaw, except the articular ends, dead and lying in the mouth, bare and ghastly, bathed in ichorous pus within its huge supplemental successor.

Shortly afterwards the necrosed jaw was removed. The operation and its sequence were both unusual. The patient was placed in a kneeling posture, with the chin on a table, and, the mouth being open, the symphysis of the jaw was split down by a chisel and mallet. The right half of the bone was then seized by large strong forceps, and wrenched from the mouth with great force. After a week the same course was adopted with the left half; but this required still greater traction. The entire bone was thus brought away, including the condyles. Ten days after the first operation the patient was seized with secondary hæmorrhage, profuse and arterial, on the *right* side from the wound, where the first portion of jaw was removed. This necessitated ligature of the right common carotid artery. The latter operation was performed by Mr. Maunder; and the patient recovered perfectly.*

The sequestra of the superior maxilla are apt to be more detached than those of the inferior—divisible and smaller, and they can be brought away piecemeal; moreover, as the upper jaw is an attached, and not, like the lower, a floating bone (with muscles ready to displace its parts when the integrity of its arch is broken), its dead portions can be removed without jeopardising the relations of the rest of the bone. Therefore a little and early surgical interference may be employed without injury, and parts brought away which, if belonging to the lower jaw, had better not be interfered with.

In the lower jaw the disease is usually so much more comprehensive, and its resultant sequestrum so solid, that patient watching and palliative treatment are all that can be adopted generally till the very close of the case. Earlier interference

* *Med. Times and Gazette,* July 5, 1862.

might disturb the relations of the supplemental bone (the *natural splint*) and the portions of jaw still living, and, by allowing the strong and antagonistic action of the muscles attached to the two halves of the latter to act separately, lead to the permanent displacement of the elements of the maxillary arch. The articular ends of the bone often, indeed in the majority of cases, though not always, escape the necrosis, when the whole of the rest of the bone may be destroyed; and this circumstance suggests a plan of treatment which may much shorten the patient's suffering. When the necrosis has evidently passed up to the neck of the condyles, the bone may be removed by sawing or nipping across the neck as high up as possible (on either side, if both sides are affected), and then dividing the body of the jaw at its symphysis, the two halves of the bone may then be withdrawn, one by one, without any external wound. Should the condyles be necrosed and follow, no harm will have been done by the previous operation, and the patient's suffering will have been much diminished and curtailed. The division of the bone may be accomplished by a Hey's saw, or some modification of it, improvised to suit the particular position of the required line of section. Variously curved bone-nippers may also be devised to accomplish the same objects. The extreme and firm closure of the mouth sometimes renders this operation very difficult.

I need not dwell upon the general treatment of these cases, as far as they are in common with those of other bone-necrosis. The particular region affected, however, involving and disabling, as it does, the masticatory function, entails some modifications. In the long tedium of their course every effort should be made to supply, by suitable food, the deficiencies which suspended mastication entails—mashed meat, eggs, cod-liver oil, and such sustainants, should be abundantly employed; and iron salts, in moderate proportion, should, if bearable by the patient, be almost a matter of daily diet rather than an occasional medicine.

CHAPTER XXII.

NECROSIS AND EXFOLIATION OF THE ALVEOLAR PROCESSES AND PORTIONS OF THE MAXILLÆ AFTER ATTACKS OF THE ERUPTIVE FEVERS.

MR. FOX, in his work on the teeth,* published at the beginning of the present century, records two instances in children in which exfoliations of the maxillæ had followed immediately upon recovery from attacks of small-pox.

In the museums of many of our hospitals and medical schools are to be found specimens of sequestra from the jaws of children, associated with a slight and imperfect history. The sequestra usually contain some of the temporary and immature permanent teeth, and, as far as the bone is concerned, are confined very generally to the alveolar processes of the temporary teeth and the subjacent bone surrounding their immature successors. These specimens are, for the most part, stated to have been obtained from children convalescent from scarlet fever; and in more than one instance I have seen the specimen labelled—"Necrosis of the jaw in a child, *produced by mercury* given in the treatment of scarlet fever": and the same explanatory description I have seen where measles has been the previous malady so treated. As I shall presently show, I believe that this condition is in no way dependent upon the mercurial treatment, but depends on the intrinsic nature of the disease itself, for which in some cases that drug happens to have been administered,—that the association has been an accidental coincidence and not a cause and consequence.

In the fourth volume of the third series of the "Guy's Hospital Reports," issued in 1858, I published a little memoir on the

* *The History and Treatment of the Diseases of the Teeth, &c.*, by Joseph Fox. London, 1806; p. 112.

morbid condition I am now considering; and this was I believe the first connected account which had been given of it and in which the relation of cause and effect had been explained. As I have but little to add to the opinions I then put forward, and less to alter, the following passages are quoted from the memoir in question:—"During the past few years I have had under my care, principally among the out-patients at Guy's Hospital, a number of cases in which necrosis with exfoliation of the alveolar processes of the maxillæ, accompanied by shedding of the contained teeth, has been one of the secondary consequences resulting from attacks of the eruptive fevers—scarlet fever, measles and small-pox. These cases have been so singularly uniform in their origin, course, and entire history, that though following different forms of eruptive disease, they would seem to have a generic identity: indeed, so similar have they been, that it would be impossible, from a mere inspection of the patient during the period of exfoliation, to have any idea as to which of the eruptive fevers had preceded the then condition—a circumstance which, while it simplifies the description of the several cases, seems to indicate that the immediate cause at least, whatever it may be, is common to the several forms of eruptive fevers after which this condition occurs.

"But though there is so complete a similarity in the cases themselves, the proportion in which they occur, as sequelæ to the previous fevers, differs very considerably." After scarlet fever I have now* (July, 1867) seen fifteen or sixteen cases; after measles about five or six, and after small-pox four. "These figures, referring as they do to sources of observation, combining private practice with the large population of poor who seek assistance at Guy's Hospital, and this extending over a period of fifteen years, may probably be taken as at least a proximate expression of what is the relative frequency with which such consequences succeed the different eruptive fevers respectively. The much more numerous examples of bone-exfoliation and tooth-shedding after scarlatina than after rubeola, especially when we consider the more general occurrence of the latter disease than the former—that almost all children

* When, in 1858, I wrote my paper for the *Guy's Reports,* the cases I had then seen were—after scarlet fever eight or ten, measles three or four, small-pox one.

have measles and that perhaps the majority escape scarlet fever—would seem to indicate that the cause of this morbid change is less common and less intense in rubeola than in scarlatina; and this idea is quite in keeping with what I believe to be the true explanation of these cases, and the nature of their essential cause. To this I shall refer more particularly presently.

As I have said, these cases are all singularly alike, and thus the narration of one case will convey a good idea of them all. Take for example the following:—

"Some years since a poor woman brought her child to me among the out-patients at Guy's Hospital, suffering from this tooth-shedding and necrosis of the lower jaw. The child's history was this: She was a remarkably healthy little girl of five years old; about two months previous she had a mild attack of scarlet fever, which had run its course, and passed off hitherto without any untoward symptoms; her recovery appeared complete, and her health restored to its usual vigour. A few days before the mother applied at the hospital, she had, for the first time, noticed that the child's breath had become offensive, and, upon examining her mouth, had discovered appearances for which she sought advice. The child now looked in remarkably good health, was rosy and robust, and all she complained of was a slight discharge from the edge of the gum on the left side of the lower jaw, at a part corresponding with the temporary molars, and of some slight pain in that region. Upon inspecting the mouth, it presented characteristic appearances with which I was quite familiar: both on the inside and outside of the temporary molars, on the left side of the lower jaw, the gum was stripped for the depth of about the eighth of an inch, leaving bare so much of the alveolus, while, from within the edge of the mucous membrane, which was red and tumid, oozed a discharge of pus; and the odour of the mouth was fetid. It was particularly observed that there was no thickening of the jaw, and no effort at the formation of supplemental bone; neither was this necrosis of bone associated with fistulæ or sinuses; the discharge of pus coming simply from the edge of the gum, where it had peeled from the alveolus. The mother of the child did not associate this condition with the previous attack of scarlatina, and was somewhat surprised when I asked her *which** of the eruptive fevers (naming them), she had recently suffered from. In answer to my query, she described the mild attack of scarlatina, which I have already mentioned.

"I directed that nothing should be done in this case beyond the occasional washing of the mouth with a dilute solution of the trishypochlorite of lime, and that the patient should see me again in a week.

"On presenting herself at the appointed day, the peeling of the gum from the alveolar process was found to have progressed considerably, not laterally, so as to involve bone corresponding to other teeth, but simply stripping more from the bone already partially laid bare. It was now found, too, that the same series of changes had commenced on the other—the right side of the lower jaw, and to exactly the same extent of lateral boundary, though as yet it had made but slight progress. This state of things gradually and uniformly progressed; the left side being in advance of the right—the discharge increasing, and the odour of the mouth becoming more offensive, till about six or eight weeks had elapsed, when the sequestrum on the left side commenced to loosen, and in a few days was readily removed by a pair of dressing forceps, accompanied by the contained teeth. After the sequestrum was removed, it was found that the base of the jaw was still entire, and the integrity of the maxillary arch unbroken; the bone having ulcerated across beneath the loculi, occupied by the forming bicuspids. The now exposed surface exhibited bleeding granulations which speedily healed. In about a fortnight the same occurrence took place on the opposite side of the jaw, without any variation in the attending circumstances."

This history may be taken as a typical example, and as illustrating the ordinary course and issue of these cases. Uniform, however, as they are in all essential particulars, they are, nevertheless, subject to considerable variations in degree of severity. Thus, in one case, which was under my care at Guy's,

* When one of these cases comes to the hospital, so characteristic are they, I always ask the parent or attendant who has charge of the little patient—"Has this child recently had scarlet fever, or measles, or small-pox?" In no one instance have I had a negative answer as to one or other of them.

not only were the corresponding sides of the same jaw attacked, but after the sequestrum and contained teeth had been cast off from the lower jaw on either side, the same occurred in the upper, so that all the eight temporary molars, and all the eight immature bicuspids, with their containing alveoli and loculi, were exfoliated. This was one of the most severe examples I have had: it was after an attack of scarlet fever. On the other hand, in a slight case, only one temporary molar was shed, with its corresponding immature bicuspid, and the bone that was exfoliated was so small in amount—a few little thin plates of alveolus—that it seemed hardly sufficient to allow the escape of the dead teeth. This case was after measles.

In the ninth volume of the "Transactions of the Pathological Society" I published a description and illustrations of several specimens of necrosed bone and teeth, which had been shed after the eruptive fevers, from which the following account has been drawn:—

The first specimen consists of the intermaxillary bones and their contained teeth exfoliated after small-pox.

Fig. 114.

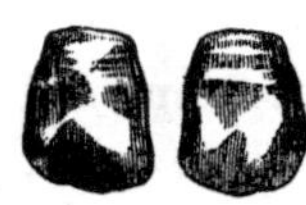

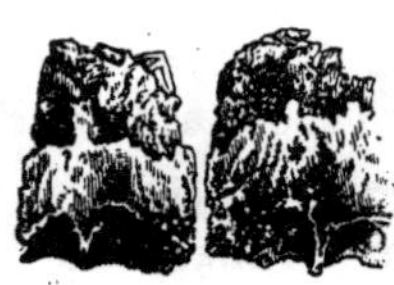

The patient from whom this was obtained was a little boy, five or six years of age, who applied to me at Guy's Hospital on February 23, 1860. His face at that time exhibited numerous dark, inky pits of recent small-pox, from which he suffered seven weeks previous: from this attack he was quite convalescent, and he seemed a healthy well-nourished child. About a fortnight after his recovery from the small-pox, the gum from the front of incisive bone on the right side was observed to recede, or ulcerate away, and this was followed in a few days by a similar affection on the left side: the mucous membrane, gradually receding from the bone till near the point where it reflects upon the lip—that on the right side being a little in advance of the left. At the same time the bone was being denuded on its palatal surface. The recession of the mucous membrane here ceased, and in a few days the right incisive bone came away of itself. This occurred early on the morning the patient came to me. When I saw the patient, the left incisive bone was so loose and so nearly detached, that I readily removed it with my finger and thumb. The temporary teeth and the immature lateral permanent incisors had fallen into the child's mouth and been lost.

The exfoliated incisive bones (fig. 114), are mere osseous shells, and contained the large crowns of the central permanent incisors: there is a partial excavation on the outer side of each incisive bone, which was occupied by the immature lateral tooth. At their lower margins are the alveolar cavities which contained the fangs of the temporary incisors.

This case is thus far analogous to one brought before the Pathological Society by Mr. Bryant—analogous in all essentials, but not in every respect the same, as his case was after an attack of measles, mine after one of small-pox. (See "Pathological Transactions," Vol. X., p. 216.) In Mr. Bryant's case the patient was unusually youthful, only three years old.

In the lower jaw I perceived, on examination, the same process was going on, though in a much less advanced stage—the edges of the gums, corresponding to the four incisor teeth, had just peeled from the edge of the bone. After this the patient did not return to the hospital, and the issue of the case, as respects the lower jaw, I did not know, nor had I an opportunity of getting the specimen. It was quite clear, however, that the same result would occur in the lower as had happened in the upper jaw, and that the incisors—temporary and immature permanent with their containing alveoli and loculi—would be shed.

The second specimen was obtained from a child who had suffered from measles, and is similar to the one which would be shed from the lower jaw of the patient I have just referred to. It consists of the central portion of the alveolar part of the lower jaw, just so much as corresponds to the incisor teeth. The temporary teeth were lost, while the bone remained in the mouth, as is generally the case; the immature dentine capsules of the permanent teeth being retained in the shed bony loculi, excepting the right lateral, which escaped and is here figured.

Fig. 115.

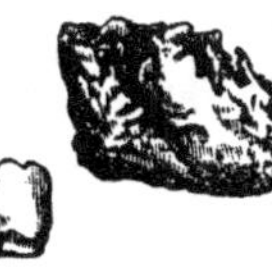

The figure (115) represents the exfoliated bone, and the crown of the right lateral inferior incisor, which fell from the imperfect sequestrum.

The crowns of the remaining immature permanent teeth remain in their bony loculi in the sequestrum.

I have no further notes of the case, than the record that the previous eruptive fever had been measles, and that the patient was a girl, four years old.

The third specimen (fig. 116) represents the superior first temporary molar and the crown of its succeeding tooth—the first bicuspid. These teeth came away with numerous minute sequestra of the alveolar processes, just sufficient to admit of their liberation.

Fig. 116.

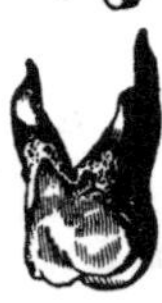

The patient was a little girl, four or five years old, and just convalescent from an attack of measles. The amount of bone lost was less than in any other example I have seen, and this has been one of the few cases that I have observed in which the mischief has been confined absolutely to one side of the jaw.

The fourth specimen was obtained from a little girl of five years old, who had suffered from a mild attack of scarlet fever about eight weeks before. The peeling of the gum from the edges of the alveolar processes had but just commenced when I first saw the patient. At this time, both on the inside and outside of the temporary molars on the left side of the lower jaw, the gum was stripped for about the eighth of an inch, leaving bare so much of the alveolus, while from within the edge of the mucous membrane, which was red and tumid, issued a discharge of pus. A week after the jaw on the other side was similarly affected, and to just the same extent. The peeling away of the gum and periosteum from the bone gradually progressed for five or six weeks, when the sequestrum was easily removed with dressing forceps. A similar sequestrum came away from the opposite side about a fortnight after.

Fig. 117.

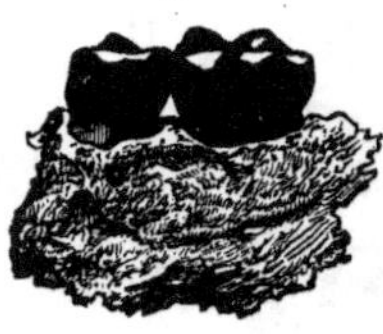

This specimen (fig. 117) consists of about two-thirds of the depth of the lower jaw, on the left side, corresponding to the two temporary molars. The sequestrum involves the immature bicuspid teeth: its jagged lower margin shows that the base of the bone had escaped necrosis.

The fifth specimen was obtained from a little girl between three and six years of age, and followed an attack of scarlet fever. It came from the upper jaw, at a point corresponding with the first temporary molar. The teeth—temporary and immature permanent—had been shed and lost. The same process had commenced on the other side of the jaw to the same extent, but I obtained no specimen from it, as the patient did not again come to the hospital.

Fig. 118.

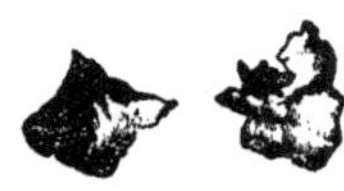

The little exfoliations (fig. 118) appear to consist wholly of thin bony walls of the loculi of the immature bicuspid: other small sequestra of bone had been previously lost.

The sixth specimen is remarkable on account of the very large amount of bone necrosed (fig. 119). It was obtained from a little girl, aged four years. She was taken ill with a sharp febrile attack on July 21, 1859. No rash was noticed, but from the ignorance of unobservant parents, who are of the lowest class, I should attach very little importance to this

Fig. 119.

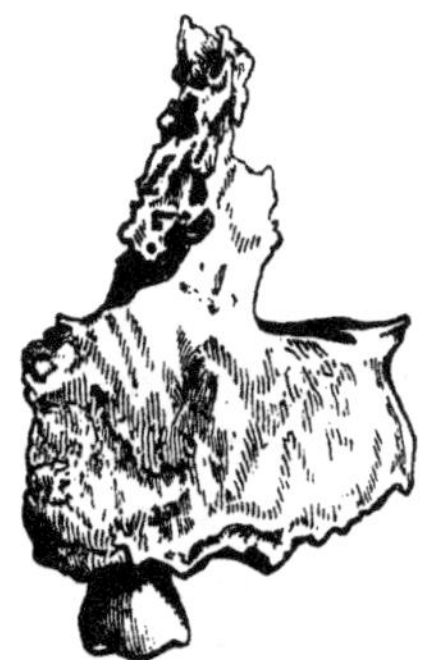

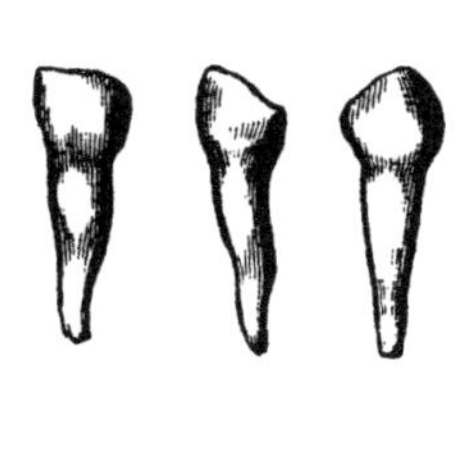

negative circumstance. The very faint evidence of eruption which is not uncommon in scarlet fever might readily escape recognition in a neglected and dirty child, as this poor little patient was. The general history of this short and sharp febrile illness coincides with that of scarlatina, or perhaps measles; however, the fact that some children in the immediate neighbourhood had scarlet fever at the same time, renders it pretty conclusive that that was the malady from which this little girl had suffered.

About five or six weeks after this febrile illness the face on the right side began to swell; on the following day two temporary teeth dropped out, and soon after another was shed. The cheek speedily became black, and a large slough from the side of the face of the dimensions of half-a-crown came away. The child had been living in squalid poverty, was very badly fed, and in a state of most imperfect nutrition.

At this time, about the middle of November, she was taken to a workhouse, and subsequently admitted to Guy's Hospital, under the care of Mr. Birkett, on January 20, 1860.

It was now found that the main portion of the right superior maxilla was necrosed and very loose; the House-Surgeon at once and very readily removed this sequestrum with a pair of dressing-forceps. The second temporary molar tooth and the tuberosity of the maxilla are all that remained in the mouth on the right side of the upper jaw.

I need not further describe this specimen, than by observing, that the great bulk of the maxilla had been involved—the nasal process, most of the palatal process, the body of the bone, with the alveoli and loculi of the temporary incisors, canine and first molar, and the four immature successional permanent teeth—the latter being retained within the bone. As the second temporary molar remained in the mouth, the loculus and pulp of the second bicuspid, and the posterior "cavities of reserve" of the permanent molars behind were probably undisturbed.

The seventh specimen (fig. 120) was obtained from the same little patient as the sixth; it consists of a portion of the left intermaxillary bone—the socket of the temporary central incisor and the loculus of the corresponding permanent tooth, the crown of which is, as yet, alone formed. The teeth came away with the bone, and with it are represented in the accompanying figure. This exfoliation took place some time before the child was brought to the hospital, but the precise date I do not know. The great disparity between the size of the sequestra from the two sides of the jaw is remarkable and very unusual; the tendency to symmetry, almost constant in these cases, is so far maintained that the jaw was affected on both sides, though it is lost in the disproportion of the amount of bone affected. It must be remembered, however, that there was an exceptional element in this case, and that the wide-spread sloughing on the right side of the face, laying bare the maxillary bone to so great an extent (very probably dependent on the cachectic condition

Fig. 120.

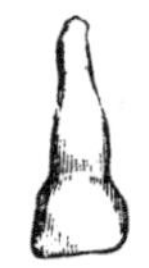

of the child), may offer a reasonable explanation of this disproportion.

The eighth specimen is interesting and exceptional: it is a blighted permanent incisor which was not shed when the temporary tooth and some necrosed bone were lost. The patient was a little mulatto girl, seven years old when I saw her. Three years before, being then four years old, she had scarlatina. Immediately on her recovery it was found that the bone in the neighbourhood of the right superior temporary central incisor was necrosed; it became exposed and in a few weeks the temporary tooth fell out; then, for the first time, small portions of bone came away, and this was going on till the child was nearly five years old. The immature permanent tooth remained; in due time it was cut with that of the opposite side; but it was excessively loose from the beginning and always remained so, being simply attached to the surface of the gum. The left central incisor was quite firm and fully developed. The looseness of the right incisor was an annoyance to the patient, so I removed the tooth. The accompanying illustration (fig. 121) represents it as seen in front and behind; *a* is the front view and *b* the back. The crown of the tooth is fully and properly formed, while a little papilla projecting up from the front of the neck, and which is deficient behind, alone represents the fang. It is clear what had happened: at the time when the child had scarlet fever, when the temporary tooth and bone were necrosed, this tooth was blighted, and though its vitality was not destroyed, it grew no more—its pulp ceased to be a forming organ.

Fig. 121.

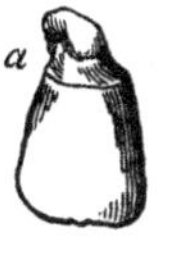

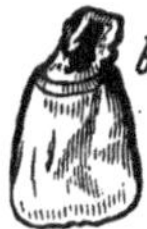

I have since seen a somewhat similar instance, in which a little patient, eight years of age, came to me at Guy's Hospital, exhibiting a deep sulcus on the left side of the lower jaw, in which lay the formed crown of the first bicuspid very loose: the first temporary molar and the surrounding bone had been lost ten months before, after measles.

I will not further dwell on individual cases and specimens, but briefly detail what have been the salient and common characters of them all, as far as my own observations have gone.

The first evidence of necrosis has always been apparent within eight or nine weeks after recovery from the eruptive fever, usually within four or five. It has seldom been preceded by swelling or pain, or accompanied by periosteal abscess; the suppuration occurring at the part where the gum peels from the alveolus, which appears to be the simple method of exposing the dead bone.

Whether in the upper or the lower jaw it usually occurs on both sides, either coïncidentally, or in quick succession; its tendency is to be symmetrical.

The severity of the previous attack of fever seems to have no relation to the extent of the subsequent exfoliation,—a very light attack of eruptive fever may lead to the loss of a considerable sequestrum, or *vice versâ*. Sometimes it is associated with other secondary symptoms, more often not; indeed, it has seemed to me to have generally occurred in very healthy children.

The necrosis is always confined to the jaws in these cases—to the bones, that is, which encompass the young teeth: the rest of the skeleton escapes.

The age at which these exfoliations have occurred is worthy of especial note. It happens during the time that the most active tooth development is going on in the jaws, and when all those parts are undergoing the most rapid nutritional changes—about five or six years of age. From three to eight are the extreme limits I have seen. Now, I believe that the necrosis and exfoliation of bone and teeth after the eruptive fevers is essentially the same as the maxillary necrosis in the victims of phosphorus fumes, and it is the result of the local application of a specific poison to the vascular parts of teeth. There is this difference, however, that in the cases we are now considering the poison is generated within the individual, but with affinities for certain structures and tendencies to action upon certain organs which give its morbid consequences an equally local character. Whatever opinions may be entertained as to the homological relations of the several tissues of the teeth to those of the general integument, there can be no question as to their being members of the dermal system, and as such we should, *à priori*, expect that they would share the consequences which attend those particular diseases, which spend their chief force on the skin. There is one circumstance however that modifies such an anticipation: it is the low state of vitality of the teeth, and the extremely slight nutritional changes which occur in them, *when once they are formed*, and which must consequently remove them to a great extent from those transient though potent influences which would destroy or morbidly affect vascular or rapid growing tissues.* But such a qualification does not apply to the conditions of the teeth during their development; from the time of birth to the eighth or ninth year the jaw bones are the seat of intense developmental nutrition in the formation of the teeth, and are among the most vascular parts of the body: about the middle of the period named, five years of age, the maxillæ contain no less than forty-eight developed teeth and developing tooth-germs. It is about this time that the poison of the exanthematous fevers appears to exert its most deadly influence on the dental system.

As far as I am aware this affection only occurs after the eruptive fevers. I have heard of one doubtful case after continued fever (typhus or typhoid); but this would form no real exception to these cases or their pathological interpretation. The continued fevers have their specific cutaneous eruptions, and their damaging influence on the tegumentary system is sufficiently attested by the falling of the hair in convalescents from them. I would not, however, be supposed to deny that jaw necrosis, associated or not with death and exfoliation of other bones, may occur in children as the result only of extreme cachexia or depressed vital nutrition.† I merely wish to assert my belief that the particular form of alveolar necrosis here described is one of the *specific sequelæ* of the eruptive fevers, and is related to its cause in the manner indicated in the foregoing page.

The issue of these cases is simply comprised in the loss of a

* I once saw a curious affection of the teeth in an adult after scarlatina. A lady about thirty-five years of age had scarlet fever badly: she had a remarkably fine set of teeth, white, large, and showy: about a fortnight after her recovery, she noticed that her two superior central incisors were becoming discoloured, and they gradually got darker and darker, ultimately becoming of a dirty pink colour. They were both exactly alike. Probably this arose from the pulps becoming disorganised during the action of the poison on the tegumentary papillæ, the colour arising from decomposed hematine permeating the dentinal tubes. None of the other teeth were affected.

† See such instances referred to in Holmes's *System of Surgery*, vol. iii. p. 642.

certain amount of bone with the contained teeth, and the consequent disfigurement. As the permanent teeth are usually lost with the temporary, the disfigurement affects the front of the mouth; but when the temporary molars and their successors, the bicuspids, suffer, the damage is comparatively slight. I have seen two examples of adults where this has happened in childhood and the alteration of the face has been wonderfully little: the first molar approaches close to the canine, and the second and third molars come well forward into the mouth, filling out the cheeks, and exhibiting no external evidence of what has occurred. In two instances, as I have mentioned, I saw the permanent teeth retained after the temporaries and the surrounding bone had been shed; but in both cases the permanent teeth were so loose as to require extraction.

Treatment.—I believe the plan of non-interference is the best in treating these cases: to let the sequestrum become perfectly loose before it is brought away. There is little discomfort; no operative interference is indicated; the extent of the necrosis appears to assert itself from the first, and cannot be curtailed. The sequestrum soon becomes loose, and may then be readily removed by dressing forceps. A weak solution of *Chloride of Lime,* or, perhaps better, of *Permanganate of Potass,* may be advantageously used as a cleansing and deodorising mouth-wash. Any general symptoms of disturbed health should be met on ordinary principles. Where the suppuration is profuse, and the bone-necrosis extensive, stimulants and tonics may be required; and in scarlet fever cases steel would be a useful adjunct; but I would observe that in the cases I have seen, the children were, for convalescents, in remarkably good health, and had, almost without exception, escaped the other secondary consequences of the eruptive fevers.

CHAPTER XXIII.

SYPHILITIC ALVEOLAR PERIOSTITIS.

I HAVE seen a peculiar affection of the alveolar periosteum and periodontal membrane, resulting in suppurative inflammation, so distinctly associated with a strong syphilitic history, that I incline to the belief that it is essentially syphilitic in its nature. The affection in question consists of a long-continued inflammation of the gums and sub-mucous structures, usually in the front of the upper jaw, with much general pain about that region. At first there is slight suppuration around the necks of the teeth, which become loose: the suppuration increases in intensity both as regards the amount of the secretion and the depth to which it enters among the roots of the teeth, till at length the whole of the region affected becomes boggy, and, as it were, undermined by the pus-discharging canals around the teeth. I may mention the following illustrative case.

A. B., a type-founder by trade, æt. 45. He states that he had suffered severely from syphilis about two years since, both with primary and secondary symptoms of a serious nature. He believes that he took mercury, but apparently not to any great extent: his mouth was never sore to a degree to cause suffering, and he is confident that he discontinued that medicine full eighteen months since. For the last year he has observed much sensitiveness of the incisor and canine teeth of the upper jaw: the teeth have become loose, and around their necks he has noticed an increasing secretion, apparently purulent. These symptoms have become so distressing that he has now applied to Guy's Hospital for their relief. At this time (June, 1860) I find the whole of the incisor and canine teeth of the upper jaw perfectly loose: around their roots there is abundant purulent secretion, which is slightly fœtid; and the secretion seems to burrow among the alveoli as though their cavities were common, by intercommunication, with each other. The patient at this time presented no syphilitic symptoms beyond a little psoriasis of the palms: all marked constitutional syphilis had ceased about six months since, but not before this affection of the mouth had established itself. As it was quite clear the teeth could not be long retained, I thought it advisable to remove the incisors and canines: I did so: the teeth were sound. The removal of the teeth gave great relief. Afterwards, within a few weeks, three or four small splinters of bone came away, and then the gum healed up firm and healthy.

I have seen four or five very similar cases: they have all occurred in hospital practice: as far as I remember all the patients have been men; and I have had reason to know, or suspect, syphilitic antecedents.

I am by no means prepared to say that these were essentially syphilitic cases, though I strongly incline to that belief. I have occasionally seen considerable suppuration around the necks of the incisor and canine teeth, which have loosened at the same time, and have been subsequently lost, and in which no syphilitic history could be discovered; but the cases I have referred to were so distinct and so severe, that, with the history of the patients, I can scarcely avoid the inference of constitutional poison which I have suggested. Still, however that may be as regards these examples, the following records certainly describe an instance in which syphilis has fallen with acute and destructive force on the alveolar periosteum and periodontal membrane.

Syphilitic Necrosis of the Alveolar border of the lower jaw: Catherine Daily, a healthy-looking Irish girl, aged 21, was admitted into Guy's Hospital, under my care, on November 5, 1859, and gave the following account of herself and her case. She stated that her health had been uniformly good: she denied having had syphilis, and she said that until the occurrence of pain in the right inferior *dens sapientiæ*, some eight months before, she had not suffered from tooth-ache or other affection of the mouth. During the previous month of April the carious wisdom-tooth caused so much pain that she had it extracted: the operation, according to her account, was performed awkwardly, and with much violence, and from this she dates all her subsequent suffering. According to her statement, great swelling occurred about the angle of the jaw in the neighbourhood of the removed tooth soon after the operation, and gradually advanced to the chin: in the former region it slowly subsided, while in the latter it increased and spread beyond the mesial line, until it reached the condition which existed at the time of her admission into the hospital. At the date on which the patient was admitted she exhibited great swelling about the lower jaw, especially in the neighbourhood of the chin, and the integument presented a bright erythematous redness, was glistening and tense; and the projection of the point of the chin, by reason of this swelling, gave a curious aspect to the continuance, especially in profile. On examining the interior of the mouth, it was found that the wound, where the *dens sapientiæ* had been extracted, was quite healed, and the gum in that region healthy; there was nothing apparent to bear out the patient's statement that the malady from which she was then suffering had arisen from the operation of extracting that tooth.

The gums in the front of the mouth and in the lower jaw exhibited intense inflammation, were greatly swollen and very red. In the upper jaw, and in the posterior regions of the lower, the gums appeared healthy; there was nothing indicating the recent operation of mercury on them, and indeed the patient denied ever having taken mercury. The teeth in the region of the lower jaw where the inflammation existed were slightly loose, and very tender when touched. It was noticed that the first right premolar was wanting, but this, the patient said, had been removed many years before.

There was no history to lead to the supposition that phosphorus-fumes had been in operation in this case. The patient had been a domestic servant in a gentleman's family: she denied ever picking her teeth with lucifer matches, and moreover there were no carious teeth in the lower jaw. As no symptoms, and as no points in the history of the case seemed to indicate anything specific in the nature of the inflammation, it was resolved to treat the symptoms individually. Six leeches were applied to the surface of the chin, and a saline aperient administered.

November 10. The patient experienced great relief from the

application of the leeches, but the pain and redness are again returning. Ordered six more leeches.

November 16. Similar relief was experienced on this occasion from the local loss of blood. The patient now complains of a painful circumscribed swelling on the side of the head over the prominence of the right parietal bone—the pain being much worse at night. Upon examining the part indicated, what appeared to be a soft syphilitic node was found. There was also a slight degree of iritis in the right eye.

Ordered four leeches to the chin to be repeated as required; and three grains of iodide of potassium to be taken three times a day.

November 23. The local affection remains much the same, but the symptoms of constitutional import are much better. The node on the head ceased to give pain on the second night after taking the iodide of potassium, and it is decreasing in size.

December 5. To-day I noticed for the first time a discharge of pus along the gum, in front of the necks of the left lower canine and left incisor teeth. This gave great relief, and the redness of the integument of the chin disappeared; the discharge is considerable. Leeches to be discontinued. From this time the discharge continued very abundant: the incisor teeth and left canine became extremely loose, and were all removed.

On April 21 a considerable mass of necrosed bone was observed protruding between the gum in the front of the lower jaw in the region which had been occupied by the missing teeth: it had long been felt by the probe, and was now conspicuously visible. It was somewhat loose, and by means of a vertical incision in front and behind it, was sufficiently detached to be removed by a pair of dressing forceps. It was a large mass, consisting of the alveolar processes of the incisors, left canine, and portions of the alveoli on either side, belonging to remaining teeth; and it extended in vertical depth to within the third of an inch of the base of the jaw.

June 21. Right second bicuspid tooth and canine were removed to-day. Small portions of bone have been coming away very frequently since the last report: and all the teeth are gone between the second left bicuspid and the right first molar—nine in all. The second right bicuspid and canine remained attached long after their sockets were lost, and I fancied perhaps they might have retained their vitality, and be permanently kept; but they became very loose and painful; so I removed them: the pulps were *dead.* There was visible, when the mouth was opened, a great sulcus in the front of the lower jaw, and this gave the patient a strange appearance when seen in profile, from the sinking in of the lower lip.

Small portions of bone again came away on June 28, and on July 2, and after that all pain in the jaw ceased, and the patient expressed a sense of relief, which she had never before experienced since the commencement of her illness.

On August 8 the patient complained of having suffered from *bone pains* for some days, which were worse at night, and the spot on the skull, where the node had been, was especially painful. There was now manifest on the forehead a single patch of copper-coloured psoriasis, of very characteristic aspect. The girl, however, still protested in her virgin purity, and declared that she had never had syphilis. Iodide of potassium was again administered with marked effect; indeed the constitutional symptoms vanished under its use.

As all loss of bone appeared now to be ended, I prepared a substitute for the missing alveoli with artificial teeth: it answered perfectly, restoring the physiognomy, speech, and mastication. Two years afterwards I again saw this girl: there had been no further loss of bone. She was then leading the life of a prostitute, which, as an evidence of character, tends to confirm (though such confirmation was not needed) my opinion as to the syphilitic nature of the case.

January 12, 1865. After losing sight of this patient for about three years, she this day applied to me at Guy's Hospital, suffering under *syphilitic impetigo* of the face. I transferred her to my colleague Mr. Bryant.

The sister of the patient called on me in the autumn of 1865 to inform me of the girl's death. She died of phthisis. I then also learnt that she had contracted syphilis early in 1859.

CHAPTER XXIV.

SALIVA: SALIVARY CALCULUS OR TARTAR.

THE fluid of the mouth, called saliva, consists of secretions from three pairs of composite glands mixed with mucus. The secretions of the three glands differ in chemical and physical characters. That of the parotid glands is limpid and watery; from the submaxillary glands it is viscid and thready, and it is still more gelatinous as secreted by the sublingual glands. It is alkaline in each case, but more so from the parotid than the other glands. The alkaline reaction, however, of the mixed fluids of the mouth is not constant. It is sometimes neutral and even acid. This latter condition varies in different individuals, and under different circumstances: it has been especially observed after long fasting and after prolonged speaking. In some persons in apparent health the saliva is always acid.

The mucus of the mouth is alkaline, but when inspissated around the necks of the teeth is apt to become acid.

The fluids of the mouth contain much nitrogenous matter, the nature of which has not been very accurately determined. The name *Ptyaline* has been given to the most intelligible albuminoid element; and this substance has an important digestive action, converting starch into sugar.

There is another remarkable substance in the spittle, *Sulphocyanide of Potassium.* This does not exist in either of the elementary secretions of the mouth, but appears after their union, and is clearly the result of some decomposition.

Saliva contains about 1 per cent. of solid matter, and of this from 7 to 21 parts in 100 are fixed salts, chiefly chlorides.

Floating in the saliva are multitudes of cast-off epithelial cells and mucus-globules. There are also numbers of extremely minute living organisms of a very low type. In their simplest forms they resemble Bacteria, but, more highly developed, constitute a sort of fungus mycelium, which has been called leptothrix buccalis. In this condition they display a mass of fibres felted together and projecting in single threads at the edge. Isolated threads exhibit an oscillatory movement.

With very high magnifying power, and the action of iodine and dilute hydrochloric acid, the threads are seen to consist of cells attached to each other in linear series; the contents of each cell are coloured by the iodine, while the septa are not affected.

The leptothrix attaches itself to the epithelium, to tartar and carious dentine. It is, I believe, universal; I have found it in every mouth where I have sought it.

The hard incrustations which collect around the teeth are true calculus, deposited from the saliva, with an admixture of certain organised elements and a small amount of matter derived from the food.

The material which most largely enters into the formation of tartar is phosphate of lime, and the organic matter consists principally of a mesh of the mouth-fungus, leptothrix buccalis.

Tartar is deposited around the teeth in situations where the saliva is at rest: on the outer sides of the upper molars, on the surfaces of teeth not used in mastication, and more especially on the incisors and canines of the lower jaw, where there is so constantly a well of stagnant saliva.

The physical characters of tartar vary considerably—it may be hard, soft, brittle, or coherent. In colour it may be green, brown, yellow, or black.

A very thin layer of tartar, of a distinctly green colour, is apt to form on the front surfaces of the permanent incisor teeth of the upper jaw soon after their appearance. It may extend to other teeth, but is mostly confined to the incisors. This form consists of a matrix of leptothrix, in which the colour seems to reside, with fine grains of calcarious deposit, epithelium and mucus cells.

Another form of tartar around the upper front teeth and sometimes the premolars consists of thin narrow bands immediately under the gum; this is usually dark brown, and very firmly adherent to the necks of the teeth.

Tartar occurring on the molar teeth is usually soft, pale buff colour, and easily detached. But the most important collections of salivary calculus occur around the front lower teeth. In this situation it forms an incrustation on the backs of the teeth, which, as it increases, fuses together and forms an even coating, connecting one tooth with another, thick at the neck of the tooth and thinning off towards the edge of the crown. In front it is less extensive, being deposited around the neck and up the sides of the teeth. But it is in this region, in front and behind, that the largest and most destructive accumulations of salivary calculus occur. These are sometimes enormous, clothing and completely hiding all the lower front teeth in one calcarious encasement.

Sections of tartar exhibit distinct lamination, parallel with the surface.

The *chemical* composition of tartar varies. It consists principally of phosphate of lime, with about 18 per cent. of organic matter and 6 per cent. of water. There is a small and variable amount of carbonate of lime. This is said to be most abundant on tartar removed from the molars opposite the discharging orifice of Steno's duct, the secretion of the parotid being also said to be richer in carbonate of lime than that of the other salivary glands. That this is so, or that there is a marked connection between salivary calculus in any one region and any particular gland, I am inclined to question. The calculus deposit derived from any particular gland probably varies very much. A salivary calculus obtained from a duct in the submaxillary gland, which was analysed by Dr. Taylor at Guy's Hospital, contained 13·6 per cent. of carbonate of lime—a most unusual proportion, and in which the parotid secretion could have had no share.

I am indebted to my friend Dr. Stevenson for the following analyses of tartar.

	Friable, Soft Calculus from Molars	Hard Tartar from Lower Incisors
Water and Organic Matter	21·48	17·51
Phosphate of Magnesia	1·31	1·31
Phosphate of Lime with a little Carbonate and a trace of Fluoride	77·21	81·18
	100	100

Upon treating tartar with strong acids and alkalis a number of insoluble minute threads are found; and these led me to suspect that silica might be detected in analysis. But Dr. Stevenson failed to discover any.

I believe that these indestructible threads are leptothrix fibres.

The *effects* of salivary calculus being deposited on the teeth vary with the degree of the incrustation and its locality. When slight in amount it occasions no injury; and, indeed, a small deposit on a faulty tooth seems to retard decay. Where it occurs around the necks of teeth in quantity, it occasions depression of the gum and absorption of the edges of the alveoli. This especially arises in relation to the lower teeth in the front of the mouth, and is the commonest cause of their loss. It frequently affects a single tooth—inferior central or lateral incisor—in the form of a fast-growing scale, rapidly depressing the gum in front and below the tooth, even with ulceration of its surface.

Sometimes the calculus forms rapidly over the whole of the lower teeth, accumulating such a bulk of deposit as to cover out of sight all the teeth and form a coherent mass. These specimens have been mistaken for bone disease, and have suggested severe surgical operations. I have seen a specimen in which the eight anterior teeth of the lower jaw were encased in a prodigious mass, leading to ulceration of the gums and absorption of the alveolar processes, so that the whole, teeth and calculus, ultimately feel from the mouth adherent together.

Ulceration of the tongue, cheeks, and lips may arise from the irritation of tartar; and I have seen a case of cancer of the lower lip associated with, and perhaps produced by, a projecting mass of tartar that exactly corresponded with the sore.

When tartar exists in any notable quantity it ought to be removed; and for this purpose a variety of instruments called "scaling" instruments have been devised. The tartar that accumulates at the backs of the lower incisors is best detached by pressing a narrow but blunt-edged blade between the necks of the teeth; and various curved blades, with different points and edges, are devised to remove the incrustations on other parts.

Superficial stained tartar may be removed by scraping; but I believe less injury to the enamel fibres is done by the momentary application of dilute hydrochloric acid, which is immediately neutralised by an alkali. The plan which I adopt is to employ a cane brush, charged at one end with the dilute acid and at the other with an alkaline powder. The acid is applied for an instant, and then the tooth is freely rubbed with the powder. The acid I use consists of one part of pure hydrochloric acid to three of water. The powder is a mixture of the finest pumice with powdered Castile soap, in the proportion of three of the former to one of the latter.

CHAPTER XXV.

EXTRACTION OF TEETH.

THE removal of the teeth is one of the most important operations which has to be performed by the dental surgeon, and one which requires both scientific knowledge and mechanical skill—knowledge of the parts involved, and a cultivated adroitness in applying the necessary forces to accomplish the intended result.

The wrenching of a tooth from its socket differs remarkably in its method from almost every other operation that the surgeon has to perform; but it is an unfortunate mistake—too often committed—to look upon it as merely involving so much strength on the part of the operator. Strength, and considerable strength, is often required; but that may be useless, and even disastrous, unless properly applied.

The forces involved in extracting a tooth are considered at length in the next chapter, and I would only remark here in reference to them that though the operator should possess all possible knowledge of the forces involved, and as far as he can the anatomical relations of the implicated tooth to the jaw, there are some forces (the *adhesion* of the tooth to the jaw and the *cohesion* of the parts of the teeth among themselves) which he can only estimate approximately. There are some general rules and observations about the extraction of teeth which may well be here enforced.

It was, I believe, an axiom of the elder Mr. Cline (and it ought to be a canon law in all operative surgery) that "every operation is performed *quick enough* that is performed *well.*" This is particularly applicable to the extraction of teeth, and is the more to be enforced, as it is so often violated, especially by young operators. The operation, if not slow, should certainly be deliberate.

In acting on a tooth for extraction the force should be applied as far as possible to the soundest and strongest part of it; and this as respects every extracting instrument. It is especially important in the use of forceps. In applying these the operator should dive or burrow as far up the roots as possible, and in holding the tooth it should be compressed but little. The operator should most carefully watch the progress of the operation, both as regards the *touch* of manipulation and as he sees its progress—never removing his eyes from the tooth till it is out of the mouth.

It is best to complete the removal of an offending tooth at once, at all events at one sitting; but this may not be possible; and it should be remembered that the breaking of a tooth, though leaving the fangs behind, is often not an unmixed evil. It may relieve pain by bleeding, and still more by opening the pulp-cavity and allowing discharge of matter. And it should also be remembered that the periosteum under the fangs of broken teeth is apt to thicken, while the sockets absorb, and thus in time the fangs become more easy of removal.

There are many *causes* which may necessitate the extraction of teeth:—

I. Toothache, in all or any of its forms, may render extraction necessary; but as such cases are often curable, the tooth, if possible, should be treated and retained.

II. Alveolar abscess may exist to such a degree and recur with such frequency as to render the sacrifice of the causing tooth necessary.

III. When a tooth occasions "abscess" of the antrum it should certainly be extracted.

IV. Trismus from pressure of the wisdom-teeth will often render it incumbent to remove these teeth, or, if they cannot be reached, the second molars.

V. Looseness, if extreme, and causing irritation, will necessitate the loss of the loose tooth.

VI. Ulceration of the tongue, cheeks, or lips, by broken or projecting teeth, often renders it proper to remove such teeth, to prevent more serious results.

VII. Epulis and polypus of the gum are causes for the same

proceeding, and there are particular reasons, especially in the former disease, why this is required. (See chapter on "Diseases of the Gums.")

VIII. Fracture of a tooth, destroying its form or exposing sensitive pulp, is another reason for extraction.

IX. The same may be said of necrosis, offensive caries, and loose stumps. And—

X. Extraction is one of the most potent means of treating irregularities.

The several instruments that are used in extracting teeth may be enumerated under the heads—

I. Forceps.
II. The Key.
III. Elevator.
IV. Fang-dividers.
V. Screw.

Forceps are adapted for seizing and wrenching the tooth from the jaw. They consist of handles, blades, and joints; and there are certain qualities about these three parts of forceps which may be enforced as common to them all.

The *handles* should fit the hand of the operator; they should be short rather than long, coarsely file-roughened, so as not to slip, and be perfectly rigid and unyielding when most tightly grasped.

The *blades* should, with few exceptions, be short, simply escaping contact with the crown of the tooth; they should be strong, but thin at the edges, though not absolutely cutting, and should be so tempered as neither to bend or break. They should be formed to fit as accurately as may be the necks, or rather the commencement of the roots of the teeth they are intended to extract; but as no two teeth are absolutely alike this can be approximate only. A molar forceps, for example, may be filed up so as to fit absolutely a typical tooth; but the next tooth will not be exactly the same; still the resemblance will be close enough for practical purposes, if a certain amount of play is allowed in the joint. It is necessary in many cases that the blades of the forceps should be bent at an angle with the handles; but this, in my opinion, should be as little as possible. A severe bend involves a sacrifice of power.

Another important point is the evenness of the edge. By

continual wear this may be damaged in two ways: by chipping and by eversion, the latter of which is fatal to a firm hold on the tooth. The edge of the blade may be kept perfectly even by the file.

The *joint* should be sound, perfectly free, and indeed permitting some lateral movement, so as to allow the blades to adapt themselves to a certain degree of variation in the form of the teeth.

As regards the varieties of forceps employed in practice, or rather, I should say, *invented* and *described*, they are endless, and have been multiplied to a needless, if not a mischievous degree. The most expert operators are those who use, within certain limits, the fewest instruments; and young practitioners will find, as they gain experience and skill, that they reduce their appliances for extracting teeth to a comparatively small number. At least, that has been my own case and that of many friends. Indeed, I believe it to be inconsistent with the perfect accomplishment of a mechanical result to be constantly changing the means of its attainment.

It is not my intention to describe at length, or to figure, the various orthodox forms of forceps.* These instruments may be divided into those for the upper and those for the lower jaw.

Upper Jaw Forceps.—Straight forceps will extract all the teeth in front of the molars; and the most expert operator with whom I am acquainted accomplishes these extractions with a single pair. It is usual to have the blades broader for the central incisors and canines than for the laterals and bicuspids, but a medium width will serve for all. Mr. Tomes urges that the section of the front blade should represent a wider arch than the back.

A very important modification of the blades is necessary where the teeth are crowded and overlap; in such case one should be narrow and the other broad, the narrow blade corresponding to the overlapped face of the tooth that has to be removed.

Molar forceps, for the upper jaw, have a particular form of blade in relation to the division of the fangs, which are three in number—one palatal and two buccal fangs. The inner blade

* Admirable sets of these instruments, of the best form and construction, are to be obtained from makers who manufacture them as a specialty: from Mr. Evrard, Messrs. Ash, or Mr. Collins.

simply clasps the neck portion of the palatal fang, while the outer blade embraces both the buccal fangs, and projects a sharp conical process between them. This latter principle originated with Mr. Snell, and was perfected by Mr. Tomes,* whose instruments have left nothing to be desired.† These forceps, of course, require to be in pairs for right and left teeth. Such instruments of ordinary blade-grasp are available for all three molars of the upper jaw, but an exceptionally small wisdom-tooth may necessitate a very small instrument of the same construction.

Lower jaw forceps are mostly of a form known as "*hawk's-bill*" forceps, in which one blade is longer than the other, and curving, more or less, over the crown of the tooth, embraces the neck on the lingual surface, while a shorter and straighter blade encircles the labial or buccal surface. These forceps are essentially the same for the incisors, canines, and bicuspids, only differing in size. Where the incisors are crowded and overlap each other, as is very common, and where regulating interference is needed, two pairs of such forceps—one with a narrow internal blade, and one with a narrow external blade—will come into requisition.

For the lower molars the forceps, of whatever nature, should have at the extremity of each blade the same arrangement as has been described on the outer blade of the upper forceps—a V-shaped process, to pass between the fangs; for in the lower jaw, the fangs being two—one behind the other—such a process will be needed on the inside as well as the out.

Other forceps are available for the extraction of the back teeth. Small parallel bladed instruments may be employed to extract the bicuspids, but they are weak and feeble in comparison.

A form of parallel-bladed forceps, known as "George's forceps," with V-shaped points, is often useful in extracting lower molars, especially in completing the removal of a lower wisdom-tooth when dislodged by the elevator.

For the temporary teeth the same instruments are required as for the permanent, but they should be smaller.

* *Medical Gazette*, 1841.

† I cannot agree, however, with this distinguished author, that the extreme elaboration of instruments, which he has recently advocated, is really necessary.

Stump forceps have been devised in endless forms. It is necessary that the blades should be long, with a gentle curve and narrow points, for the extraction of simple isolated stumps.

The Key-instrument is now very generally and very properly abandoned; but I still think there are a few cases in which it may be employed with advantage—namely, where the first or second lower molar tooth is very carious on the outer edge, the decay descending below the gum and leaving an unsound surface for forceps, and with a neighbouring tooth standing on each side. To these narrow circumstances I think the use of the key should be confined. If a tooth is wanting on either side the elevator can easily dislodge the offender, and the forceps withdraw it, but where there is not this favouring condition I believe that the use of the key will be a readier and less painful proceeding in the particular case I have mentioned. I need not enter into a description of this instrument; but there is one point in its construction which I would urge, namely, that the fulcrum should have a rotating plate; this prevents the laceration and much of the crushing of the gum, though the pressure of course remains.

The Elevator.—This is one of the most useful of instruments for extracting teeth, and it is capable of application in a larger number of cases than any other. By it any tooth or fang may be removed under certain circumstances.

The forms of the elevator have been multiplied almost indefinitely, but that which is usually adopted, and which I find best, consists of a blade and a shaft, as figured in the illustration, where the instrument is displayed in face and in profile (fig. 122), attached to a substantial "balloon" handle. The blade should be flattened on one face and convex on the other, and the shaft should be short and very strong.

Fig. 122.

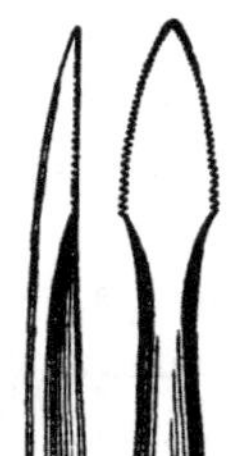

Another point which I have found of great advantage, and which originated with myself, is to have the edges of the blade serrated; it prevents the instrument from slipping, and it bites the neck of the tooth, or side of the fang acted on, with marked tenacity.

As its name implies, the instrument is used to elevate or lift the tooth out of its socket: it is employed as a lever acting against the offending organ, the socket of which or a neighbouring tooth being the fulcrum. In using the elevator the flat surface of the blade is forced against the tooth to be removed, the convex surface towards the fulcrum, and as the wedging, digging force is continued the instrument should be slightly rotated, the convex surface moving over the fulcrum, while the lower sharp edge of the blade clings to the neck of the tooth and lifts it. Where the fulcrum is a standing tooth the instrument should be held with slight obliquity from a horizontal direction; where the socket is the fulcrum the position should be nearer a vertical one.

It is always desirable in using the elevator to direct the pressure against the tooth to be extracted so that it should rise out of the socket, where there is most space, and not against an obstacle.

The casualties that may arise in the use of this instrument, and the precautions necessitated, are discussed in the next chapter.

Fang-dividers or *splitters* are most useful instruments under certain circumstances—when the crowns of molar teeth have broken in attempted extraction, while the fangs remain coherent and firmly impacted by contiguous obstacles. I am surprised that these instruments are not alluded to in text-books on dental surgery, nor generally adopted.

Fang-dividers are something like bone-nippers, with strong blades, having cutting edges and points which meet. I employ two forms, one in which the blades are but slightly bent obliquely on the handles, and the other nearly at right angles—the former for the upper jaw, and the latter for the lower. The handles should be strong and rigid and the joint round.

There is often much difficulty in extracting fangs of broken teeth when united together and supported by contiguous teeth. It has been proposed to trephine the side of the alveolus in such cases, and I have invented a small trephine for severing the roots by cutting away the central portion that held them together; but I have found these fang-dividers much more practical and efficacious.

In using the instrument it should be forced home by the side of the fangs till they are embraced, and then they should be nipped asunder. When thus separated they are loosened at the same time, and the elevator or forceps easily completes their removal.

The Screw.—This is a very valuable instrument for a few exceptional extractions, namely, in those cases where the single fanged upper teeth have become very carious and hollow up the pulp canal, so as to be more or less like open funnels. In such cases the roots will not bear the pressure and traction of forceps. This condition is not infrequently seen in old pivoted teeth.

The screw is of conical form, so as to fit as accurately as may be the hollow of the fangs. I have several screws in which the expansion of the cone varies so as to suit different hollows; and in my instruments I had the worm of the screw so cut as to point backwards to the hand of the operator (as is seen in the figure, 123), by which means the hold upon the fang is firmer. The handle and shaft of the instrument may be the same as those of an elevator. In using the screw the cavity should first be scraped out, to remove all soft dentine, and then the instrument cautiously introduced and screwed on till it can no longer be turned with ease. A quick sharp pull will readily bring away the fang.

Fig. 123.

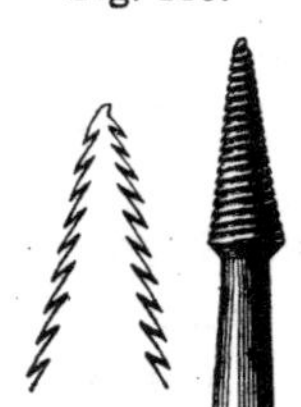

In America the screw has been associated with forceps in one instrument: this has appeared to me unnecessary.

The screw is really a valuable resource, and for the want of it I have known the alveolar process at the front of the jaw seriously injured, in removing some very hollow incisor fangs. A gentleman had long worn pivoted central incisor teeth; the fangs had become mere hollow funnels; serious abscesses occurred in connection with the fangs, and their removal became necessary. The dentist failing in his efforts, took his patient to an eminent London surgeon, who placed the gentleman under chloroform, and proceeded to extract the fangs by removing the alveolar process in front of them; this was chiselled away till they were fully exposed; and the roots being long, the bone was taken away on either side to near the root of the nose. The symptoms were relieved; but the loss of bone was such as to produce a deep depression on either side of the centre of the upper lip, much injuring the expression. These tooth-fangs could have been easily removed by the screw without damage to the jaw.

The forces employed in extracting teeth consist of pulling in all cases, and, associated with it, rotation or torsion, or a swaying from side to side; these modifications of the pull being determined by the particular tooth operated on.

Teeth with conical fangs are first dislodged by twisting; those with compressed fangs or with more than one fang are started from their sockets by a lateral movement, and in some cases the two may be combined.

The *incisors* of the upper jaw have roots which are typically conical, and they are readily dislodged by torsion, and may then be removed. The same applies to the upper *canine*, but its fang is apt to be somewhat compressed, and it twists with less ease.

The *upper bicuspids* should be dislodged by a very slight lateral movement, and then drawn nearly downwards, or with a little inclination outwards. From the extreme brittleness of these teeth the operator must be careful to grasp them as high as possible on the fang, and to use a minimum of compression.

The *upper molar* teeth are best detached from their sockets by being seized high up, the outer blade of the forceps being pressed well in between the two buccal fangs, and the instrument then swayed firmly, but *slowly* and *slightly*, outwards and then inwards, till the attachment is felt to give way. This is frequently attended with a cracking of the alveolar process. The tooth should be drawn downwards and decidedly outwards.

The *upper wisdom-tooth* is extracted with peculiar ease by an extreme outward traction. If the tooth is simply seized and drawn directly outwards into the cheek, almost at right angles to the jaw, it slips from its socket with singular facility. In cases where the wisdom-tooth has been long extracted I have noticed that the same proceeding applies, although in a less degree, to the second molar. This does not appear to have been observed previously.

The *lower incisors* are so flattened in the fang from side to side that rotation with them is scarcely possible. They should be slightly dislodged by a forward and backward movement, and then drawn vertically upwards. The forceps to accomplish these extractions should be narrow hawk's-bills, with very little bend, the lingual blade being slightly curved and a little longer than the labial, while the handle should be bent only sufficiently to escape the upper teeth. Where it is necessary, with overlapping teeth, to use forceps with a narrow blade on one side especial care should be taken to prevent that blade from slipping aside between two teeth and forcing them apart.

The *inferior canines* and *bicuspids* may be extracted with similar instruments of somewhat larger size, and used in the same manner, the operator standing well over his patient, so as to draw the tooth vertically upwards, or nearly so.

The *lower molars*, first and second, are best removed by strong and stout hawk's-bill forceps. These are usually made too curved upon the joint, by which power is lost. In employing them the tooth should be swayed from without inwards, and the reverse, till its attachments are felt giving way, when it should be drawn upwards, outwards, and a little backwards. If it is drawn too much outwards the external plate of the alveolus is apt to break and come away. With "George's" forceps this is not so liable, but they have less power than the hawk's-bill.

The lower *wisdom-tooth* is best extracted by the elevator, with or without the subsequent assistance of forceps. The backward bent fangs of the third lower molar present peculiar physical difficulties for extracting the tooth by ordinary methods, yet this very circumstance renders its removal very easy with the elevator. If the instrument is brought to bear on the front of the neck of the tooth, using the second molar or the alveolus as a fulcrum, and the crown of the tooth is then turned backwards towards the ascending ramus of the jaw, the tooth slips out of its socket, curling backwards in the axis of the fang's curve. Should the tooth not be quite free, it is easily brought away with forceps.

Stumps of teeth are easily removed if single, tolerably coherent, and of some long standing, and they may be extracted by instruments suited for corresponding teeth. Isolated fangs of molars may be withdrawn by long narrow-bladed forceps slightly curved. When single fangs to be removed are the result of recent fracture it may be necessary to dislodge them first with an elevator, and then extract them with forceps. But when the fangs are those of molars, and are still united together at the neck, especially in cases of recent fracture, the matter is one of more serious difficulty. Three courses are open to the operator. If there is a vacant space next to the broken tooth, the elevator may dislodge the whole *en masse* in that direction, and it may then be lifted from the socket by forceps. If it is hemmed in by standing teeth on either side, then either the fangs must be separated by a fang-divider and removed singly, or they may be extracted collectively by forceps specially devised to meet such cases. This principle originated with the late Mr. Arnold Rogers. Two such instruments are figured in the accompanying illustrations, and are known respectively as "Baly's,"* and "Stevens's"† forceps. In the first

Fig. 124. Fig. 125.

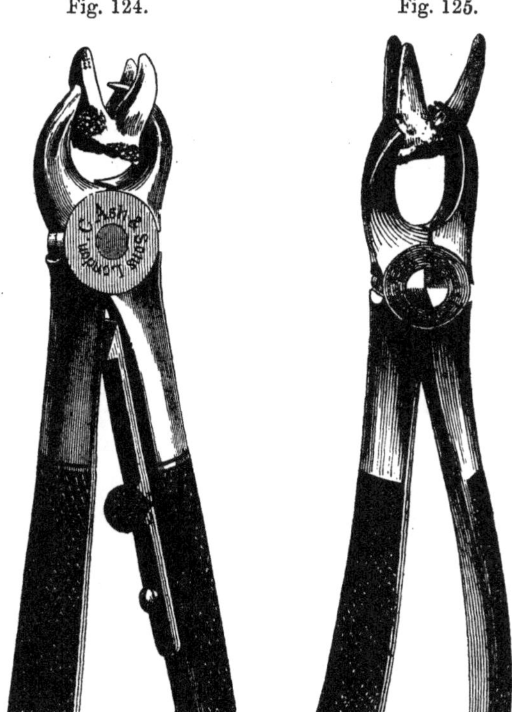

(fig. 124) a thin palatal blade, roughened to prevent slipping, embraces the inner fang, while a strong, pointed, curved blade pierces the gum and alveolus, and forces its way between the buccal fangs. In Stevens's forceps (fig. 125) the palatal blade is divided into two points, which pierce the alveolus and firmly hold the inner fang. These are powerful instruments for ex-

* *British Journal of Dental Science,* vol. xiv. p. 55.
† *Ibid.* p. 180.

traction, but they frequently act as fang-dividers, and then the roots have to be removed in detail. A similar instrument, with two piercing points, is made for lower molars.

It occasionally happens that the roots of double teeth are so entangled with the bone of the jaw that their attempted removal is either attended by fracture of the jaw or of the tooth. These casualties are fully considered in the next chapter. The best chance of extracting the remains of teeth broken under these circumstances is to split the fangs asunder and try to remove them separately. If this cannot be accomplished, I agree with Mr. Tomes that it is better to "allow the extremity, or even the lower third to remain, unless it is clearly the subject of disease."

Cases may arise, however—such as an outward-opening alveolar abscess—in which every vestige of the tooth must be got rid of, even if necessitating the removal of a portion of the jaw.

CHAPTER XXVI.

ON THE CASUALTIES WHICH MAY ARISE IN THE OPERATIONS OF TOOTH EXTRACTION.

THE literature of the profession contains very little bearing on matters discussed in this chapter, and in legal investigations where blame is charged there is much difficulty in quoting authorities. Here and there isolated instances of misfortune or unexpected and unsuccessful results are frankly recorded: but where shall we find the whole matter considered in a concrete form? Or where can counsel point to those *literæ scriptæ* which the Court, in judicial enquiries, always looks to as guiding, if not governing, in special matters of professional knowledge and practice?

It is but fair for practitioners of all professions whatsoever to record their failures as well as their successes. Not only is it right as a matter of abstract truth, but it is just that younger and less experienced men should feel that matters do not always go well with their seniors; that others who have had far longer and wider experience than themselves have at times to regret untoward and unsuccessful operations. Of course those who have had most experience and are naturally gifted with mechanical dexterity will have the largest average of success; but I trust that, in our profession, no one will shrink from acknowledging that success does not always attend his best efforts.

There are special reasons why the possible casualties, that may fairly arise in tooth extraction, should be affirmed and acknowledged by the heads of the profession. Legal proceedings of the most unjust character have been instituted and carried into court, to the great cost and injury of innocent defendants;

and the facility given by our County Courts, for suing *in formâ pauperis*, affords tempting opportunities to unscrupulous people to hazard a legal process, which cannot entail loss on them, and which may possibly issue in gain by award of damages.*

Few professional men are likely to be so exposed to these misfortunes as practitioners of dental surgery.

Practical experience, involving that of the largest hospital and medical school in London, and extending now to twenty-three years' duration, has brought under my notice many and varied disasters, in some of which I have been an unintentional and most unwilling agent.

My own note-book, circumstances which have been authenticated to me, and such few records as have been published, enable me to make the following enumeration :—

I. Breaking of tooth.
II. Breaking of jaw.
III. Taking out wrong tooth.
IV. Taking out two teeth instead of one.
V. Removing capsule of growing permanent tooth in extracting its temporary predecessor.
VI. Tearing gum.
VII. Wounds produced by slipping of elevator.
VIII. Extracted tooth falling into the air-passages.
IX. Extracted tooth falling into the pharynx and being swallowed.
X. Crushing the inferior maxillary nerve.
XI. Dislocating the lower jaw.
XII. Breaking one tooth in extracting another.
XIII. Cutting lip in removing a jagged extracted tooth.
XIV. Forcing tooth or tooth-fang into the antrum.
XV. Forcing tooth-fang into an abscess-excavation in maxilla.

In estimating the casualties which may arise in extracting teeth it is well to consider the essential nature of the operations themselves. They are different from all or nearly all other surgical proceedings. In removing a tooth the operator wrenches or tears an organ from its living connection with the rest of

* For the legal questions which may arise on these points the reader is referred to *The Medical Practitioner's Legal Guide*, by Hugh Whiteman Esq., Barrister-at-Law. Chapter IV. p. 36.

the body, frequently by the exercise of great force. And this force is often applied with little intelligence—the operator being necessarily ignorant, from the hidden and varying nature of the parts, of many of the conditions with which he has to deal. How different is all this from what usually attends operative surgery—how different from the keen cutting of sharp instruments, where force is at a minimum in comparison with results attained; and from the intelligent proceedings of a careful dissection, where the removal of disease is accomplished by manual precision based upon the exact knowledge of elaborate anatomy.

I would not for a moment imply that the extraction of teeth does not require the application of dexterity to anatomical knowledge: but, where great force has to be applied, that *per se* is adverse to mechanical delicacy. The force which the operator has to expend in removing a tooth is often very great indeed: occasionally one has to exercise the whole muscular power of the hand and fore-arm. It would be difficult to estimate, in measure of so many pounds, what is the force thus sometimes employed, but it must be immense; and, with the exception of the reduction of dislocations of the larger joints, is probably in excess of that which is used in all other operations of surgery.

Now, this active force on the part of the operator is applied in opposition to certain static forces latent in the parts implicated, namely—the *co*-hesion of the parts of the tooth between themselves, the *ad*-hesion of the tooth to the jaw, and the *co*-hesion of the elementary structures of the jaw where it embraces the tooth.

These static forces may vary indefinitely, both absolutely and relatively; and it is their *relative* variation which mainly causes uncertainty in the issue of an operation of tooth extraction, and which, where that variation is abnormal, may lead to some of those casualties which I propose now to consider. The adhesion of the tooth to the jaw is normally the weakest of the three static forces indicated, and this it is which the operator seeks to violate. But the circumstances may be otherwise. Thus, while the adhesion of the tooth-fangs to the alveoli may be very strong, the cohesion of those parts of the tooth which can be grasped by the operator may be very weak, and in such case the tooth will break and its fangs remain in the embrace of the socket; or, while the tooth adheres with much firmness to the jaw, it may be dense and coherent in its structure, and thus, the operator pushing the traction he employs to an issue, the cohesion of the parts of the jaw may prove the weakest point, and then the tooth will be brought away with more or less of the alveolar process adhering to it. And these conditions are mainly if not wholly hid from the operator till the catastrophe has declared them. That which comes most obviously within the observation of the operator is the cohesion of the parts of the tooth; and its holding together or its fracture may be to some extent predicted; but even here he may be deceived.

I. The *breaking of a tooth* in attempted extraction may arise from its intrinsic brittleness, or from the nature of its connection with the jaw. Unquestionably caries is the commonest cause of that fragility which leads to tooth-fracture; but there is a marked difference, independent of decay, in the frangibility of teeth in different individuals; and I am inclined to think that the easy breaking of teeth apparently sound, and those which fracture when but little decayed, sometimes arises from that imperfect calcification of the dentine which leaves a large amount of interglobular material unimpregnated with earthy matter. The structure of the tooth is thus soft at parts, and, not being homogeneous, is not coherent.

The connection of the tooth to the jaw may lead to tooth-fracture by close *adhesion* properly so called; or by *entanglement* of bent or divergent fangs among the bone of the jaw.

The adhesion is sometimes wonderfully close, and plates of alveolus are found so firmly attached to the fangs of extracted teeth as to lead, at a superficial observation, to the idea of anchylosis: but I believe true anchylosis never occurs between the jaw and tooth in man. I have sought for it in vain and made many sections for the microscope in endeavouring to find it; but in every instance a fibro-vascular tissue has intervened between the bone and the crusta petrosa.* Still, practically, the adhesion is equivalent to anchylosis.

* The absence of anchylosis as an occasional pathological condition in man is a remarkable circumstance, considering the great similarity between the crusta petrosa and true bone in such close contiguity, and considering also that the layers of crusta petrosa of neighbouring fangs often become fused

The entanglements of fangs may be very various, and where they diverge, and, then converging, embrace masses of bone, constitute the most potent causes of tooth-fracture.

But in all these conditions of possible accident, how often can the operator fully comprehend beforehand with what he has to deal? And how can blame be fairly brought home to him for a consequent tooth-fracture? Unquestionably many teeth are broken in attempting to extract them, which ought not to be broken; but in many other instances no amount of forethought, or experience, or mechanical dexterity could have avoided a disaster, the circumstances producing which having been beyond the ken, or the possible prevention of the operator.

II. *Fractures of the jaw* involve the same series of forces, though with differently varying proportions, as those which occasion tooth-fracture. The adhesion of the tooth to the jaw, and the cohesion of the parts of the tooth, must be superior to the cohesion of the jaw-bone; and so the latter gives way.

I believe that perfectly innocent fracture of the jaw, where there is no excess of adhesion of the tooth to the bone, and where none of the latter is removed, is very common indeed. When an upper molar with wide-spreading fangs is brought away quite clean and free of any attached bone, fracture of the alveoli has nevertheless very often taken place. If the operator will place the finger and thumb of the left hand on either side of the alveolus during the operation he will be conscious of the fact—the spreading of the plates of bone and their breakage are quite palpable. But here the fracture heals "by first intention" and is harmless. Indeed, *simple* fracture of the jaw in tooth-extraction where circumscribed is scarcely to be looked upon as a casualty of any moment. In persons, however, of unsound or tainted constitution, it may be the starting-point of very disastrous results.

together. In fish, batrachians and reptiles true anchylosis of teeth to jaw is a frequent condition; and in them the disparity of uniting tissues is often considerable. The nearest approach to a union of skeleton-bone to tooth tissue in man with which I am acquainted, was described by myself in the *Transactions of the Pathological Society* for 1854. In this case processes of periosteum passed through minute foramina in the tooth near the neck and, at a corresponding part within the tooth, was a mass of bone exactly like cancellated skeleton-bone organically united to and continuous with the surrounding dentine.

In looking through books on dental surgery I have been struck by the conspicuous absence of narrative cases in which some part of the jaw has been seriously fractured in tooth extraction, though such casualties have probably happened to very many practitioners: and where allusions to these accidents are made they are usually so expressed as to imply blame or malpraxis in others. Surely this is not fair.

At a trial which, a few years since, I attended as a witness, the main question raised was the culpability of an operator in breaking a portion of the jaw while extracting a tooth; and the best authority that could be quoted for the defence was Heath "On Injuries and Diseases of the Jaw."

Mr. Heath remarks—"Fractures of the alveolus, however, are often unavoidable during the extraction of the molar teeth even in the most skilful hands, since the position assumed by the fangs is occasionally such that extraction without displacement of the bone to some extent is impossible." This is very just, but it is insufficient; and the very sensible remarks and the interesting case,* which he quotes from Dr. J. Richardson immediately after, would have warranted a wider and a far more serious reference to unavoidable and unblamable disasters.

I have had many cases in which more or less of the jaw has broken in extracting teeth; but the following are the records of the most severe instance that has occurred under my hands:—

A. B——, a lady's maid, came to me in August, 1864, to have the two superior central incisors removed for unsightly decay, with the view of their replacement by artificial teeth. She was about thirty-five years of age; the jaw bones were large and thick, and the teeth above average size. The superior laterals were wanting and had never appeared, the result being a decided gap between the neighbouring teeth, and the incisors themselves were seperated. I first extracted the right tooth, which was very firm and required the exercise of much force to remove it. It held immovable for some time, when suddenly, with a feeling of socket-fracture, it came away; and I found the whole of the front plate of the alveolus firmly attached to the unusually broad fang from neck to apex.

* Published in the *Dental Cosmos* and reprinted in the *London Dental Journal,* August, 1863.

In proceeding to remove the left incisor I placed the patient's head under my left arm, and firmly grasped the front of the jaw on each side of the tooth between the thumb and forefinger of the left hand, and then applied the forceps. The tooth was very firm, and I used great force certainly in my efforts to extract it, but not more than I have frequently employed without harm both before and since. Suddenly, with a crunching sound and sensation, I felt the jaw-bone give way to an extent that was quite alarming. I instantly desisted from pulling and endeavoured to soothe my patient, who was conscious that some disaster had occurred. Upon examining the parts I found the whole mass of bone corresponding to the intermaxillary bones had broken away and was merely held in place by the soft tissues. A vertical fracture extended from the side of the canine up to the root of the nose, then nearly horizontally across to the opposite side, being connected there with another vertical fracture.* The lesion passed completely through the jaw from before backwards, and there was a wound in the palate three quarters of an inch from the alveolar border, through which there was considerable hæmorrhage. This state of matters caused me some anxiety, though I felt I could not blame myself for what had happened. The severance of the bone was so extensive and complete that I naturally looked for necrosis as a probable result. But the issue of the case was most happy: the fractured bone united at once, without an untoward symptom. I afterwards levelled the decayed tooth to the neck; and the patient has now worn the artificial substitutes for years without discomfort. How different might have been the result! Had I pulled for another second the bone would probably have torn through the soft parts and have come bodily away; or in a cachectic patient necrosis might have followed; and I might have had endless blame for a disaster which I could neither foresee nor prevent; and which was brought about by performing an operation in a perfectly legitimate manner.

This is the most serious fracture that has occured to me; but I have recently heard of one still more severe example. In this

* It has occurred to me as just possible that this fracture may have been determined by the presence of that condition—so very rare in the human subject—the existence of a suture between the intermaxillary and maxillary bones.

case the operator broke the horizontal ramus of the lower jaw completely through: and the character of the practitioner is such, and his ability so far beyond dispute, that the question of blame or error could scarcely be raised.

III. The *accidental extraction of a wrong tooth* is a very rare occurrence indeed in the hands of a qualified and capable operator. But I fear, among students and young beginners, it occurs more often.

That most practitioners have sometimes taken out a wrong tooth from error in judgment is probably too true. It is not always easy to decide which is the offender where the symptoms may depend upon one of two or more teeth, and the operator may, after the most careful scrutiny, decide upon the wrong one. And again, in regulating teeth, such errors of judgment, though less excusable, are certainly not less common. Indeed I fear that a want of due attention to the common sense principles of tooth-thinning in crowded jaws leads to the sacrifice of many good teeth that might be retained. However, it is not on such cases that I desire here to dwell: they are errors of judgment, not accidents—the operator intends to take out a certain tooth and he does it. But the disaster of taking out a wrong tooth accidentally is exactly the reverse of this—the operator seeks to do one thing which he fails to accomplish, and he does another which he never intended. Now, to take out a sound tooth, which had in prospect years of usefulness, and to leave behind a decayed one, which the patient sought the operator's aid to remove, is the most unqualified calamity that can occur in tooth extraction; for, though other accidents may be of more serious consequence to the patient, still this is without mitigation—it is misfortune on both sides.

I am thankful to say it has never occurred to me; and this perhaps on account of the early warning I had in seeing it happen in the days of my pupilage to one of my companions, and that from a cause which appeared to me at the time very evident and easily obviated. I believe that three circumstances may conduce to this untoward result:—

a. The slipping of the instrument after application and before traction;

b. Application of the instrument to a wrong tooth by a short-sighted person; and *c.* The sudden plunge of a frightened patient during the operation itself.

The first is essentially the accident of the student; and how often have I seen a nervous young beginner set about the operation as though courting such a result—grasping the tooth with the forceps and then, turning away his head with an eager, anxious face, commence tugging lustily without ever again assuring himself that he still pulled at the tooth he had chosen. The early example of this disaster to which I have referred occurred in the first days of my pupilage, when I was articled to a general practitioner in the country. One of my fellow pupils, somewhat older than myself, was a reputed expert at tooth-drawing, and great was the execution which he did, with a certain rough dexterity, among the decayed teeth of the poorer people of the parish, and great was the reputation he was gaining, till one day a disaster occurred and his character collapsed very suddenly. Mr. K. took out teeth boldly and without hesitation; but then he had the student's trick—he applied the instrument and everted his head, and his glance only returned when the proceeding was completed. I well recollect the calamitous morning when a neighbouring linen-draper's assistant came to the surgery with a swollen face and a dreadfully inflamed gum to have his decayed and aching right lower first molar " drawn." He was seated in the especial chair; the key (Mr. K.'s favourite instrument) was duly clothed with lint, and operation commenced. The claw was applied to the tooth and my friend everted his gaze. Presently something gave way; the instrument started from the patient's mouth and a tooth rolled on to the floor. But it was not the carious molar. There upon the carpet lay the second bicuspid—sound, white and spotless; while the cause of all the patient's sufferings was just where it had been before. The poor man left the surgery much worse off than when he came—his tooth-ache was terribly exasperated, his tender gum bruised and lacerated by the fulcrum of the key, and his jaw minus a sound tooth. There was a great disturbance: legal proceedings and damages were talked about; but unexpected circumstances put an end to the matter. About a week after the catastrophe the patient had violent hæmoptysis, and a few days after he died in a second attack.

But the lesson I learnt that morning has never been lost upon me, and many a Guy's student has had the benefit of it; for I lay it down as a *canon law* in my first precepts on tooth extraction—

When you have applied your instrument to the tooth keep your eyes on both till the tooth is in your hand. And thus I trust I have taught young operators from yielding to what seems to be an almost instinctive dread of watching the violent disseverance of a tooth from the jaw.

The *application of the instrument to a wrong tooth by a short-sighted person* is, I believe, the explanation of this disaster sometimes occurring. An instance of it happened within my own knowledge not very long since, in which it thus arose—at least that is the interpretation which I should place upon it. I would not however have it implied that men who are short-sighted are, from that circumstance, disqualified from operations. On the contrary some of the most skilful and most successful of surgeons, whether practising in the narrow field of dental surgery or the wider one of general surgery, have laboured under this defect, and have had to seek the assistance of glasses to establish just vision.

The *slipping of the instrument through the fault of a nervous patient* is no doubt an occasional cause of the extraction of a wrong tooth, and this may be considered as shifting the blame from the operator to his patient, or at all events of relieving the former; but still all extractions of teeth, whatever force may be needed, should be conducted with the closest observation of its progress, and with such reticence of power as will enable the operator to suspend proceedings in an instant.

Whatever excuse may be made, the extraction of a sound tooth when the removal of a diseased one was intended is, for the dentist, the most injurious accident that can occur, and one which he would have great difficulty in explaining away before a jury, should the patient seek pecuniary compensation for his loss.

IV. The *removal of a sound tooth with an unsound one in extracting the latter* is a very regrettable circumstance, but it is not, like the former, an unmixed evil; a loss has been sustained, but a gain has been achieved as well. Many circumstances may conduce to this result:—

a. Misapplication of the instrument; or its shifting by the careless hold of the operator, or by the nervous movement of the patient;

b. A narrow space through which the tooth has to pass, caused by the overlapping of its neighbours;

c. The organic union of contiguous teeth;

d. The starting of a fulcrum tooth in employing the elevator; or

e. The fibrous connection of neighbouring temporary teeth.

The causes which I have first mentioned are the same as those which have been alluded to as leading to the extraction of a wrong tooth, and need not be farther dwelt upon.

The *narrow space* which is sometimes left by the convergence of teeth on either side of the one to be extracted furnishes conditions amply sufficient to bring about this disaster; and I regret to say that many years ago I myself had the misfortune to remove a sound tooth with a carious neighbour from this cause. It occurred long since, when I was practising surgery generally, and before I had adopted a special branch, and I did not then know how to meet the difficulty. It happened thus:—A young lady came to me with a carious aching second lower bicuspid on the right side. The tooth projected inwards towards the tongue, and the first bicuspid was directed somewhat backwards towards the first molar, and was partially received in the carious hollow of the second bicuspid. With a narrow hawksbill forceps I pulled the tooth outwards, hoping it would slip through its neighbours; but it caught the first bicuspid, and, this having a short and conical root, sprang from its socket and was out in an instant.

I was very much disconcerted at the misfortune, as may be imagined; but my patient accepted it more philosophically, and congratulated herself that one less tooth remained for future pain. Still it need not have happened. A few passages of a dividing file would have removed the projecting edge of the carious cavity which evicted the sound tooth: or I might have extracted the offender from the opposite side across the mouth. In either plan I should now add the precaution of placing my thumb on the crown of the first bicuspid while extracting the second.

The *organic union of contiguous eeth* inevitably leads to

the sacrifice of both when one has to be removed. And the operator may or may not know this beforehand. If the union of the two teeth is congenital (having arisen from their development in one sac and with coherent pulps), in which case the union is by dentine, the operator is usually aware of the circumstance before the extraction, the union being sufficiently extended into the crown to be apparent. But where it occurs in after-life, as the result of hypertrophy of crusta petrosa, soldering the fangs together in a common envelope, nothing is known of it till the teeth are out of the jaw.

I have removed united teeth under both these conditions.

In one instance, which was congenital, a little boy had the left lateral and central incisors of the lower jaw united by dentine, and the union was quite apparent. The lateral was carious and was so dreadfully painful that I determined to extract it, and, having told the parents that the central tooth would come with it, I did so. The union was very complete: the pulp cavities communicated, and there was pus in that of the central incisor.

An example of the other kind occurred to me in 1867, and I find it thus recorded in my note-book:—"A maiden lady came to me to-day (June 24) to have her jaws cleared of stumps and decayed teeth preparatory to wearing artificial substitutes. She was forty years of age. I had extracted several, all coated about the fangs with excessive cement, when I removed the first upper biscuspid root on the right side: with it came away the root of the second biscuspid: they were united together by a common cemented sheath. The gum was so full, and the tongues of gum passing up between the two buried fangs were so complete as to mask this union entirely."

This is a cause of accident which entirely exonerates the operator.

I have known the *fulcrum tooth* (sound) *slipped out of its socket* by the pressure of the elevator in extracting a tooth next to it. It occurred to a student. Though I have never entirely removed a tooth thus, I have (as, I suppose, has happened to others) occasionally loosened one in this way. Where the fulcrum tooth is in the least jeopardised I always place the thumb of my left hand hard upon it during operation.

The fibrous tissue connecting temporary teeth, usually by

their necks, is sometimes so strong, after the union of the teeth to the jaw has been loosened by absorption, that the extraction of one brings away another attached to it.

I find the two following cases in my note-book:—

"Upon extracting a temporary right lower canine tooth this day (February 3, 1868) I brought away with it the first temporary molar. They were not united by dentinal or osteal tissue, but were encased in a common sheath of periosteum. The molar was carious, and had apparently led to absorption of alveolus, so that its adhesion to the socket was very slight and the septum between the teeth had probably vanished. At the same time there appeared to be periosteal hypertrophy around the fang. The canine was sound and its fang but little absorbed. The child's age was a little over eight. (This tooth was extracted for regulation: incisors pushed forward, underhung jaw threatened.)"

The other case is recorded as follows:—"I this day (May 6, 1869) at Guy's Hospital extracted the right first permanent lower molar (carious) from a little boy—a small backward child, eleven years old.

"The first and second temporary molars were in their places in front of the tooth. Upon extracting the permanent molar both the temporary teeth came away with it—the three being connected by a continuous fibrous cord around the necks. The connecting link is very firm, especially between the permanent tooth and the second temporary molar."

Fig. 126.

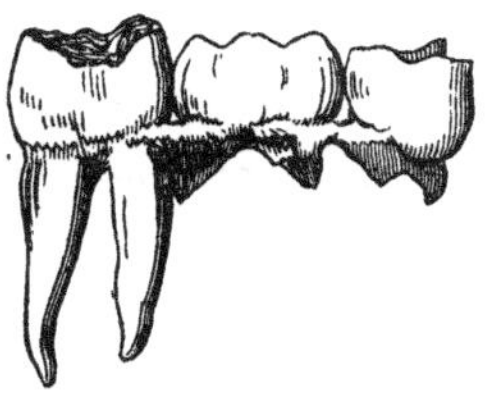

My late brother, Dr. Hyde Salter, made a sketch of the teeth *in situ*, and from it the above woodcut was executed (fig. 126). I have thought the specimen sufficiently remarkable to deserve this permanent record.

Such cases are curious and interesting rather than important. They involve neither blame to the operator, nor material injury to the patient.

V. *Removing the capsule of a growing permanent tooth in extracting its temporary predecessor* is a very rare accident indeed. Still, it does sometimes occur; but I believe, as far as experience has yet gone, only affecting the second temporary molar of the lower jaw and the immature bicuspid below it. This casualty has not occurred to me, nor have I ever heard of a case among my professional friends. Many years ago I saw a specimen in the musuem of the late Mr. Durancé George, in which an extracted lower second temporary molar tooth held, within the embrace of its fangs, the capsule of the immature second bicuspid tooth, and the label attached to the bottle recorded the specimen as an example of the casualty I am considering.

Mr. Tomes * mentions two such cases as having come within his knowledge, and his remarks are accompanied by some speculations as to the probable cause of the accident; but, unfortunately, he has given no critical description of the specimens themselves, which would have been highly interesting.

Mr. Spence Bate has published and figured an example of this casualty. † The temporary molar was removed on account of painful caries.

It may be rather a matter of surprise that this accident is not more common, considering the close developmental connection between the temporary tooth and its forming successor. Dr. Blake ‡ long ago showed that there exists a fibrous pedicle connecting the temporary tooth with the capsule of its successor in early development, and, though this attachment becomes reduced, by the increase of bone between the two as growth progresses, the pedicle is still connected with the fibrous tissue around the neck of the temporary tooth and with the summit of the capsule of the permanent tooth beneath. In exceptional cases this connection may be unusually strong. Again, the inflammatory action arising from caries in a temporary tooth may cement that union by the development of organisable lymph, and by the absorption of the intervening osseous tissue, just as I have shown it occurred between a temporary canine and first molar, and thus the capsule of the bicuspid may have a fatal adhesion to the temporary tooth above it, which is obliged to be extracted for painful caries.

These pathological conditions may combine, or may separately

* *A System of Dental Surgery*, p. 580. London, 1859.

† *Med. Times and Gazette*, vol. iv. fourth series, p. 561.

‡ *An Essay on the Structure and Formation of the Teeth in Man*, &c. By Robert Blake, M.D., p. 38, pl. ii. Dublin, 1801.

and alone lead to the casualty; but in no instance, as far as I can see, would it be possible for the operator to anticipate such a result, or to prevent it.

VI. *Tearing the gum* in extracting a tooth is usually a very small matter, and I should not have alluded to it but for a single serious instance which came under my care.

Formerly it was the custom to "lance the gum" around a tooth about to be extracted; but this proceeding, while it increases the ceremony and prolongs the patient's suffering and painful anticipation, does little good in most cases. Still, bits of gum are sometimes brought away with the tooth, and worse results have happened, which lancing would have prevented.

The case I refer to was that of a young lady, nineteen years of age. She had suffered much from a carious *dens sapientiæ* in the lower jaw, and induced the general practitioner, who attended the family, to extract it. There was no difficulty in getting out the tooth, which was done with parallel-bladed forceps; but when it was out of the socket the surgeon found it was still attached by a long riband of gum and mucous membrane, extending almost to the centre of the soft palate in front of the tonsil and uvula. This was cut across, rather indiscreetly, close to the tooth, and the flap of mucous membrane still hung into the mouth when I saw the patient, and it caused much tickling and irritation of the fauces. I snipped it off with scissors. There was more bleeding from the raw surface than one would have expected, and much swelling and painful deglutition followed. The surgeon was blamed; but I think unfairly. He performed the operation against his wishes, as he avoids interfering with teeth as far as possible; and I do not see how he occasioned the result by malpraxis.

VII. *Wounds produced by the slipping of the elevator.*—The elevator is no doubt capable of doing serious mischief in the hands of a reckless or inexperienced operator; but where employed with caution it is safe as well as most useful. The wounds produced by the elevator are occasioned by the slipping of the instrument from the sudden giving way of the obstacle against which it is pressed; but no sudden yielding of the tooth need lead to such a result if the force applied be of proper character. It is an indiscriminate, unguarded push, or plunge that leads to injury of the soft parts in the mouth; whereas, if the instrument is applied with a firm hand and reticent power, the operator is able to suspend all force the instant the tooth is dislodged.

I recollect many years ago, when I was house-surgeon at King's College Hospital, a poor man came to the out-patient room to have a molar tooth extracted, and a student essayed to do it with an elevator. The instrument slipped, and, having traversed the mouth, pierced the cheek on the opposite side, and apparently divided the transverse-facial artery. I was sent for, and found the patient bleeding copiously from the wound within the cheek; the blood was arterial and flowed with considerable energy. I applied pressure to the wound, and then the cheek became considerably infiltrated with blood. As the case seemed important I admitted the man into the house and watched him. The bleeding gradually ceased, and the swelling of the cheek from extravasated blood, though considerable, did not enlarge after the first hour. The artery was probably completely divided, so it contracted and closed. I discharged the man the next day with a swollen and livid cheek.

I have seen the tongue pierced and considerable bleeding follow from the slipping of the elevator.

A few weeks ago a gentleman came to me to have the fangs of a lower wisdom tooth extracted: he had been operated on by a surgeon who attempted to extract the tooth with the elevator. The crown had broken off and the instrument slipping backwards completely transfixed the soft palate close to the tonsil. No harm resulted; but had the wound been half an inch further outwards it might have been a serious matter. When I saw the patient the wound was still scarcely healed.

The elevator is particularly adapted for the extraction of the lower wisdom teeth; but in this operation the surgeon should recollect the very important nature of the contiguous soft parts, and especially the proximity of the internal carotid artery, which is just behind the tonsil and often in actual contact with it.

I may here mention a singular disaster which occurred many years ago to the late Mr. Joseph Fox, who more than half a century since was surgeon-dentist to Guy's Hospital. In those days it was not uncommon to extract teeth with a punch struck by a mallet, just as farriers take out horses' teeth now.

On the occasion in question Lady H—— went to Mr. Fox to have a molar tooth extracted, and he essayed to move it with the punch. The instrument slipped and the blow must have been a hard one, for the punch, traversing the mouth, completely transfixed the opposite cheek and protruded an inch or so outside the face. The case has not been recorded, but it certainly occurred.

VIII. *Extracted tooth falling into the air-passages.*—This is beyond comparison the most disastrous accident that can arise in extracting a tooth. Fortunately it is of very rare occurrence: but the general adoption of anæsthetics is likely to increase its frequency.

It must arise from a tooth getting loose from the grasp of an extracting instrument, then being caught in the current of an inspiration, and thus drawn through the glottis. But usually the irritability of the mucous membrane at this portal of the respiratory passage would arrest its ingress and lead to its immediate expulsion from the mouth. Still, even during perfect consciousness and complete nervous irritability, the foreign body may slip through the *rima glottidis* and enter the trachea. When, however, the patient is under the influence of an anæsthetic the protective function of the glottis is greatly reduced, and it not unfrequently happens that blood passes from the mouth into the lungs under such circumstances. I have long felt that this additional risk attends the employment of anæsthetics, and have been on the look-out for such casualties.

It behoves the operator, when extracting a tooth for a patient thus unconscious, to take particular care to remove it with all speed and certainty from the mouth. And this especially applies to cases where the elevator is used, as that instrument takes no actual hold on the tooth it dislodges.

The following is the history of a case in which the falling of a tooth into the respiratory passages terminated fatally.

It occurred in Ireland and is recorded by Mr. Houston in his Catalogue of the Museum of the Irish College of Surgeons:—

*Falling of an extracted tooth into the respiratory passages, Bronchitis, Pneumonia—Death.**—" A molar tooth of an adult

* *Descriptive Catalogue of the Preparations in the Museum of the Royal College of Surgeons in Ireland.* By John Houston, M.D. Vol. ii. p. 160. Dublin, 1840.

man, which had passed through the larynx into the trachea, on the instant of its extraction by a dentist. On the first application of the instrument, a fragment of the crown was chipped off and removed from the mouth by the operator. By a second attempt the tooth was started from its socket; but, on being loosened from the claw of the instrument, it suddenly passed down the throat, during an effort of inspiration, and was not seen afterwards by either the patient or operator. The man felt, at the instant, a momentary, sharp, pricking pain at the top of the windpipe. This was instantly followed by a severe fit of coughing, which soon went off, but recurred again several times without any evident cause, and at each time with less and less severity, until, after a few hours, it ceased to produce any further annoyance. He complained also that, from the moment of the operation, he could not get rid of an undefinable uneasiness in the chest; a sensation of weight in breathing, and a tendency to draw heavy sighs, which haunted and kept his mind in a continual state of inquietude. Occasionally he coughed up a little frothy mucus. He had no hoarseness, no acceleration of breathing, no pain in any part of the chest; and no difference in the relative facility with which he took in or breathed out the air. In twenty-four hours after the accident the following stethoscopic signs existed:—A mucous rattle in the lower part of the trachea; both sides of the chest gave an equally clear sound on percussion; but, notwithstanding their similarity in this respect, there was a marked difference in the intensity of the respiratory murmur, that of the right side being more feeble than that of the left. These signs were fixed, and uninfluenced either by position of the body or by violence in efforts of respiration. A difference of opinion, on the part of the gentlemen who saw him in consultation, as to the nature of the affection—the case being novel and involved in much obscurity—caused a delay in any attempt at operation, until symptoms had gone so far that no good could result from the use of the knife. The man died on the eleventh day after the occurrence of the accident, having passed successively through the several stages of bronchitis, pneumonia, and pleuritis, first of the right and secondarily of the left lung.

"The *post-mortem* appearances exhibited all the lesions attendant on these affections; and the obnoxious tooth was discovered lying in the right bronchial tube about one inch below the bifurcation of the trachea; the fangs were directed towards the lung, and the broken crown looked up towards the larynx. The tooth lay loose in the tube: it had two long fangs; and, when tested with the splinter which had been broken off in the first attempt at extraction, was found to fit in most accurately, and to make by the junction a perfect tooth. Both fragments are exhibited in the preparation." *

Mr. James Bate, of Tiverton, has kindly sent me the particulars of a case which occurred in his own practice. A young lady, twenty years of age, had a tooth removed under the influence of bichloride of methylene. She was very nervous and screamed hysterically during the whole proceedings. In removing the forceps from the mouth the tooth escaped its grasp, and in a convulsive inspiration she drew it back into the windpipe. After a considerable time the patient gave a violent cough and ejected it.

Mr. Braine has recorded a case in which a patient inhaled a tooth-fang during anæsthesia from nitrous oxide:—

"S. L——, aged twenty-four, while under the influence of the gas, appeared to swallow an upper molar root of large size, which had been removed from its alveolar cavity and had fallen into the mouth; she coughed occasionally and complained of pain in the chest till 11 o'clock at night, when, during a violent fit of coughing, the piece of tooth came into her mouth, and was thus happily got rid of." †

The term "swallowed" here used is evidently a mistake. If the fang had been really swallowed into the stomach, it would, on being returned, have been vomited; but after so many hours that would be very improbable. However, it was *coughed* up and must have come from the air-passages clearly. In reply to inquiry, Mr. Braine has kindly informed me—"My impression is, that in the case you allude to, the root of the tooth lodged in the ventricle of the larynx, and that it was dislodged from its position during a violent fit of coughing, and with the expiratory gush of air from the lungs was carried into the mouth." Wherever located, this tooth-root was got rid of on very easy terms. Teeth or broken fangs are likely to present forms and

* See also the *Dublin Journal of Medical Science*, vol. v. p. 42.

† Case recorded by Mr. Braine, in *Trans. Odont. Soc.*, vol. iii. p. 36.

edges very suited to firm impaction in the bronchi, and in any case might resist all efforts at expulsion, and again lead to fatal results.

IX. *An extracted tooth falling into the pharynx and being swallowed* is a comparatively trivial matter. But it is sufficiently undesirable nevertheless, for the operator ought to be able to show the result of the operation; and a patient may well object to the passage of a hard indigestible body through his alimentary canal. A tooth however is not likely to do harm, and indeed the temporary teeth, especially in the lower animals, are not infrequently swallowed with the food, when they are shed, and they produce no ill results whatever.

I recollect this little misfortune having twice occurred to me. Once when a bicuspid, with apparently a very short and conical root, sprang from its socket upon the mere pressure of the forceps and, falling into the throat, was instantly gulped down.

In the other instance a little nervous girl would only allow me to take out her loose tooth with my finger and thumb. It slipped from my grasp and was instantly swallowed.

In neither case did any harm arise. Indeed these cases are only worth mentioning to complete the list of casualties.

X. *Crushing the inferior maxillary nerve.*—I am surprised that this circumstance is not alluded to in text-books on dental surgery, as an occasional result of extracting wisdom teeth of the lower jaw. I have however never met with any description of it.*

Four instances have occurred in my own practice, and my relative, Mr. Bell, tells me that he has met with four.

When we consider the close contiguity of the fangs of the lower molar teeth to the inferior maxillary nerve, especially those of the *dens sapientiæ*, it is remarkable rather than otherwise that such an accident is not more common, and still further so when it is remembered how often a deeply impacted tooth has to be dug for and prized out.

The most severe example of this casualty with which I have met is recorded in my note-book as follows:—

"Baron T——, a gentleman connected with the turf, about twenty-five years of age, had been under my care occasionally

* Since the above has been in type an interesting example of this casualty has been described by Mr. Holden. See *Trans. Odont. Society*, vol. vi. (New Series) p. 224.

for some months, on account of tardy and painful wisdom tooth eruption, especially on the right side. In the early spring of 1865 he had been exposing himself to cold on Newmarket Heath, and had an attack of tonsillitis and inflammation of the fauces and velum palati. This condition of the soft parts very much exasperated the pain produced by the impacted right *dens sapientiæ*, and his brother brought him up to town, distracted with pain, and insisting on the immediate removal of his tooth. This was no easy matter as it was deeply imbedded behind and below the second molar, and I had the greatest difficulty in getting hold of it. However, with a pair of long-bladed hawksbill forceps, I at length grasped the tooth, and with the exercise of much force dislodged it. It had barely passed the patient's mouth when he sprang from the chair, and, placing both hands upon the right side of his mouth and chin, exclaimed in the wildest excitement, 'What *have* you done? what *have* you done? You've torn away my lip; my lip is gone.' We tried to pacify him, and then, as we brought him to something like reason, he seemed bewildered, for he was able to feel his lip and chin with his fingers, though he could not feel his fingers with his lip and chin. It was quite clear what had occurred, and by degrees the patient explained what he felt, or rather what he did not feel. All the teeth of the lower jaw on the right side were dead to sensation, and the whole area of the lip and chin, supplied by the mental nerve, was absolutely numb."

The extraction of the tooth was in other respects satisfactory, and the patient was quite relieved of the painful symptoms caused by the impaction, but the sentient paralysis caused him much alarm.

About six weeks afterwards the patient came to me, and at that time there was scarcely any return of sensation. Six months having elapsed I again saw him: he could then feel when the skin of the lip and chin were touched; but it was not a natural sensation, being a feeling of "formication," or what is popularly called "pins and needles." From that time to the present he has been often under my hands, and I learn that sensation of the parts has never been completely re-established.

This is the most severe case I have had, and the only one in which the injury has been permanent.

Two other examples have occurred to me from extracting

wisdom teeth; they were slighter and the patients soon completely recovered sensation. One of these is recorded in the "Guy's Hospital Reports," third series, vol. xiii. p. 92. A fourth case arose in extracting a first lower molar: it was an enormous tooth, with fangs the $\frac{13}{16}$ of an inch long; these diverged and converged, involving bone, which broke and came away with the tooth. The operation was performed while the patient was under the influence of nitrous oxide gas: upon recovering he complained of numbness of the right side of the lip, chin, teeth and jaw. It occurred in January, 1871. I subsequently learnt that sensation had completely returned.

In all the four cases that occurred in Mr. Bell's practice the numbness passed off in a few days; and this must be considered as the ordinary sequence of the accident.

I believe it would not be possible to predict or to prevent this casualty; and no blame can attach to the operator.

XI. *Dislocating the lower jaw.*—This is a very rare accident attending tooth extraction; and occurs much less frequently than one would, *à priori*, expect. There are very few recorded examples of it, and I have never heard any of my professional friends mention the disaster as having occurred in their practice.

The articular surfaces of the temporal bone, which receive the condyles of the inferior maxilla are very little cupped in the human subject, and have consequently but a slight grasp upon the articular head of the bone. The principal cause of the dislocation of the lower jaw is wide opening of the mouth, as in yawning and laughing, when the condyles slide forward on the *eminentiæ articulares;* the movement being excessive the condyles slip altogether beyond the articular surfaces and are then drawn up into the zygomatic fossæ by the temporal muscles. The mouth is thus *fixed* wide open—the jaw dislocated. Now, when we consider how wide the mouth is often stretched open in tooth-extraction, and how much traction is applied to the jaw by reason of the firm adhesion to it of the tooth to be extracted, it really is remarkable that the accident of dislocation is so rare.

The earliest recorded case of this casualty with which I am acquainted is given by Mr. Joseph Fox:*—

* *The History and Treatment of the Diseases of the Teeth,* &c. By Joseph Fox M.R.C.S., p. 167. London, 1806.

"It was in attempting to extract a tooth that I had an opportunity of attending to this accident. Last summer, in passing through Dorchester, I called to see a gentleman, who, after the customary salutations, informed me there was a lady of his acquaintance who wished to have a tooth extracted, and was at that instant upon the point of going to Weymouth to consult a dentist from London, who was on a visit there. He immediately introduced me to her. I found that this lady had several times been the subject of luxation of the jaw, and she was in fear lest the accident should again be occasioned by the operation. The tooth she wished to be extracted was one of the *dentes sapientiæ* of the lower jaw. I consented to attempt the operation, but wished that Mr. Arden, the surgeon, who had reduced her jaw two or three times before, should be present.

"I had scarcely fixed the instrument upon the tooth, when, by a spasmodic action of the muscles, the jaw slipped forward, and became luxated. Attempts were made, first by Mr. Arden and then by myself, to reduce the jaw by the usual method of pressing down the back part of the jaw with the thumbs, and raising the chin with the palms of the hands; but neither of us could succeed, although very considerable efforts were made.

"I then happened to recollect a statement once made to me by M. de Chament, of his having been frequently applied to by a person at Paris, who was subject to this accident; and that he always succeeded in reducing the luxation immediately by making use of a lever of wood, as recommended by Dr. Munro. I inquired for a piece of wood which I could employ in this way, and was so fortunate as to be furnished with a piece of about an inch square and ten or twelve inches long, which was used as a flat ruler. I introduced this into the mouth, so that the extremity lay upon the under molars, and then, by raising the other end with the hand, the teeth in the upper jaw became the fulcrum. The jaw on that side was then depressed at the posterior part, when the condyle immediately passed over the edge of the eminence. I then applied the lever to the other side of the jaw, and disengaged that in like manner, when the muscles instantly drew the jaw back into its proper situation."

Mr. Fox mentions another case:*—"I have been informed

* Loc. cit., p. 169.

by Mr. Heaviside that he was lately sent for to reduce a luxation of the jaw which had occurred to a lady, from merely opening her mouth widely to have her teeth scaled."

An instance of this accident is recorded by Dr. Harris.* It occurred to a young lady seventeen years of age, in an attempt to extract the first right inferior molar. Both condyles were luxated: the dislocation was easily reduced; and afterwards, by supporting the jaw with the left hand, the tooth was successfully removed.

This casualty never occurred to me in extracting a tooth; but it did once happen, when I was taking a model of the lower jaw. Some years since an old lady came to me to have an entire set of teeth. She was about seventy years of age; she was infirm, and her tissues generally seemed flabby and lax. Her mouth was toothless. I took the upper model first; and then, having taken that of the lower jaw and removed it, I noticed that she did not shut her mouth—it was fixed wide open. The patient did not seem alarmed or distressed, but pointed to her mouth and attempted to explain to me what I already saw very clearly. Her jaw was dislocated on both sides. The condyles had slipped forward noiselessly, and I was not aware of it till I saw she could not shut her mouth.

I reduced the dislocation with the greatest ease. Placing my thumbs within the mouth as far back as possible, and pressing down the angles of the jaw on either side, I tilted up the chin with the points of my fingers, and the condyles went back into their places in an instant.

The patient then told me that she frequently "put out" her jaw in yawning and laughing.

Had I known this beforehand I should certainly have endeavoured to prevent the accident by supporting the chin and not opening the mouth very wide.

This is an accident that may occur to any one, and I am surprised it is not more frequent. But where the tendency to luxation is known, preventive measures ought to be adopted; and the plan recommended by Mr. Fox seems to me to be a very good one. He says:—"To prevent this accident from happening in the extraction of a tooth, to persons who have

* *Principles and Practice of Dental Surgery.* 9th edit. p. 440. Philadelphia, 1866.

been previously subject to a luxation of the jaw, I have contrived a bandage, which will ensure the safety of the patient during the operation. The bandage consists of a piece of leather, formed so as to receive the chin, and a strong cap, that may be placed upon the top of the head, which are connected by two straps on each side; it is to be fixed when the mouth is opened to a certain degree, with the condyles as far back as possible; the cap is then to be put on the posterior part of the crown of the head, and, the leather being applied to the chin, the straps are to be buckled tight, when it will not be possible by any effort to advance the jaw so much as to endanger its luxation, and the tooth may be extracted with safety." *

Probably an efficient apparatus on the same principle might be improvised out of a piece of calico.

XII. *Breaking one tooth in extracting another* sometimes happens; and it may arise from the lateral slipping of the instrument wrenching off a portion of a contiguous tooth in the same jaw; or, by the sudden giving way of a tooth under extraction, a blow may be struck by the instrument upon a tooth in the opposite jaw. It is only in this latter way that I have seen a serious tooth-fracture accidentally arise in the operation of extraction, and only once have I seen it. The misfortune occurred in the hands of a student. He was extracting a lower first molar with a pair of George's forceps, and was standing opposite the patient.. Suddenly the tooth gave way and the back of the instrument, striking the left upper lateral incisor a violent blow, broke across the crown and exposed the pulp. The root was extracted afterwards, and no doubt the gap closed up, as the patient was but a lad and the teeth were rather crowded.

The student had had but little experience and probably was unaware of the yielding of the tooth previous to its final severance from the jaw, and thus too far prolonged great force of traction. I doubt if it could have happened in well-practised hands. Still it is just possible that such a casualty may occur to any one.

XIII. *Cutting the lip in removing a jagged extracted tooth* has sometimes occurred, where the adhesion of the tooth to the

* Loc. cit., p. 170, pl. ix., fig. 5.

jaw has yielded very suddenly and the tooth has passed out of the mouth with a jerk. I have never seen a serious case of this kind myself, though two or three slight ones have come under my notice.

XIV. *Forcing tooth or tooth-fang into the antrum.*—A most interesting example of this casualty is recorded by Mr. Catlin,* in which the fang of a first upper molar tooth passed into the antrum in an attempt to extract it. And considerable difficulty was subsequently experienced in removing it, from the circumstance that the antrum was partially divided by a septum behind which the fang became pocketed. The reader will be amply repaid by perusing Mr. Catlin's interesting paper.

This casualty occurred to me very recently. A lady required several stumps removed from the upper jaw. I succeeded in extracting all on the right side very satisfactorily with stump forceps, but upon applying the same instrument to the buccal fangs of the left first molar they both, one after the other, slipped from my grasp and passed into the antrum. I had not the slightest reason to anticipate such an occurrence. The palatal fang came away easily, being firmly supported by a bony socket while I burrowed for and seized it. I briefly searched for the missing stumps in vain. So, as the patient had undergone a good deal of pain and distress, I requested her to come and see me again in a week. Before that time, however, had elapsed she called on me saying she could still feel the remains of the tooth with her tongue, but she had suffered no pain or inconvenience. Upon inspecting the mouth I found both fangs free in the wound where the operation had been attempted: they had gravitated into wound and were held in place by a clot that surrounded them. With a pair of common dressing forceps I picked them from the mouth, and the wound soon healed. It is clear that in this case there had been very extensive absorption of the floor of the antrum around the outer fangs of the first molar, so that the osseous tissue was wanting there entirely. Considerable absorption of this kind is by no means uncommon; but the accident of pushing a tooth-fang into the maxillary sinus, in the endeavour to extract it, is certainly a rather rare occurrence.

* "On the Form and Size of the Adult Antrum," &c. In *Transactions of Odontological Society*, vol. ii. p. 31.

I only recollect having had this accident on one other occasion; and, judging from these instances, I think it could scarcely be predicted or prevented.

XV. *Forcing tooth-fang into an abscess-excavation in maxilla.*—I enumerate this casualty from the recollection of a single example that occurred to myself. Many years ago a surgeon, a neighbour, came to me with very great swelling of the front of the upper jaw on the right side. It was occasioned by the remains of the lateral incisor tooth, which had decayed and broken off level with the gum. There had been repeated discharges of pus; but the abscess sac appeared undiminished: it was as large as a chestnut. In endeavouring to lay hold of the fang with stump forceps it slipped away into the sac and could not be recovered. There was a large gush of pus at once, and I imagined the sac would collapse; but it remained scarcely diminished for a considerable time, and the fang could not be reached. It was then determined to lay open the sac and remove the fang. This I did very easily; and I doubt not the parts would soon have returned to a healthy condition, but the patient died a few days afterwards of typhus fever.

CHAPTER XXVII.

HÆMORRHAGE AFTER EXTRACTION OF TEETH.

Long-continued and obstinate bleeding after the extraction of teeth is an occasional and troublesome complication of this operation. It is not a common consequence; indeed it is very rare, considering the enormous numbers of the operations, and how seldom in proportion continued bleeding follows them: hundreds of teeth are daily extracted, and yet it is rare indeed that the surgeon is called in to arrest persistent bleeding which supervenes upon the operation.

The troublesome hæmorrhage from the wound of an extracted tooth is of a peculiar character; it is not a rapid arterial discharge immediately following the vascular rupture which the tooth-extraction causes, but a continuous, abundant flow of blood welling-up in the empty socket, and developing itself into a serious and sometimes alarming symptom, usually many hours after the operation. The profuse pouring-out of vivid arterial blood, which sometimes follows the drawing of a tooth, has no relation to the circumstance we are considering; that generally lasts but for a few minutes, and then ceases; though it may in some instances occur to an extent, and for a continuance, that startles the patient, and may cause syncope, as I have more than once seen following the extraction of loose teeth associated with very vascular, spongy gums.

The continued hæmorrhage is not the discharge of any considerable arterial trunk that may have been wounded, as was formerly supposed, but the passive bleeding of the entire disrupted surface, from an inability of the vessels to accomplish the curative closure of their broken ends. In the majority of the recorded cases there has been distinct evidence of the hæmorrhagic diathesis existing in the individual affected; and in not a few, the patients have themselves been aware of the tendency, from having experienced similar consequences attendant on the previous extraction of other teeth. Indeed some persons (I have such patients of my own) refuse to have any more teeth removed, preferring rather to suffer any amount of tooth-ache, on account of the alarming hæmorrhages which have followed the operations before.

A very interesting example of this distressing consequence of tooth-drawing, showing its constitutional nature, was under my care some years since. A clergyman from one of the midland counties came to town to me on account of the hæmorrhage which had followed the extraction of a lower molar tooth three or four days before, and was still continuing. He was reduced to a pitiable condition of exhaustion and bloodlessness. All the local means usually adopted had been tried, but without success: the bleeding, however, speedily ceased under the use of large and frequently repeated doses of *tannin*. The history of this gentleman and his family is curious and instructive. As a boy, from the most trivial accidents, such as a cut finger, he sustained prolonged and almost irrepressible bleeding: during his whole life, the slightest blow or bruise would cause a large and very disproportioned ecchymosis: a few years before, he had sustained a week of hæmorrhage, after the extraction of a tooth. This gentleman has three married sisters, all of whom suffer from terrible floodings at the birth of each child. He has a little boy, as liable to bleeding from a trivial wound as he himself was in his childhood.

In the month of May 1864, a very interesting case of alveolar hæmorrhage came under my notice, in which the patient, after the arrest of the tooth-socket bleeding, died a few days subsequently from sanguineous apoplexy.

Mr. R——, a city merchant, about 60 years of age, required an inferior incisor tooth extracted. He left me a few minutes after the operation, the bleeding having ceased. Shortly afterwards rapid and continuous hæmorrhage supervened, and, having continued for thirty-six hours, he came back to me in a very exhausted condition. I then plugged the cavity with cotton wool (which, by the way, makes an admirable plug), and the bleeding was restrained. A fortnight after this the patient, while dressing in the morning, was seized with sanguineous extravasation in the brain, and died in a few hours. He had never previously suffered from hæmorrhage of any kind.

I am not acquainted with any recorded examples where this casualty has followed the extraction of teeth in children. Two such instances have occurred in my own practice.

Miss C——, a young lady of healthy appearance, 11 years of age, was brought to me by her father to have a first lower permanent molar tooth extracted. Its removal was not followed at the time by more than usual bleeding. A few hours afterwards a slight sanguineous oozing developed itself, and during the night became a rapid and abundant hæmorrhage. She had returned to her home in Berkshire, and was then obliged to seek the assistance of the family medical attendant, who plugged the cavity, and for a time arrested the flow of blood, but it recurred again and again for three days, when it finally ceased.

Master W——, a puny little boy, 10 years old, at school in the neighbourhood of town, was brought to me to have his teeth regulated. I found it necessary to extract two lower temporary incisors. The bleeding ceased, and he left my house: in an hour it recurred, and continued obstinately for three days and nights. It then yielded to internal astringents and plugging.

It is of especial importance to bear in mind the general and diathetic nature of alveolar hæmorrhage, in devising its proper treatment. Anything which would increase the wound, or add a fresh one (such as the cautery or the ligature of an arterial trunk), is contra-indicated. A fatal example of alveolar hæmorrhage, in which both these means were adopted, is recorded in an early number of the "Medico-Chirurgical Transactions." * The previous history of this patient is singularly like that of the clergyman whose case I have just mentioned, in the hæmorrhagic diathesis manifesting itself in childhood, and his having sustained a terrible loss of blood—the bleeding lasting for twenty-one days—when another tooth was extracted before. In the treatment of this fatal hæmorrhage, the actual cautery produced only a temporary arrest of bleeding; it was then determined to tie the carotid artery: the operation was

* "A Case of Fatal Hæmorrhage from Extraction of a Tooth," by Richard Blagden, *Med.-Chir. Trans.* vol. viii. 1820.

performed by Sir B. Brodie, without any relief to the original symptoms; the wound in the neck only furnished another bleeding surface, and evidently hurried on the fatal catastrophe. In another recorded case where the cautery was used, the edge of the lip was accidentally burnt, and the surface thus cauterised soon commenced bleeding profusely, and continued to do so till the fatal termination of the case, which was hastened by it.

There is a particular form of this kind of hæmorrhage which, though involving a constitutional condition, does not imply hæmorrhagic diathesis. In women when menstruation is imminent, or in process, the extraction of a tooth may be, and sometimes is, followed by a vicarious discharge of blood from the wounded alveolar surface. I have myself had two such cases. In one the patient was a young lady, about 20 years of age; menstruation was just about to commence, as I subsequently learnt from her mother. After the extraction of the tooth, a lower molar, the bleeding ceased; but in about ten hours it recurred, and then became continuous and obstinate, and it lasted for two days, so as to occasion considerable anxiety. It was obstinately impressible by local means. Under the influence of hot hip-baths and aloetic purgatives the catamenia were induced, and the hæmorrhage immediately ceased. I have since had a very similar instance in a married woman.

I have at the present time under my care for mechanical assistance a lady's-maid (Mrs. S. O.), who many years since, while a patient of Mr. Bell's, had some teeth removed just as she was about to menstruate. The operation was followed by protracted hæmorrhage, which lasted during the whole of the catamenial period, and ceased when she was no longer unwell. The bleeding was not alarming, and she had no professional assistance, but its coincidence with menstruation, and the fact of the catamenial being imperfect at that time, suggested to her own mind the compensatory nature of the sanguineous evacuation.

In these cases, doubtless, the bleeding was the vicarious manifestation of the periodic function.

The *treatment* of alveolar hæmorrhage after tooth-extraction divides itself into local and general; the local treatment consisting in the application of styptics, with continuous pressure upon the bleeding surface; the general treatment, in the rapid and abundant administration of internal astringents.

The local plan of a plugging compress, recommended by Hunter, is that now universally adopted: "In general it will be sufficient to stuff the socket with lint, or lint dipped in oil of turpentine, and to apply a compress of lint, or a piece of cork thicker than the bodies of the adjacent teeth, so that the teeth in the opposite jaw may keep up a pressure.

"It has been advised to stuff into the socket some soft wax, on a supposition that it would mould itself to the cavity, and so stop the bleeding: this, perhaps, may sometimes answer better than the other method, and therefore should be tried when that fails."*

The restoration of the extracted tooth to the socket has also been tried with success. I have found cotton wool an exceedingly good plug, being easily fitted by pressure into the socket to its very extremity. For the purpose of forming a plug of lint, a strip should be cut of an elongated wedge-shape, and this should be introduced, the pointed end first; the extremity should be pushed into the bleeding socket, and driven well home to the bottom; the strip of lint should then be folded and re-folded upon itself, so as to make the plug very solid, pressing on the entire superficies of the socket. When the compress of lint or cork has been put over this, the mouth should be closed and the jaws kept permanently together, so as to exert considerable and persistent pressure by means of a broad bandage tied under the chin and over the head. Where the opposing teeth in the other jaw are wanting, it may be difficult to keep up the compress-pressure by the mere closure of an edentulous jaw upon the bleeding alveolus. To meet such a difficulty, apparatus, called *alveolar tourniquets*, have been devised. Mr. Higginbottom, of Nottingham, was, I believe, the first to invent an *alveolar tourniquet*.† It is an instrument consisting of two blades, or shafts, united at one end, and capable of approximation and compression by means of a screw, and free at the other extremities; these latter are armed with pads, one applying to the compress in the mouth, and the other to the exterior: where the bleeding is in the lower jaw, the blades

* *A Practical Treatise on the Diseases of the Teeth*, p. 92. By John Hunter. London, 1778.

† "On Arrest of Bleeding after Extraction of Teeth," by J. Higginbottom, F.R.S., *Prov. Med. Jour.* vol. iv. 1842.

are nearly equal, the exterior one simply passing under the base of the horizontal ramus; for the upper jaw the instrument is less applicable, and the outer blade requires a long curved sweep so as to grasp the top of the head. I doubt, however, if an alveolar tourniquet would answer in any case as well as a compress within the mouth. Where there are no teeth in the jaw opposite that from which the bleeding takes place, a piece of cork or wood might be hollowed so as to fit the surface of the edentulous gum: this, resting on a piece of lint, would not injure the mucous membrane, and, by its means, firm, steady pressure could be kept up: the mouth would be closed, and the patient comparatively at his ease, which could not be the case during the employment of the tourniquet. Various local astringents have been recommended in conjunction with the lint-plug; matico has been highly spoken of: I have found an alcoholic saturated solution of tannin answer the purpose very well; but probably the old remedy, turpentine, has never really been superseded.

I would suggest that, in any very obstinate or alarming case, *pressure* on the common carotid artery on the side where the hæmorrhage is occurring might arrest it, or at least assist in the treatment. I am induced to make this suggestion by an interesting case that recently occurred in the practice of Mr. Maunder, at the London Hospital. A man had sustained a severe comminuted fracture of the lower jaw, lacerating the inferior dental artery: there was a wound into the mouth through which profuse and alarming arterial hæmorrhage occurred. Ligature of the carotid was contemplated: when it was found that pressure on the artery in the side of the neck by means of the thumb, or points of the fingers completely controlled the bleeding. Upon removing the pressure the hæmorrhage immediately recurred. Several of the students undertook to keep up the pressure, relieving each other from time to time, and it was thus sustained for two hours and a half, when it was found that the bleeding had finally ceased. A similar course should, I think, be tried in any very obstinate case of alveolar hæmorrhage. The application of extreme cold in the form of ether spray would probably assist in suppressing obstinate hæmorrhage. I have not had an opportunity of trying this treatment in a diathetic case of continued bleeding; but, experimenting after ordinary cases of extraction, I have found that it exerts a marked effect in checking the flow of blood.

I am convinced, however, that it is a great mistake only to treat these cases topically: they are obviously manifestations of constitutional vice, and require a corresponding general treatment. Astringents should be had recourse to at the earliest stage: they can do no harm, and may be suspended at any time, while in the majority of instances they will be most beneficial. These cases often extend over so long a period that there is abundant time to bring constitutional treatment into full operation. Tannin and turpentine have been the most successful of internal remedies in recorded cases: with the latter drug steel might be advantageously combined, especially in the form of the muriate tincture.

I would suggest either of the two following prescriptions as likely to be of service.

Vitelli Ov. ij.
Olei Terebinth. ʒiſs.
Sacchari ʒij.
Tinct. Ferri Ses-Chloridi ʒiij.
Aquæ ℥viij.

A table-spoonful to be taken every hour: or—

Tannin gr. v.
Spt. Vini Rect. ʒſs.
Aquæ ℥jſs.

To be taken every hour. As tannin is apt to produce nausea when taken on an empty stomach, I would recommend its association with some (non-albuminous) food. In the irritability of sanguineous exhaustion, opiates may become necessary in large doses.

Other circumstances require attention; the patient should occupy a cool apartment, and local icy applications may be beneficial. The upright posture is to be preferred; or if the patient goes to bed, he should be bolstered up in as elevated a position as possible, while the circulation in the lower extremities should be encouraged.

In women during the menstruating period of life, it should not be forgotten that the hæmorrhage may be associated with suppressed menstruation, and constitute a vicarious discharge; and remedies should be adopted to meet this contingency.

CHAPTER XXVIII.

CLEFT AND PERFORATE PALATES.

Lesions of the palate are naturally and very truly divisible into *accidental* and *congenital*: the former the result of accident or disease; the latter produced by a suspension of fœtal development. In most instances accidental lesions of the palate consist of perforations, more or less irregular, by loss of bone, of the hard palate; while congenital lesions nearly always consist of a cleft involving the soft palate, are more or less symmetrical, and have a definite relation to the elementary parts of which the mouth is formed. But *cleft* palate *may* be accidental, and *perforate* palate *may* be congenital. Again, in either case they may be simple or compound; *simple*, involving only one, hard or soft palate; *compound*, involving more or less of both. In congenital cases the lesion may vary from a mere central division of the uvula to a complete and wide separation of the true maxillæ—the intermaxillary bone being tilted forwards on the end of the vomer as a distinct osseous tubercle—and a total deficiency of the soft palate. In accidental cases there may be an aperture no bigger than a straw, or the whole of the floor of the nose may be lost, soft as well as hard.

Congenital defects of palate involve the most curious and interesting considerations of morphological development, and are susceptible of an obvious explanation.

All congenital defects of the mouth may, I believe, be traced to suspended development at some early period of fœtal life—this suspension being only local and often very partial; but establishing and retaining as a permanent condition the separation of some parts which are originally developed from distinct centres. And thus that, which should have been but temporary and transient, becomes a permanent condition.

These facts have long been appreciated by philosophical surgeons; and an excellent account of the literary history of the subject will be found in the article on *Hare lip* * in Dupuytren's "Leçons Orales."

In the earliest condition of fœtal existence—as soon, that is, as the embryo is sufficiently developed for examination—it is found that the oral and nasal cavities form but one, and are common. The superior maxillæ develope as two lateral masses, and by the extension inwards on either side of horizontal processes the palatal portions are formed, as regards the maxillæ proper and the palatal process of the ossa palati. At the same time the septum narium is in process of development; and at its anterior inferior apex a tubercle is formed which constitutes the incisive or intermaxillary bones; and these are from the first (generally at least) united together. Thus there are three elementary parts which go to form the palate—the palatal processes of the maxillæ proper and of the ossa palati, on either side, and the palatal portion of the intermaxillary bones forming a central part in front. These three elements are separated by a trifid or Y-shaped division that may be traced in the bones up to a time beyond the middle of intra-uterine gestation: the stem of the Y corresponding to the separation of the right and left palate and maxillary bones; the fork with the divisions between the latter and the ossa incisiva. The velum palati is also formed by the union in the middle line of two lateral halves, and appears to be the last part to unite. It is by the fusion of these several palate elements that the cavity of the nose is divided from that of the mouth. And it is by the persistence of the separation, or some part of it, that congenital cleft palate is established. It will be found in after-life that the lateral separation on either side corresponds in the alveolar arch with the interval between the lateral incisors and canine tooth.

Based upon these considerations, Mr. Pollock, in his admirable article on "Cleft Palate," &c.,† has divided these malformations, according to the progressive changes that occur, into—

* "Du Bec-de-lièvre congénital:" *Leçons Orales de Clinique Chirurgical*, par M. le Baron Dupuytren. Paris, 1839. Tome iii. p. 470.

† "Diseases of the Mouth, &c." in *Holmes's System of Surgery*, vol. iv. p. 88. 1864.

"1. The most extensive, a double cleft of the alveolus; a fissure running on either side of the median line, in the course of the lateral sutures already described, unites with the opposite one and opens into an entire cleft of the hard and soft palate.

"2. A single cleft of the alveolus, on one side or other of the median line; running back and into an entire cleft of the hard and soft palate.

"3. The alveolus entire; the cleft of the palate complete from that process backwards.

"4. The cleft running as far forwards as the middle of the palate-processes of the superior maxillæ, or through the palate bones only.

"5. Fissure of the whole of the soft palate, or only implicating the uvula.

"Between the extreme of one and the other every gradation of extent may occur."

Sometimes, but not commonly, there is a congenital *perforation* of the palate, a hole either circular or oval communicating between the nose and mouth. When present it is usually towards the back of the hard palate, and Mr. Pollock has pointed out that in such cases "the median line of union is very plainly marked on the under surface of the soft palate and the uvula by a distinct straight thin cicatrix,* showing the union of the sides of the soft palate completed, although the palate bones, in consequence of their defective development, were unable to perfect the naso-oral septum in their immediate neighbourhood."

Where the intermaxillary bones are separated on both sides from the maxillæ, the tubercle which they constitute together is very apt to be tilted forwards with much projection—a condition which I think may be met with a special mode of mechanical treatment to be described hereafter. The separation of the intermaxillary bone from the maxilla is often associated with a suppression of the lateral incisor tooth on that side.

Where the cleft in the front of the mouth is single it is nearly always on one side, corresponding, that is, to the interval be-

* I have twice seen a similar *congenital* cicatrix in the upper lip. In one instance it was associated with cleft-palate. In the other there had been a narrow escape of cleft-palate: there was a slight notch in the jaw between the lateral incisor and canine; and the incisor teeth on that side were displaced and irregular in position.

tween the intermaxillary bone and the maxilla, for it seems that the intermaxillary bones of the two sides are far more prone to unite together, and accomplish that union earlier, than these bones are to fuse with the maxillæ proper, though the ultimate union of the former is by suture and the latter by a complete continuity of tissue.

Very rarely indeed the fissure in the front of the mouth may be single and central, either from the total absence of the intermaxillary bones, or from a fissure between them.

The former condition* is described by Rokitansky: and there is a specimen of it in the Museum of the Royal College of Surgeons, London.

The latter, cleft between the intermaxillary bones, I have once seen in my own practice. In this instance the right bone was slightly deficient, and the right central incisor was wanting; but the lateral was present in contact with the canine, separated by a deep fissure from the incisors of the other side.

Accidental lesions of the palate, clefts or perforations, may exist to any degree or in any form; and they may be caused by constitutional disease, by violence, or by surgical operation.

By far the most common cause of accidental lesion of the palate is constitutional syphilis, leading to bone disease, in which the hard palate is very prone to suffer. A certain portion of the bony palate becomes specifically inflamed, is necrosed, and then exfoliated, leaving a perforation into the nasal cavity. The same may happen from scrofula. Losses of portions of the palate, requiring the supplemental aid of the dental mechanist, are among the contingencies of gun-shot wounds, occurring in battle; and I have seen an instance of attempted suicide, in which a pistol-ball perforated the palate, and went no further, leaving a permanent hole in the floor of the nose. Again, the surgeon may find it necessary to remove more or less of the upper jaw, leaving the restoration of lost parts and the occlusion of the nose from the mouth to mechanical appliances devised by the dental surgeon.

Now, the evil consequences of a defect in the naso-oral septum are of a very marked and distressing character. A little

* I have seen this condition in the sheep. In a newly born lamb, which died from inability to suck, I found a complete cleft, central in front; and there was no vestige of the intermaxillary bones.

child with a cleft palate cannot suck properly; where the nose and mouth cannot be completely separated, a person is unable to articulate intelligibly; in eating and drinking, food passes from the mouth to the nose, and deglutition is very imperfectly and painfully performed.

To meet these serious inconveniences, great mechanical ingenuity has been brought to bear.

Nearly as far back as surgical literature extends we find notices of mechanical devices to repair lesions of the palate. An elaborate account of the literary history of this subject, to which I am much indebted, is given at the commencement of Mr. Snell's *Memoir*, "On Obturators or Artificial Palates," and to that work I beg to refer those who are interested in curious surgical literature.*

Without going into tedious detail it may be mentioned that the still-common obturator for perforations of the hard palate —consisting of a disc of metal with a sponge passing into the nose—was invented by Ambrose Paré,† an eminent French surgeon who flourished about the middle of the sixteenth century.‡ He also devised another apparatus, consisting of a similar disc of metal to close the orifice on the oral surface of the palate: from the upper surface of this plate projected a short process, a movable pivot, surmounted by an oval button: by the rotation of the latter, when *in situ*, a quarter of a circle, its ends were rested on the nasal surface of the palate and so the obdurator was kept in place. Both these apparatus involve the same objectionable principle—the sustentation of the mechanism by means of pressure of some kind on the walls of the orifice.

* *Observations on the History, Use, and Construction of Obturators or Artificial Palates*, by James Snell, M.R.C.S., London, 1824. Mr. Snell's valuable work has long been out of print, but the historical part of it seems to have been pretty closely copied by Mr. Sercombe in his paper "On the Treatment of Cleft-palate," published in the first volume of the *Odontological Society's Transactions*, which is accessible to everyone.

† *Les Œuvres d'Ambroise Paré*. Lyon. 1541.

‡ Mr. Sercombe is mistaken in describing Jaques Guillemeau as the inventor of certain obturators, and also as being antecedent to Ambroise Paré. Paré was born soon after the year 1500 and died at a very advanced age in 1590. Guillemeau was born about half a century after him, and died in 1612. Guillemeau translated Paré's works into Latin, and derived what he knew of obturators, &c., from Paré.

The true principles upon which obturators should be constructed were first laid down by M. Bourdet,* an intelligent French surgeon, who devoted his attention to the diseases of the teeth, and who practised about the middle of the last century.

M. Bourdet appreciated the great injury that is done in the treatment of perforations of the hard palate, by the passage of processes through the orifice into the nose for the support of the obturator. He advocated the plan of arching over the vault of the palate by thin sheet metal, supported by attachment to the teeth on either side, and thus completing the septum between the nasal and oral cavities, where loss of bone had made it incomplete:—"Those which are more complex, and one piece of which enters the hole in the palate to form a *point d'appui* of the plate, have a great inconvenience. This piece is an insuperable obstacle to the cicatrisation of the orifice; and the contraction of the granulating edges is entirely prevented by the presence of this foreign substance: they can never meet, and the patient is obliged to wear the obturator all his life. So unless the loss of the bones of the palate be prodigious, or the holes formed by the necrosis of an extraordinary diameter, the simple plate which I propose is to be preferred." "This plate ought to be of silver or gold, and should never be applied till all the necrosed bone has been removed from the roof of the palate."† Bourdet appears further to have been aware of the curative effect of the use of this simple obturator. He states as his experience that the perforation in most cases closes more or less completely when thus treated in about six months: in not a few instances healing altogether.

In 1786 M. Pière Fauchard‡ described obturators combined with artificial teeth; which appears to be the first time that this was accomplished. His apparatus retained the vicious principle of pressure within the nasal fossa by a process through the orifice.

M. Touchard§ published an account of an apparatus not only to supply palate and teeth, but a large portion of the maxillary

* *Recherches et Observations sur toutes les parties de l'Art du Dentiste*, par M. Bourdet, Dentiste, reçu au Collége de Chirurgie. Paris. 1767.

† Bourdet, loc. cit., tome second, p. 278.

‡ Le Chirurgien-Dentiste. Paris. 1786.

§ *Description d'un obturateur dentier présenté à la Société de Médecine de Paris; suivie de remarques sur les dents artificielles.* Paris. 1814.

bone, which, with nearly the anterior half of the bony palate, had exfoliated. The large mass of lost substance was restored by hippopotamus ivory, and the whole retained in place by elastic gold bands attached to the teeth that remained.

Hitherto all the attempts at restoration had been of hard parts, and it is not until we come to the writings of M. Delabarre* that we find any account of artificial soft palates.

M. Delabarre was much impressed with the fact that in congenital cases of deficient palate the most constant want was of *soft* velum: hard palate might be defective, but, if so, the soft palate was more so. And he conceived the happy idea that soft palate might be supplied by the adaptation of a pliant elastic sheet of material resisting the action of the saliva, and which might be attached to an artificial hard palate where that was employed, or to some firm line across the back of the mouth, where the artificial hard palate might not be needed.† Sheet caoutchouc furnished the necessary physical conditions, and this he employed, as have his followers, with marked success. He describes a case in which he supplied the hard palate, a row of artificial teeth in front and the velum with a uvula behind as one apparatus: and others, where the soft palate alone was wanting, in which a C-shaped arch of metal, fastened by bands to the molar teeth, formed the fixed line to which the india-rubber velum was attached.

Delabarre laid great emphasis on the use of an artificial uvula as necessary to give proper *timbre* to the voice, and to assist in the act of deglutition. He more particularly enforced the latter use, stating that the uvula acts as a "bolt" while pointing downwards, as it rests on the posterior wall of the pharynx—thus preventing the velum from doubling upwards in the act of swallowing.

Mr. Snell was the first person in this country who practically understood the mechanical appliances which were available for the treatment of congenital deficiencies of the palate, and his essays upon this subject, and upon the employment of obturators, have never received the attention and acknowledgment which they deserve. I have already alluded to their

* *Traité de la partie mécanique d'art du Chirurgien-Dentiste.* Par C. F. Delabarre, tome premier. Paris. 1820.

† Loc. cit. tome premier, p. 316.

historical completeness: their practical merits are of an equally high order.

The apparatus devised by Mr. Snell was in all essentials similar to those employed in the present day. A firm palate of ivory or gold, to which was attached a flap of sheet india-rubber stretching from the pillars of the fauces on either side and held firmly against them, so as to follow their movements and be entirely under their control, by a gold (spiral) spring attached to the artificial hard palate and the false velum. There were two elements in Mr. Snell's apparatus which more recently have not been thought of essential value—namely, an artificial uvula attached to the end of the velum, and a supplemental vomer passing up from the dorsal (nasal) aspect of the hard palate, and in the form of two thin gold plates, embracing the imperfect natural bony septum.*

The same principles as those advanced by Delabarre and Snell have been carried out with more or less modification by Mr. Stearns † and Mr. Sercombe ‡; but there have not appeared to me any modifications in their apparatus of sufficient importance for historical recognition.

In December 1864, Dr. Kingsley, of New York, read an account, before the Odontological Society of London, of a new form of artificial palate,§ consisting of a vulcanite hard palate, to the posterior part of which is attached an elastic india-rubber velum. On either side of the artificial hard palate is a groove which receives the edge of the palatal process of the cleft. This apparatus is supported by wedging into the fissure, and resting by a ledge of vulcanite upon the nasal surface of the cleft palate. It will be observed that in this plan the interval of the fissure is occupied by the false palate, and support gained by material passing into the nose and resting on the floor of the

* Loc. cit., pp. 27, 28, 29. Also "Case of Congenital Division of Hard and Soft Palate, &c.," by James Snell, M.R.C.S., in *London Medical Repository*, vol. xx. p. 365. London. 1823.

† "A New Instrument designed to Remedy the Imperfection of Speech consequent upon Congenital Fissure of the Soft Palate," by C. H. Stearns. *Lancet*, vol. ii. 1845, pp. 7, 260, 284, 310.

‡ "Cleft-palate; its Surgical and Mechanical Treatment," by Edwin Sercombe, M.R.C.S. *Transactions of Odontological Society*, vol. i. London. 1858.

§ "On the Treatment of Congenital Cleft Palate," by Dr. N. W. Kingsley, in *Transactions of Odontological Society*, vol. v. p. 195. London. 1865.

nasal fossa, thus reverting to the objectionable principle adopted previous to the time of M. Bourdet.

In any case where there is a lesion of the palate, the question may naturally arise, whether the treatment shall be surgical and radical, or merely supplemental and mechanical: whether, that is, the surgeon shall endeavour to restore the natural parts to a normal continuity, or the dentist shall supply, by foreign material, an equivalent of what is deficient.

Most forms of perforate and cleft palate, unless of extreme severity, are susceptible of radical cure by means of plastic surgical operation. I beg to refer the reader who would seek further information on this subject to Mr. Pollock's exhaustive essay in "Holmes's System of Surgery" already referred to.

The relative advantages of treating clefts and perforations of the palate by mechanical appliances and by operation, have been much discussed, and I cannot help thinking with some unfairness on the part of the dentists.

It has been argued by them that the operations of staphyloraphy are attended with a notable amount of danger to life; by an excessive amount of pain during their performance, and further, that the resultant soft palate produced by the union of the natural parts is less effective for articulation than one supplied by a foreign material.

The first of these objections—that the operation is dangerous to life—itself shows the spirit of special pleading which has been directed against the surgical treatment of these cases; for the gentleman, who advanced this objection, was able to adduce but one solitary instance of a fatal result. Of how few equally important operations could this be said!

As regards the pain of the operation, how incomparably less distressing than the tedious processes of the mechanist's manipulations constantly to be repeated through life, and these coupled with the abiding sense of dependence upon another's help, which the unfortunate patient must ever feel!

In stating the comparative advantages of surgical and mechanical treatment, this dependence upon the mechanist has never been sufficiently appreciated, as it seems to me, by those who espouse the palliative and supplemental help of the dentist. I cannot but look upon it as the great and overwhelming objection to false palates, where they can possibly be avoided—

where they can be substituted, that is, by surgical cure—that the sufferers of this malformation should be dependent upon another individual for the service of speech ; that, if an accident befall his artificial mouth, he is helpless and practically dumb, till the artificer again makes good his mouth deficiencies. I will illustrate this by what is taking place at this very time with one of my own patients.

A young English gentleman is in Switzerland for his education. He has a complete fore-and-aft fissure, dividing the soft palate, the palatal bones and true maxillæ; the intermaxillary bone is separated from the maxilla on one side. He wears an artificial palate, hard and soft, with which I have supplied him. Recently an accident has broken his artificial help, and he is unable to use it. Where he is he can get no assistance. This has necessitated his sending the apparatus to England for repair, and some ten days or a fortnight must elapse before he can talk or swallow properly. How far better to have had the fissure closed by operation, which in his case might have been done.

The evils which arise from cleft or perforate palate are, difficulty of sucking and swallowing in infancy, and imperfection of articulation through life. The first two have long ceased to be operative when the patient comes into the hands of the dental surgeon; but the latter remains of serious import, and of much interest in the practical treatment of these cases.

The effect which cleft or perforate palate has upon articulation, the alteration that it produces in the pronunciation of certain letters, depends upon its preventing the closure of the nasal passages. When the mouth is closed in effecting certain articulate sounds, the sound, instead of being completely stopped, as it is in the natural condition of the parts, is continued on through the nose: letters, therefore, that require for their pronunciation a complete and absolute stoppage of the air, cannot be pronounced with cleft palate, but become converted into certain other letters, which correspond to them, and are effected in exactly the same way, except that the sound, stopped at the lips, or elsewhere, is continued on through the nose. This will be better understood, and more easily illustrated, if we examine for a moment the method of formation of the sounds involved.

There are three points at which complete closure may be

made by the organs concerned in articulation—three straits, or points of stricture, where the passage of air and sound may be suddenly shut off at will, or suddenly started; where, therefore, vocal sounds may be closed or commenced, viz. at the lips, the teeth, the soft palate; the closure at these several points, produced by the apposition of the lips, by the pressure of the margin of the tongue against the upper alveolar arch, and by the contact of the root of the tongue with the dropped soft palate. The letters that are formed at the first point are called labials, those at the second dentals, those at the third palatals. But at each of these three points the method of closing or starting a vocal sound may be varied in three ways, and thus we get altogether nine sounds, or letters. 1st. The stoppage may be complete with gentle breathing (spiritus lenis); 2nd. with aspirate breathing (spiritus asper), and 3rdly, the stoppage may be complete only at the mouth, the passage of air and the sound being continued through the nose. If I produce closure at the lips with the gentle breathing, I pronounce B; if with the aspirate breathing, P; if, the lips being closed, the sound is continued on through the nose, I pronounce M. If I produce closure by the apposition of the tongue to the upper alveolar arch with the gentle breathing, I pronounce D; if with the aspirate breathing, T; if, the edge of the tongue being apposed to the alveolar arch, the sound is continued through the nose, I pronounce N. If I produce closure at the palate with the gentle breathing, I pronounce G hard; if with the aspirate breathing, K; if, palatal closure being produced, the sound is continued through the nose, I pronounce NG. This will perhaps be clearer and more intelligible when tabularly expressed, in the following way:—

	Lenis.	Aspirate.	With nasal continuation.
Labials . . .	B	P	M Labio-nasal.
Dentals . . .	D	T	N Denti-nasal.
Palatals . . .	G hard	K	NG Palato-nasal.

Now what cleft palate does is to change the letters of the first and second columns into the corresponding ones of the third—the mutes B, P, D, T, G hard, and K, into the nasal semivowels M, N, and NG. For by destroying the integrity of the party-wall between the mouth and nose, by establishing between them a community of cavity, it renders it impossible for any oral closure to bring the escape of air, and of sound, to an absolute stop; arrested at the lips, or alveolar arch, it continues to escape through the nose. That this is the true explanation of the articulation of cleft palate is proved not only by the physical necessities of the case, and by the kind of change of letters that we find, but by the fact that pinching the nose, so as to close the nostrils, restores to a person affected with cleft palate the power of pronouncing labial and dental mutes.

The way that cleft palate modifies speech will be at once recognised by a few examples:—

"Both brothers drove in a gig to Dorsetshire," would become "Moth mruthers nrove in a nging noo Norsenshire;" "David caught a bad cold," would become "Navin ngaaughn a mân ngoln." "Bride" would become "Mrine," "Bad" would become "Man," "Tape" would become "Name," "Dagger" would become "Nanger;" &c.

This is exactly the reverse for what takes place with a cold in the head, or in a person with nasal polypus. There, from the stoppage in the nasal passages, the sound cannot be continued through the nose after it has been stopped at any of the oral straits. The nose being already stopped, the stoppage of the mouth stops everything, and thus the nasal semivowels are converted into their corresponding mutes—M into B, N into D, and NG into G hard. Thus "The afternoon was fine, though the morning was rainy," would become "The afterdood was fide, though the bording was raidy."

Artificial apparatus for remedying perforations and clefts of palate, and for restoring other lost parts of the mouth, may be conveniently divided into—

I. Obturators;

II. False palates;

III. Various supplemental arrangements, comprising the two foregoing, with or without artificial teeth, and masses compensatory of lost portions of jaw.

In illustrating the *Practical Treatment* of these cases of

palate lesion, it may, I think, be best accomplished by defining their general principles, and, by narrating typical examples, describing the means adopted for their relief.

The object is to restore the parts, by mechanical aids, to that which was their normal condition, as far as possible, and so to establish their functions.

In congenital cases, where the patient has never had a complete oro-nasal septum, the normal physical condition may be closely approached; but it is long before the patient can use it with advantage; it is a new education to speak, and to eat, and to swallow, with the large common cavity now divided by a septum. In congenital cleft palate, the tongue becomes large, and is used as a plug to fill the hiatus in the back of the mouth in speech and in other functions. It is long before it recovers from this curtailment of room. How different is it in accidental cases: the instant the perforation is closed in them, the voice and all the functions, which had been performed from birth till the lesion occurred, are restored with scarcely a defect.

But in making these restorations one point is to be particularly remembered—the condition of the damaged parts should not be further injured in giving temporary relief. Probably the simplest and, for the time, the most convenient method of relieving a perforate palate, is Paré's Obturator—a disk of metal and a sponge in the nose; but it is most injurious to the unfortunate patient's future condition, as the pressure of the expanding sponge causes progressive absorption of the margins of the orifice to an unlimited extent. Any plug kept in position by tight fitting acts in the same manner.*

There is a preparation in the museum of St. Bartholomew's Hospital (Ser. I. No. X. 232) of the scull of a person who lost a portion of the palate, probably from syphilis, and who obtained temporary relief by stuffing the oro-nasal aperture with a large cork, gradually adding to the size of the plug, to meet the requirements of the ever-increasing orifice, till the whole of the hard palate had disappeared; the palatal processes of the ossa palati, as well as those of the maxillæ, being lost. The

* It is a remarkable fact that in the Exhibition of 1862, where many apparatus for the relief of perforate and cleft palate were exhibited, the great majority were constructed on this vicious principle. Upon this I made a special report. See *Reports of the Juries*, 1862, class xvii. p. 12.

progressive absorption under this continually advancing pressure had removed the vomer, the inferior turbinated bones, and the nasal walls of the maxillary sinuses. Such a specimen is an eloquent commentary on this reprehensible plan of treatment.

And that which applies to a perforate palate, applies also to a congenital cleft palate. I cannot conceive that an apparatus consisting of a hard wedge, passing forward into the cleft, and resting upon the nasal surface of the palate, can be worn without an increase and expansion of the fissure; though, no doubt, for the time being, Mr. Kingsley's arrangement may be very comfortable and very firm, as is the case with Paré's Obturator. As regards the latter, there has been abundant time and opportunity to appreciate and realise its ultimate evil consequences. Mr. Kingsley's apparatus has hardly yet been sufficiently long in use to declare its real effect upon the parts of a defective palate; but as long as pressure occasions absorption, I cannot conceive that this mode of treatment will fail to maintain, and probably increase, the existing deformity.

In taking models for obturators (and this still more applies to those for false palates, involving the soft parts) it is often necessary to have a special tray, or model-spoon, made for the particular case to be treated, as in the ordinary symmetrical spoons the wax is not brought to some part of the palate where it is essential to have a correct impression. To accomplish this, I have been in the habit of first taking a mould approximatively true, and then of having a model-spoon constructed of ordinary tinned sheet-iron, so as to fit pretty evenly over the variously modified surface of the malformed or diseased palate. A handy mechanist will easily extemporise such an appliance, or with explanation it may be entrusted to a common tinman.

M. Préterre, who displayed at the Great Exhibition of 1862 (Class 17–1756) a large collection of well-made specimens of artificial palates, &c., explained to me that he took his models with spoons which he made at the time of thin sheet-lead. He showed me some of these: the lead was about the thickness of No. 8 sheet-gold. He beat the lead pretty nearly to the form of the mouth, and, having filled it with wax, took his impression. It appeared a ready and rapid method, but I thought the lead hardly firm enough for the purpose.

Two advantages are gained by thus making special model-spoons for each case: perfect adaptation and even pressure upon the surface that is to be moulded, and the absence of any superabundance of wax. Where too much wax is used, and extends, after the impression has been taken, much over the edges of the spoon, it is very apt to drag the model out of shape upon its withdrawal.

There is one source of fallacy in taking these models, which it is difficult to guard against. The front of the palate is hard and fixed: the back of the palate (even in front of the velum) is soft, and more or less mobile, yielding under pressure. When the wax is applied to take an impression, it is rigidly embossed by the general form, and by all the inequalities of the front of the palate, while the softer structure behind yields, rising upwards under the same force. The resultant model is therefore too vaulted behind. The posterior edge of the false palate or obturator made upon such model is consequently apt to cut the soft mucous membrane, especially on either side of the middle line, where it passes off to the pillars of the fauces. To obviate this, the wax should be as soft as possible, and the force of pressure principally applied to the front of the mouth. But even with these precautions, the back edge of the obturator frequently cuts; and, in that case, it is necessary either to bend away the posterior margin of the palate after it is made, or to thicken the model at a part corresponding to the injured mucous membrane, and re-stamp the plate.

To prevent the wax from passing into the nasal cavity through a perforate palate, a piece of muslin, or fine net, may be placed over it, immediately before the introduction of the model-spoon into the mouth.

I. Obturators.—Obturators etymologically signify *stoppers*, and the term is correctly enough applied to such instruments as were employed by Paré; but it hardly conveys a just idea of the improved apparatus which was inaugurated by Bourdet.

Obturators are properly constructed to *cover over*, on the oral surface, perforations of the palate, usually the hard palate alone, which may be congenital or accidental. They should be composed of some thin material, which will very little encroach on the oral cavity. Thin sheet metal is the best substance to use —gold, platina, or dental alloy (an alloy of platina and silver). The first is perhaps the best; but I have recently used the dental alloy very largely in hospital practice, with very good results. Vulcanite (indurated sulphuret of caoutchouc) is frequently employed; but it is bulky and brittle, and, I think, inferior to metal. As it is desirable to have the material as thin as possible, I employ metal plate—No. 6 of the gold-flatter's gauge—and, when I use gold, it is 16-carat alloy, so as to be rigid and not easily bent.

After taking a good model, the plate is to be struck up as in the making of plates for artificial teeth. Care should be taken that the adaptation immediately around the orifice should be very accurate; but there should be no projection whatever into the hole. The support of the obturator is easily effected by collars or clasps around suitable teeth. Frequently, there are spaces where teeth have been extracted, which facilitates the adaptation of the collars; but if not, then, with a dividing file, intervals may be made for the purpose. When all the teeth are lost, the same effect may be produced by an arrangement adapted to the lower jaw, and connected with the upper by means of spiral springs which keep the upper piece—plate, teeth and obturator—in proper position. Such arrangements remove all the defects, and supply all the requirements at once—appearance, articulation, and mastication are all restored. I cannot conceive any condition in which it is necessary to support an obturator by processes passing into the nose; and I am convinced that any, and every other, arrangement is preferable to that plan.

In accidental cases, where the perforation of the palate is occasioned by the loss of diseased bone, it is a matter of the greatest importance to apply the obturator as soon as possible after the sequestrum has come away, and while the wound is still in a state of active granulation; for the presence of the obturator is not negative, when it spans over the perforation. An orifice which, when allowed to remain open, will continue *in statu quo*, or very little diminish, will rapidly contract when the passage of air and of fluids between the oral and nasal cavity is prevented, and when the granulating edges are supported and protected from being bruised by the food. This, though evidently understood by Bourdet, has not, I think, been sufficiently appreciated of late; but it is of the utmost importance in treating these cases. It is surprising how the granulations will stretch across the upper surface of the obturator and close up the orifice; and, in more advanced and neglected cases, the same condition may be imitated to some extent, by frequently scarifying the edges of the perforation, always taking care to restore immediately a well-fitting obturator. I have seen an opening as large as a shilling contract, under this treatment, so that at the end of a few months a probe could be barely pushed through it.

Occasionally, a portion of the floor of the antrum is lost by necrosis in cases of severe "abscess" of that sinus, and its cavity becomes common with that of the mouth, by an aperture of variable size. The orifice should be immediately closed, or rather spanned over, by a plate (upon which substitutes for lost teeth may, or may not, be fixed), and the result will be, in many instances, the development of a membranous growth supplying the lost bone, completely scaring over the wound, and forming a floor to the sinus.

Fig. 127.

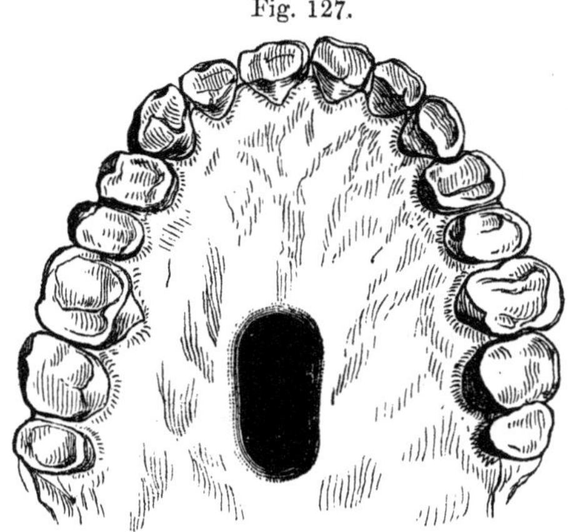

The accompanying illustration (fig. 127) represents the palate and upper jaw of a man who lost a portion of the palate from syphilis. The patient was about forty-eight years of age when he came under my care at Guy's Hospital. He had been a sailor, and in early life had contracted syphilis, with slight secondary symptoms.* He had not seriously suffered till about a year before he came to me. At that time, he was in a state of destitution, and became much reduced in health and strength.

* I have applied obturators for perforations occasioned by tertiary syphilis, inherited syphilis, scrofula, pistol-shot (attempted suicide).

An abscess formed in the roof of the mouth, and in a few months a piece of bone, about the size of a man's thumb-nail, and involving the whole thickness of the palate, came away. When the patient applied to me, six months afterwards, the orifice into the nose was of the form and size indicated in the figure. The damaged articulation and other inconveniences were as usual in such cases. I took a model of the mouth, and filed an interval between the first and second bicuspid teeth, on either side, so as

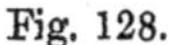

Fig. 128.

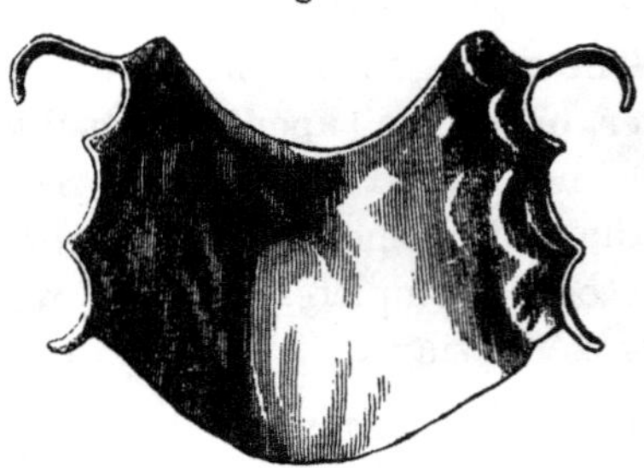

to admit a flattened wire for fastening. An obturator of dental alloy was then made, as represented in figure 128. This fitted accurately, and completely restored the oro-nasal septum. The patient was surprised at his articulation being again perfect; and, as he sucked a vacuum in his mouth, he exclaimed with glee, "Ah! now I shall be able to smoke again." I saw him three months afterwards, when the orifice had decreased about a third of its original size.

II. False or Artificial Palates.—Under this heading I desire to treat of those appliances which compensate for loss of soft palate, and frequently of hard palate also—usually of both—whether such defects are congenital or accidental. In the great majority of instances these cases will be found of congenital origin.

Just as a rigid plate is required to replace a defect in the hard palate, so a structure which is pliant and elastic is needed to supply the deficiencies of the mobile soft palate. Caoutchouc fulfils these requirements remarkably well; and in some form it is the substance which is now universally adopted.

But cases may arise in which a soft artificial palate would be a useless appendage. The artificial soft palate is purely passive and mechanical, and is dependent on the action of the muscles of the fauces for the performance of its articulating and deglutory functions. Unhappily, in some cases of disease—never, I believe, in congenital cases—the whole of the soft muscular parts at the back of the throat are lost; and then the artificial soft palate becomes a useless and unmeaning addition to the hard oro-nasal septum. These remarks are based upon the observation of an unusually severe case of tertiary syphilis under my care, in which the whole of the hard palate was lost; all the soft palate likewise, and every indication of the tonsils and pillars of the fauces had disappeared, and left only a common smooth cicatrix on each side of the back of the mouth. Here a soft elastic flap served no office of the velum pendulum palati, and after trial it was removed; but a thin gold disc, separating the nose from the mouth, for the anterior five-sixths of the cavities, was of much comfort to the patient.

With the firm conviction that no portion of a false palate (as in the case of an obturator) should pass into the nasal cavity, I believe the best form of apparatus is some modification of those which were devised by Bourdet and Snell; and the accompanying illustrations of a cleft palate, with the artificial restoration I adopted, will best display and explain the plan which, I venture to think, is most properly adopted in the treatment of these cases.

An artificial palate, then, supplying both the hard and the soft parts, consists of a plate o metal, or other hard substance, and a mobile flap, either itself elastic, or, if rigid, rendered elastic in its movements by a spring; or, again, the action of the flap may consist of its own elasticity, combined with the stronger motor power of a spiral recoiling spring. Indeed, the latter combination is the one now usually adopted, and I believe is the best. It is the plan which, after some experience, I now always employ.

My friend, Mr. George Parkinson,* who has had large experience in these cases, uses a flap, or representative soft palate, composed of *indurated* vulcanite, a hard un-pliant disc, whose movements are regulated by the faucial muscles, opposed by an elastic coil spring. This flap is attached to the artificial hard palate by a hinge. The adaptation of this rigid velum to the ever-changing form of the faucial walls, must, at times, be im-

* "On the Adaptation of Artificial Palates," by George Parkinson, M.R.C.S., *Lancet*, 1867, vol. i. p. 41.

perfect; and the action of the hinge-joint, in some movements, must leave an interval between the hard and soft palate; but, in effect, Mr. Parkinson says, these defects are rendered nugatory by the mucus which fills up the gaps. Certainly, a velum which does not undergo destruction by the action of the saliva, and so require occasional renewal, is very desirable; and, if such an appliance can be effected without loss of mechanical function, it is a valuable achievement.

In supplying the soft palate, it is generally found that, at first, the contact with the fauces occasions retching, and even sickness. In practice, it is best to supply a very small flap at the beginning, and increase the size every few days: by this means the irritability is soon and effectually overcome. The soft palate should ultimately be ample.

Fig. 129.

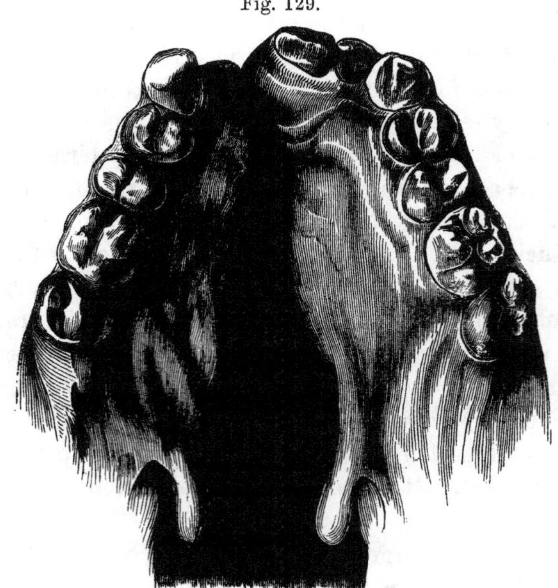

The accompanying illustration (fig. 129) represents the upper jaw of a man in whom there was a complete fore-and-aft cleft of the palate: the right incisive bone was scarcely represented, and both the incisor teeth on that side were wanting.

A hard palate was fitted to the roof of the mouth; and, when fairly adapted, a soft palate was added. An incisor tooth was placed in the interval between the existing central incisor and the right canine. Being a hospital case, dental alloy was used for the hard palate.

Fig. 130 represents this artificial palate as seen on the oral surface, and fig. 131 the same in profile.

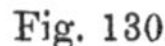

Fig. 130.

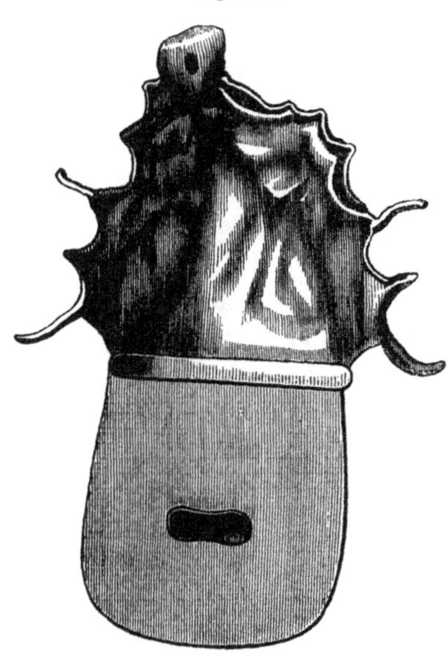

As regards the support of these artificial palates, the same remarks apply, in every respect, as those already made regarding the support of obturators. But to prevent the dropping of the

Fig. 131.

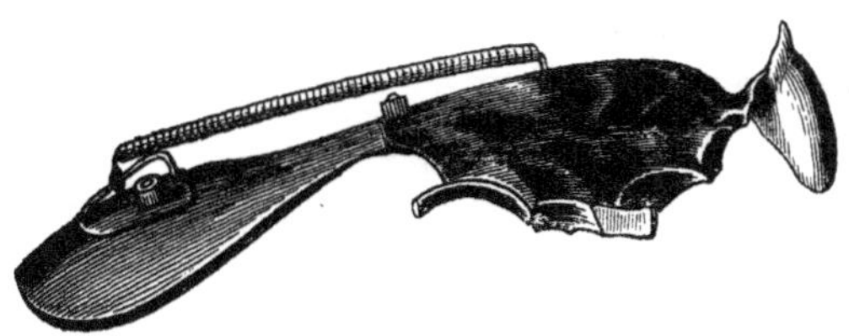

hinder part of the arrangement, it is well to have fine thin clasps extended round the back molars. These effectually resist the depressing action of the muscles of the fauces.

The attachment and movements of the elastic flap—the soft palate—are important considerations. The contact with the pillars of the fauces should be constant, and the elasticity of the moveable artificial velum should be only just sufficient to accomplish this, the power of the muscles being feeble. This requires some nicety. Doubling the thickness of caoutchouc at its attachment may answer; but the best plan, I believe, is an extremely delicate elastic coil of gold-wire, attached at one end and moving free, by a ring embracing a horizontal wire at the other, as seen in fig. 131. This latter arrangement prevents all *traction* on the coil lengthwise when the flap is much depressed, and thus equalises the elastic action of the spring at all degrees of bend.

The soft palate is attached to the hard by means of nuts and screws; and an intelligent patient can easily adjust new india-rubber flaps when necessary. Unindurated vulcanised rubber becomes sodden and soft in time, and requires renewal.

As regards the period of life at which false palates can with advantage be applied, I agree with Mr. Parkinson, who says:—"I do not think artificial palates can be adapted with advantage to children under twelve years of age, and that ordinarily sixteen is quite young enough" (loc. cit.). Those who are practically acquainted with the influence which regulating-plates, when worn very early while there are still temporary teeth, have upon the order and regularity of second dentition; or have watched the results in after-life of rigid unyielding masticatory apparatus in restraining those changes of maxillary form which would otherwise have occurred, must feel the desirability of postponing, as far as possible, any mechanical hindrance to the evolution of the permanent teeth and the jaw-bones.

In cases of cleft palate, in which the intermaxillary bone is tilted forward as a tubercle on the end of the septum narium, I think, with Mr. Pollock,* that the bone should not be removed, but forcibly pressed into its right position; and, if done after the teeth are cut, it may be retained there by apparatus such as is described (p. 49) in treating V-shaped jaw.

III. Various Combinations.—Teeth, palates, and masses compensatory of lost portions of jaw, may be made in endless variety. I may mention a few examples that have been under my own treatment within a recent period, by way of illustration.

* *Holmes's Surgery.* 2nd Edit. Vol. iv. p. 418. 1870.

Supplemental right upper maxilla, palate, and teeth.—This apparatus was to supply the mass of the right upper jaw, which Mr. Bryant had removed for *osteochondroma.** The whole of the right upper jaw was removed, excepting the orbital plate, on May 4, 1869, and on the 20th of the following October I supplied the deficiency by a large massive apparatus, composed of vulcanite, and bearing artificial teeth. It was necessary to construct a special wax-spoon for taking the model; but this was readily done.

The loss of bone had completely opened the nasal cavity, and all the troubles of mastication, deglutition, and speech, which occur in such cases, were very marked. When I took the model I found that the right cheek had fallen in very considerably, and there was much difficulty in getting a sufficient bow to the arch. Moreover there was but an imperfect attachment for the artificial piece, the teeth of the opposite side forming the only support. Still, in effect, that was found sufficient; and, though the edge of the convexity of the vulcanite at first caused some discomfort, and even ulceration of the cheek, this soon passed off. The ultimate result was most satisfactory, all the functions of the mouth being perfectly restored.

Apparatus to restore considerable loss of upper jaw, double perforation of palate, lost teeth, &c.—A poor woman came to me at Guy's Hospital suffering from secondary syphilis, which had affected the palatal and alveolar processes of the upper jaw. The two upper central incisors, the left lateral, and canine had been shed, with the containing alveoli, and a considerable mass of necrosed bone, reaching to the root of the nose, had been exfoliated. Two portions of the hard palate had also come away necrosed, leaving two separate orifices between nose and mouth, each about ⅜ths of an inch in diameter. The loss of front teeth and contiguous bone caused much disfigurement, and the perforations in the palate entailed all those difficulties in speech, mastication, and fluid-swallowing which have already been described. The accompanying illustration (fig. 132) shows the condition of the mouth, minus the dotted lines, which indicate the restorations. The two bicuspids had been lost by caries many years before the attack of secondary syphilis.

* *Guy's Hospital Reports*, vol. xv., third series, p. 262; plate III., fig. 2.

The case presented opportunities of restoring three lost elements of the mouth—teeth, a mass of alveolar process and

Fig. 132.

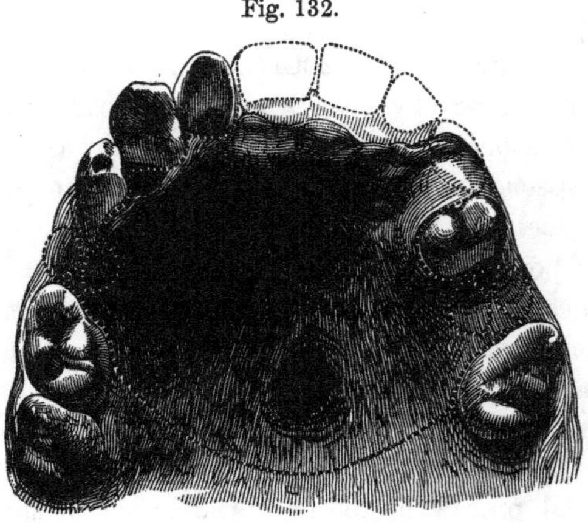

bone, and the occlusion of the nose from the mouth by false palate. This was accomplished by the piece exhibited in fig. 133. It was composed of vulcanite, in which teeth were

Fig. 133.

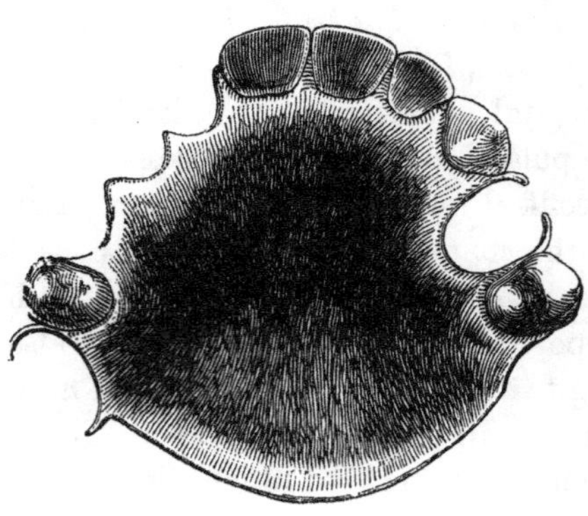

embedded. The arrangement completely restored the form and functions of the mouth. The holes into the nose rapidly contracted, and after three months would barely admit the passage of a straw through them.

Supplying deficiency in upper jaw, with perforation into front of nasal cavity.—This also was a syphilitic case: it occurred to a cabman who, after many years' subsidence of secondaries, had disease of the palate and alveolar border of the front of the upper jaw. The result was loss of bone, involving the four incisive teeth, and leaving a perforation into the nose just under the upper lip. An apparatus of vulcanite was made to supply the lost jaw-substance and teeth, closing also the perforation into the nose. The latter, which at first would have admitted the passage of the little finger, closed completely in two months.

Obturator for perforate palate, with entire set of artificial teeth.—In this case the patient was a gentleman who had early led a libertine life. Syphilis had perforated his palate, and mercury had loosened and shed his teeth.

When he first came under my care, he was wearing one of Paré's obturators—a disc with a sponge in the nose. The hole in the palate was then nearly the size of a florin. He showed me a collection of these obturators, some twenty in number, which had been used and cast off as the orifice enlarged. The perforation through the palate was originally not larger than a threepenny-piece, but the distending action of the sponge had increased it to its present area. The patient's teeth were at this time very loose indeed, and many of them had fallen out sound. I was obliged to remove the remainder, and then constructed for him an entire set of artificial teeth on gold plates, making an obturator of the upper plate completely spanning over the perforation. The apparatus was kept in place by spiral springs, connecting the upper and lower plates. The orifice did not materially contract; indeed, after long standing, I believe, the tendency to contraction ceases. But the patient wore the arrangement with perfect comfort for many years—mastication, deglutition, and articulation being completely restored.

Restoration of the bulk of lower jaw.—An engineer soldier was recently under my care at Guy's Hospital, suffering from necrosis of the greater part of the lower jaw, the result of a kick from a horse, which ended in his losing the whole of the alveolar border and all the teeth; but the arch of the jaw was in no part broken through, though in some places not more than the sixth of an inch thick. Several teeth were wanting in the upper jaw. This case admitted of very simple and effectual treatment. A mass of vulcanite, set with teeth, was moulded to replace as nearly as possible the lost bone, &c.; and spiral springs connecting this with an upper frame, also set with teeth, held the whole in place. The action of this apparatus has been quite satisfactory.

It would be useless to enumerate other similar cases, which, however, might be done almost indefinitely. Large numbers of persons, who daily follow the ordinary avocations of life, are wearing, unknown to those around them, some form of these mouth restorations, without which they would be incapacitated and quite unpresentable. The comfort of these supplemental apparatus is unspeakable; and, as I have remarked, they may be constructed to meet almost every conceivable lesion of the mouth.

INDEX.

LONDON: PRINTED BY
SPOTTISWOODE AND CO., NEW-STREET SQUARE
AND PARLIAMENT STREET

www.ingramcontent.com/pod-product-compliance
Lightning Source LLC
LaVergne TN
LVHW011156110826
845150LV00006B/1238

* 9 7 8 1 4 2 5 5 4 6 2 5 0 *